FOUNDATIONS
OF
MENTAL HEALTH COUNSELING

FOUNDATIONS OF MENTAL HEALTH COUNSELING

Second Edition

Edited by

WILLIAM J. WEIKEL, Ph.D.

*Professor and Chair
Department of Leadership and Secondary Education
Morehead State University
Morehead, Kentucky
and
Eastern Kentucky Counseling and Rehabilitation
Services*

and

ARTIS J. PALMO, Ed.D.

*Bethlehem Counseling Associates
Bethlehem, Pennsylvania*

With a Foreword by

Edwin Herr, Ed.D.
*Pennsylvania State University
University Park, Pennsylvania*

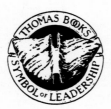

CHARLES C THOMAS • PUBLISHER, LTD.
Springfield • Illinois • U.S.A.

Published and Distributed Throughout the World by

CHARLES C THOMAS · PUBLISHER, LTD.
2600 South First Street
Springfield, Illinois 62794-9265

© *1996 by* CHARLES C THOMAS · PUBLISHER, LTD.
ISBN 0-398-06669-8 (cloth)
ISBN 0-398-06670-1 (paper)
Library of Congress Catalog Card Number: 96-21358

Printed in the United States of America
SC-R-3

Library of Congress Cataloging-in-Publication Data

Foundation of mental health counseling / edited by William J. Weikel,
Artis J. Palmo ; with a foreword by Edwin Herr. — 2nd ed.
        p.   cm.
    Includes bibliographical references and index.
    ISBN 0-398-06669-8 (cloth). — ISBN 0-398-06670-1 (pbk.)
    1. Mental health counseling—Practice. 2. Mental health
counseling. I. Weikel, William J. II. Palmo, Artis J.
RC466.F68   1996
616.89—dc20
                                                        96-21358
                                                          CIP

CONTRIBUTORS

EDWARD S. BECK
Private Practice

STEPHEN L. BENTON
Kansas State University

JAMES A. BOYTIM
Private Practice

DAVID K. BROOKS, JR.
Kent State University

LINDA BROOKS
University of North Carolina, Chapel Hill

DUANE BROWN
University of North Carolina, Chapel Hill

MICHAEL N. CEO
Private Practice

RODNEY K. GOODYEAR
University of Southern California

DOUGLAS R. GROSS
Arizona State University

KATHLEEN H. JONES
Lehigh University

SHARON E. ROBINSON–KURPIUS
Arizonia State University

STEVEN P. LINDENBERG
Private Practice

DON C. LOCKE
North Carolina State University, Asheville

JANE E. MYERS
University of North Carolina, Greensboro

ARTIS J. PALMO
Private Practice

LINDA A. PALMO
Private Practice

DEAN W. OWEN, JR.
Morehead State University

ROBERT H. RENCKEN
Private Practice

E. DUANE RIEDESEL
Private Practice

GAIL P. ROBINSON
Private Practice

MARY B. SEAY
Allentown College

THOMAS A. SEAY
Kuntztown University

GARY SEILER
Private Practice

LINDA SELIGMAN
George Mason University

MICHAEL SHOSH
Private Practice

HOWARD B. SMITH
Northeast Louisiana University

WARREN THROCKMORTON
Grove City College

DAVID VAN DOREN
University of Wisconsin, Whitewater

MOLLY VASS
Barry University

WILLIAM J. WEIKEL
Morehead State University

To our wives, Vanessa Weikel and Linda Palmo, who came into our lives at a time when we needed a stable rudder to guide us personally so that we could be better professionally.

FOREWORD

Foundations of Mental Health Counseling is a unique book. In one volume it comprehensively charts the antecedents to, the present status of, and the future trends for the newest group to claim competence in mental health care: Mental Health Counselors.

The uniqueness of this book lies in its contributors and in its content. It is unusual in our sophisticated age of professional imperatives and boundaries to witness a relatively small cadre of competent and dedicated persons lead a systematic crusade to have their specialty recognized as deserving parity with older and established professions. Yet, that is precisely what unfolds in these pages. The reader is a witness to the creation of a reality; to the testimony of those who attended the birth of a professional identity, gave it life, and energized its impact on the world of mental health care. Thus, in many parts of this book one reads original material, first party accounts, of what it means to sense and act upon a historical moment of readiness, of need, of opportunity.

The content of this book is also, in many ways, unique. It draws together from a spectrum of sources, historical tracings, rationale, conceptual models, descriptions of clientele and settings, as well as a wide-ranging view of the interventions of significance to mental health counselors. As such, the contributors' chapters converge to provide a unified structure to mental health counseling which is not typically found in edited books. At the same time, the various chapters probe with insight some of the major contemporary issues facing the mental health professions today. Among them are such concerns as cross-cultural counseling, credentialling, training, ethics, and third-party reimbursement, chapters which can be read with profit by any mental health provider, not only mental health counselors.

A further valuable dimension of Foundations of Mental Health Counseling is its grasp of the emerging settings and behavioral foci to which mental health counselors can apply their skills. The highlight sections as well as the chapters which discuss mental health counseling in sex positivism, gerontology, thanatology, hospital and clinic settings, hospices, business and industry, alcohol and drug abuse, and consultative arrangements are comprehensive analyses of the locations and the behavioral domains which represent current environments and populations at particular kinds of risk. Inherent in such analyses is the important notion that mental health counselors possess "elastic" skills; skills which are not limited to specific populations or institutions but are generalizable to a broad array of primary, secondary, and tertiary mental health purposes.

Finally, *Foundations of Mental Health Counseling* reflects the elements of an activist credo. In its format and substance, it stakes out the claims of mental health counselors to recognition as fifth-core providers, and it provides the challenges—political, legislative, economic, functional—to which the long-range planning of the profession must be committed. This important book takes scholarly aim at the historic delivery of mental health services and the traditional core providers of such services—psychiatrists, psychologists, social workers, psychiatric nurses—in the United States. Every counselor will be enriched by the book's lucid statement of the need for new approaches to mental health care and of the ability of mental health counselors to serve such needs.

EDWIN L. HERR
The Pennsylvania State University
State College, Pennsylvania

PREFACE TO THE SECOND EDITION

The second edition of this book coincides with the twentieth anniversary of the mental health counseling profession. In the twenty years since the founding of the American Mental Health Counselors Association in 1976, the profession has matured and the term *Mental Health Counselor* has entered the health care lexicon. Universities throughout the United States routinely prepare mental health counselors and forty-one states now have legislative recognition of counseling professionals!

We were aware of the need for this book in 1986, since, at best, current texts devoted only a chapter to the mental health counseling revolution. We hoped it would be adopted by training programs and were pleased by its widespread acceptance and utilization by working counselors and researchers. Now, ten years later, we offer an expanded and updated version for students, practitioners, and researchers, written by frontline professionals and experts in their various areas of mental health.

We would like to thank all of our contributors for their time and talents and our publishers at Charles C Thomas for their patience and guidance. Most of all, thanks to the men and women who have nurtured this profession and made it the fifth force core provider in the mental health care system!

William J. Weikel
Artis J. Palmo

CONTENTS

SECTION V—ASSESSMENT, RESEARCH, ETHICS, CURRICULUM, AND TRENDS IN MENTAL HEALTH COUNSELING

FOUNDATIONS OF
MENTAL HEALTH COUNSELING

SECTION I
MENTAL HEALTH COUNSELING
IN AN HISTORICAL PERSPECTIVE

Chapter 1

MENTAL HEALTH COUNSELING: THE FIRST TWENTY YEARS

David K. Brooks, Jr. and William J. Weikel

In an organized sense, mental health counseling is a very young discipline, at the time of this writing, almost two decades old. It is also a dynamic discipline, one within which there is still active debate about professional identity, role, function, and professional preparation. Furthermore, most of its practitioners believe that mental health counseling has a bright future and choose to focus most of their energies in that direction. When the history of mental health counseling is written in a more definitive fashion than is possible in 1996, the present generation of activists and true believers may discover that their professional careers have paralleled most of the profession's significant milestones and that they have had a hand in shaping their own destinies and that of their profession. Practitioners in few other fields have been able to make this claim. Thus, the history of mental health counseling is still very much in the process of becoming.

Mental health counseling did not emerge full-blown in 1976 with no previous history. A number of necessary antecedents led to the founding of the American Mental Health Counselors Association (AMHCA) in that year, and certainly there were many individuals who were practicing as mental health counselors (MHCs) before they began to apply the title to themselves and their work. These antecedents do not form a traceable and purposeful historical path, but each may be considered an essential thread, without which the fabric of the profession would be less than whole.

HISTORICAL ANTECEDENTS

The beginnings of contemporary approaches to the treatment of mental and emotional disorders are usually traced to the late 18th century. Prior to that time, persons suffering from mental and emotional disorders were either confined in asylums with wretched conditions and no systematic treatment or lived as itinerant paupers, driven from town to town. Earlier still, mental illness had been viewed as a spiritual disorder resulting from demonic possession and curable only by exorcism or by burning at the stake.

Moral Treatment

The event usually credited with bringing about a change in attitude toward mental illness was the appointment in 1793 of Philippe Pinel as director of the Bicetre, the largest mental hospital in Paris. The French Revolution was in full flower and Pinel brought the principles of "liberty, equality, and fraternity" to his new task. One of his first acts was to release the inmates from their chains. To the surprise of his critics, Pinel's reforms worked. He forbade corporal punishment and used physical restraint only when patients presented a danger to themselves or others. He introduced his methods to the Salpetriere, a hospital for women, when he was made director there in 1795. Pinel later wrote an influential book on institutionalized treatment in which he developed a system for classifying various disorders and advocated the use of occupational therapy as an adjunct to treatment. He kept detailed statistics on the patient populations in his charge and his claims of cure rates resulting from his methods are impressive, even by contemporary standards (Murray, 1983).

At about the same time, William Tuke, a Quaker, founded the York Retreat in England. While this was in many respects a utopian community, the Retreat focused on providing a restful, orderly environment in which those suffering from emotional disorders could return to normal functioning.

During the first half of the 19th century, in the United States, a number of reformers, most notably Dorothea Dix, were successful in founding private asylums and state hospitals operated on humane principles similar to those advocated by Pinel and Tuke. These highly structured environments emphasized the removal of distressed persons from their families or other accustomed settings, manual labor, regular religious devotions, and systematic educational programs aimed at redirecting thought patterns and teaching self-control. This combination of what would be known today as milieu therapy and psychoeducational programming represented a significant alternative to both the medical and the custodial models of treatment. Crucial to the success of these institutions was the role of the attendants as models of appropriate behavior (Sprafkin, 1977).

Following the Civil War, however, there was a dramatic change in patterns of institutionalized care. The state asylums were required to accept a broader range of patients, including alcoholics, the criminally insane, and apparently deranged immigrant paupers. The generation of antebellum reformers had done an inadequate job of choosing and training their successors. Thus, as they retired or died, new hospital superintendents were installed who were unfamiliar with the humanitarian ideals of their predecessors. Levels of funding declined from both public and private sources. Furthermore, the medical model of treatment reasserted itself as medicine became a more organized discipline. As Sprafkin (1977) points out, these factors combined to seal the doom of moral treatment approximately 75 years after it began.

During the next half century, conditions related to the care of the institutionalized mentally ill declined steadily. For all intents, state hospitals and most of the private asylums were little more than warehouses for society's castoffs. Once committed, patients rarely emerged to reenter anything resembling a normal life. A significant and most fortunate exception to this pattern was Clifford W. Beers, who had spent much of his youth and early adulthood in a series of institutions. In 1908, Beers published *A Mind That Found Itself,* an autobiographical account of his experiences in mental hospitals. The heightened public interest created by his book led Beers to found the National Committee for Mental Hygiene in 1909. This organization acted as an advocate for the humane treatment of the mentally ill and was the forerunner of the present National Mental Health Association. These groups have had a powerful, positive impact on public policy related to mental health issues in the ensuing 85 years.

Clifford Beers' early efforts in the area of mental health reform occurred during the Progressive Era, a period of American history characterized by intense activity in a variety of social concerns. Progressive reformers directed their energies toward improving public health through federal inspection of food processing, toward economic justice by the passage of antitrust legislation, and toward improving the lot of the urban poor by the founding of settlement houses, among other activities. Beers' ideas fell on fertile ground during this period.

Vocational Guidance

Youth unemployment was a major problem at the turn of the 20th century. Frank Parsons, another Progressive reformer, focused his energies in this area, working first at the Bread Winners Institute, which was operated by a settlement house, and later founding the Boston Vocational Bureau. Parsons was one of the first to be aware of the tremendous change in occupational choices presented by rapid industrialization coupled with the social dislocation created by the movement of entire families from failed farms to the burgeoning cities. This experience was particularly bewildering for older boys who had been accustomed to working on the farms and whose potential wages were needed for family support, but who found themselves lacking both skills and the needed orientation to an industrialized workplace (Whiteley, 1984).

The purpose of the Boston Vocational Bureau, founded in 1908, was to work with young men to match their interests and aptitudes with appropriate occupational choices. Parsons described his procedures in *Choosing a Vocation* (1909), a short and straightforward work that details a process of interviewing, rudimentary motor skills testing, and providing information about various occupations. Frank Parsons died shortly after founding the Vocational Bureau and before his book was published, but his efforts led to the first national conference on vocational guidance in 1910, sponsored by the Boston Chamber of Commerce (Whiteley, 1984). Later, in 1913, the National Vocational Guidance Association (NVGA) was founded to foster vocational guidance services in schools and to encourage the advancement of this new profession by providing a forum for the exchange of ideas among practitioners.

Moral treatment and vocational guidance are the two major historical antecedents of the mental health counseling movement. Moral treatment is crucial for its emphasis on the potential of disturbed persons for recovery and its early anticipation of psychoeducational methods as viable treatment modalities. Vocational guidance is important for its establishment of the role of the professional counselor, although much of that original role has changed and expanded in the years since. In the same sense that the Progressive Era's settlement houses gave birth to the profession of social work, the early vocational guidance programs often found in these same institutions were the incubator of modern mental health counseling.

ANTECEDENTS IN PROFESSIONAL PRACTICE

In addition to moral treatment and vocational guidance, there were a number of other antecedents necessary to the development of mental health counseling. Among these were advances in testing and assessment technologies, the emergence of nonmedical approaches to psychotherapy, research and theory building focused on normal human development, innovations in group counseling and psychotherapy, and the development of psychoeducational approaches to treatment. Each of these antecedents in professional practice will be sketched briefly in this section.

Testing and Assessment

Prior to the early years of the 20th century, estimation of human abilities and aptitudes was based largely on speculation about the relationship between intelligence and heredity. Educational achievement of the time was more closely related to socioeconomic status than to intellectual ability, with the "sons of riches" (Green, 1985) almost always receiving a superior education regardless of their level of mental ability.

Two French psychologists, Alfred Binet and Theodore Simon, were commissioned by their government to study ways of detecting measurable differences between normal and retarded children so that placement into special education programs would be facilitated for those who needed such experiences. Their work resulted in a series of standardized tasks that could be performed by children of different mental ages. The concept of mental age led to the development of the intelligence quotient (IQ) as a standard measure of intellectual ability.

This was the beginning of widespread and sustained activity in testing and assessment that has continued throughout the years since. Group intelligence tests emerged with the United States entry into World War I and became a fixture in the public schools shortly thereafter. Tests of specific aptitudes were first developed for selection of streetcar motormen in 1912 and now measure everything from musical ability to clerical speed. Vocational interest measurement achieved statistical respectability and acquired greater utility through the work of E. K. Strong and G. Frederic Kuder.

Personality assessment is yet another area in which measurement specialists have been extremely active. The first objective personality test was developed by Edward Elliott in 1910. The publication of the

Minnesota Multiphasic Personality Inventory (MMPI) by McKinley and Hathaway (1940) paved the way for the systematic application of standardized measures to the diagnosis of mental and emotional disorders. Another category of personality measures is projective instrumentation, the most prominent of which are the Rorschach inkblot test, first published in 1921, and the Thematic Apperception Test (TAT), initially developed in 1938.

Advances have been made in clinical assessment as well. Despite the present sophistication of both objective and projective measures, mental health practitioners in several disciplines have found that such approaches are often insufficient to adequately diagnose a client's difficulties. The multiaxial scheme presented in the fourth edition of the Diagnostic and Statistical Manual of Mental Disorders (DSM–IV) is widely used, as are a variety of behavioral assessment procedures.

Perhaps the most challenging assessment issue confronting mental health counselors (MHCs) and allied professionals involves evaluation of treatment outcomes. Demonstrated therapeutic effectiveness is being demanded by government funding sources, by private insurance carriers, and by managed care plans. Research that has been underway for nearly two decades continues to attempt to more accurately describe what happens in the process of behavior change and to measure its progress in both process and outcome dimensions.

Nonmedical Approaches to Psychotherapy

Prior to World War II, psychotherapy was practiced almost exclusively by psychiatrists or by nonphysician therapists who relied on medical models of treatment. *Counseling and Psychotherapy* (1942) was the first of several works in which Carl Rogers, a clinical psychologist by training, advocated client-centered therapy, now known as the person-centered approach. Rogers had no use for diagnostic labels or prescriptive methodologies. It was his conviction that individuals, regardless of how bizarre their symptoms might appear, have within themselves the resources for positive behavior change. He stressed that the conditions of the relationship between counselor and client are the primary medium through which such change occurs. It is difficult to imagine an approach to psychotherapy that is more at variance with the traditional medical model.

The various behavior therapies have been almost as influential as

Rogers, although they differ considerably from his basic tenets. Based on principles of learning and conditioning, the behavior therapies view emotional disorder as the result of faulty learning. Since maladaptive behavior has been learned, it can be unlearned and replaced with new behaviors that are more advantageous to the individual. A more recent version is cognitive-behavioral therapy, which emphasizes the role of cognitions as mediators between stimulus and response.

The postwar era has witnessed the propagation of a number of other nonmedical approaches. While none of these has had the widespread impact of the person-centered approach or the behavior therapies, each of them claims a substantial number of adherents. Among these are reality therapy, gestalt therapy, humanistic-existentialist therapies, transactional analysis, rational-emotive therapy (a type of cognitive-behavioral therapy), family systems approaches, neurolinguistic programming, narrative therapy, and solution-focused brief therapy.

Theories of Normal Human Development

The emergence of psychology as a scientific discipline in the late 19th century was accompanied by increased research and theory building in the area of abnormal human behavior. Normal development, with the exception of inquiry into sensation and perception, was not regarded as worthy of scientific study. Even though Sigmund Freud (1905/1953, 1923/1961) posited the first comprehensive theory of human development, his interest was in psychopathology, not in normal behavior.

Jean Piaget (1896–1980) was a Swiss developmental psychologist whose work forms the basis of much of what is currently accepted about normal human development. Most of Piaget's research was concentrated on the cognitive development of young children, but more recent investigators have applied some of his basic principles to other areas of human functioning as well as tracking developmental processes across the lifespan. Examples of this activity include Kohlberg's (1973) stages of moral development, Perry's (1970) formulations of intellectual and ethical development in college students, and Selman's (1976, 1977) studies of social perspective-taking in young children.

Closely related to the cognitive-developmental school is the work of Jane Loevinger (1976) in ego development. Focusing on the ego as the "master trait," Loevinger's research has resulted in the identification of ten stages of ego development.

According to Rodgers (1980), cognitive-developmental theorists (including Loevinger) focus on the "how" of human development, while psychosocial developmental theorists concern themselves with the "what." Erik Erikson was the best known theorist of the psychosocial group. For him, life span development consisted of eight developmental crises, each of which involves resolution of a crisis of polar opposite dimensions in an individual's life.

It should be apparent that there is much diversity of opinion among the various theorists as to what constitutes normal development. There are some common elements or themes that tend to tie the various schools together. Most of the theorists agree that the interaction between person and environment is critical to satisfactory development in virtually all dimensions. There is also general agreement about the presence of a motivating force or organizing structure at work within the individual. With respect to the nature of the developmental process, most theorists agree that within normal individuals, development is relatively orderly, sequential, generally stage-related but not necessarily age-related, cumulative, and proceeds from simple to complex structures and/or operations (Brooks, 1984). These common themes allow the sketching of a rough model of normal human behavior that is descriptive of development at various points along the life span, depending upon which theory one is using as a referent. Practitioners may thus assess their clients according to multiple dimensions of functioning.

Group Counseling and Psychotherapy

Like several of the antecedents discussed so far, the origins of group counseling and psychotherapy can also be traced to the early years of the 20th century. According to Gazda (1982), the earliest application of the group medium for treatment purposes was in 1905 when J. H. Pratt used group meetings to instruct tuberculosis patients in hygienic practices. Although Pratt originally began this practice to save time, he noticed that the effects of group interaction tended to increase the attention patients paid to his instructions. Another American pioneer was L. C. Marsh, who used a variety of group techniques to treat hospitalized schizophrenics. Marsh's motto, "By the crowd they have been broken; by the crowd they shall be healed" (quoted in Gazda, 1982, p. 9), summarized the beliefs of many pioneers in group counseling and psychotherapy.

It might be expected that the Viennese psychiatric schools would have contributed to the early development of therapeutic group work and, indeed, this was the case. As early as 1921, Alfred Adler, who had previously broken with Freud and established his own system of psychotherapy, was conducting therapeutic interviews with children before audiences of his fellow therapists. Although he initiated this practice for purposes of training, Adler noticed differences in the progress made by his young clients in the presence of a group. He began to involve the group more in the interview process and developed what would today be known as multiple therapy, e.g., more than one therapist working with a client simultaneously. Adler's followers in the United States have modified his practices to incorporate family therapy into the group interview process.

Jacob Moreno was another Viennese therapist who began his work with groups of prostitutes. Emigrating to the United States in 1925, he was extremely influential in the development of modern group therapy, coining the term in 1932 (Gazda, 1982). Moreno is principally known for his work in psychodrama, "an extension of group psychotherapy in which there is not just verbalization but the situation is acted out in as realistic a setting as possible" (Moreno & Elefthery, 1982, p. 103). Although Moreno's name is synonymous with psychodrama, he has only recently been given credit for his influence in the development of a number of other approaches to group work.

There are at present group applications for virtually every major system of individual counseling and psychotherapy. There are, however, no individual therapy applications for such group work techniques as sensitivity training, encounter groups, or psychodrama. The range of therapeutic possibilities open to counselors and clients is thus expanded by the tremendous activity in the group work arena over the past 80 years and particularly those developments of the past three decades.

Mental health counseling has been especially influenced by developments in group counseling and psychotherapy because much of the research, theory building, and practice of the last 30 years has been done by individuals primarily identified with the counseling profession. The work of George Gazda, Merle Ohlsen, Walter Lifton, Don Dinkmeyer, and Gerald Corey is standard reading in virtually every graduate counseling program.

Psychoeducational Approaches to Treatment

As was shown to be the case with group counseling and psychotherapy, it is difficult to pinpoint the exact beginnings of psychoeducational approaches to treatment. Most writers agree that such approaches did not exist in the professional literature prior to the 1960s. Several commentators (Authier, Gustafson, Guerney, & Kasdorf, 1975; Gazda & Brooks, 1985) emphasize the impact of Carl Rogers and his associates (Rogers, Gendlin, Kiesler, & Truax, 1967) in specifying the conditions under which behavior change is most likely to occur. Authier et al. (1975) also recognize the role played by Skinner and his fellow behaviorists in providing the basis for the technology of psychoeducational approaches.

Regardless of their origins, psychoeducational approaches are different from other approaches to treatment in that they emphasize the client as learner rather than as patient and cast the role of the mental health professional as teacher rather than as healer. In other words, such approaches are the antithesis of the medical model. Often called "training-as-treatment," these approaches assume that the client is merely deficient in skills needed for effective living, rather than being sick and in need of cure. The counselor's task, therefore, is to teach the necessary skills in a systematic way so that they can be applied not only to the presenting problem, but generalized to other areas of the client's life as well.

An impressive array of skills training programs and packages has emerged in the last 30 years. Included among these have been programs in interpersonal communication skills (Carkhuff, 1969a, 1969b; Egan, 1982; Gazda, Asbury, Balzer, Childers, & Walters, 1984; Ivey & Authier, 1978), assertiveness training (Alberti & Emmons, 1970; Galassi & Galassi, 1977; Lange & Jakubowski, 1976), relaxation training (Bernstein & Borkovec, 1973), and rational thinking (Ellis & Harper, 1975).

Professionals identifying themselves as mental health counselors were not involved in the development of any of these training programs, but the impact of these programs on the practice of mental health counseling has been profound. It would be difficult to find mental health counselors, except perhaps those of an orthodox psychoanalytic orientation, who did not use psychoeducational methods in their work with clients. This is not to say that these approaches constitute even the major component of a mental health counselor's skills, but they have found favor in dealing with such client issues as stress management, low self-esteem, and poor social interactions. There is little doubt that the practice of mental health counseling would be very different if psychoeducational skills training methodologies had not been developed.

LEGISLATION AND PUBLIC POLICY

So far, this chapter has traced historical and professional practice precursors that were necessary for the emergence of mental health counseling in the 1970s. These antecedents were the result both of societal trends and movements and of professional advances within the mental health disciplines. To have major impact, however, both societal phenomena and significant shifts in treatment must find expression in political actions. It is therefore safe to say that mental health counseling would probably not have developed at all had it not been for a series of legislative initiatives spanning more than a half century. It is almost equally certain that the future development of mental health counseling depends to a considerable extent on the outcome of future legislative decisions.

Legislation Affecting the Development of the Counseling Profession

Professional counseling received its initial legislative mandate in the Smith-Hughes Act of 1917. The National Vocational Guidance Association had been founded four years earlier and youth unemployment was still a major social priority. The Smith-Hughes Act, like its predecessors, the Morrill Acts of 1862 and 1890, represented a major federal excursion into education funding, a matter traditionally left exclusively to the states. While the intent of Smith-Hughes was focused on funding vocational education programs, a section of the law provided for vocational guidance programs in public schools. Vocational guidance was supported by at least three other vocational education acts prior to World War II. Among the key provisions of these acts was funding for vocational guidance leadership positions within state departments of education. Such funding was continued well into the 1970s. Following World War II, Congress enacted legislation providing for veterans' educational benefits that included funds for vocational guidance services. These benefits were later extended to veterans of the Korean conflict.

Federal legislative initiatives in support of vocational guidance were important for the future development of mental health counseling because such acts reinforced the professionalization of counseling and provided funds for the delivery of counseling services. The fact that counselors focused almost entirely on vocational issues during this time is less important than the emergence of counseling prior to 1950 as a unique human services profession.

The impact of counseling in educational settings was further enhanced by the passage of the National Defense Education Act (NDEA) of 1958. This act provided a major funding source for school-based counseling services and for university programs to train counselors. Passed in part as a reaction to the launching of the Sputnik satellite by the former Soviet Union, NDEA was designed to help the United States overcome what were perceived as serious educational deficiencies. Of particular concern was the relatively low number of youth expressing interest in careers in mathematics and the physical sciences. Remedies supported by NDEA included a testing program to identify students with math and science ability. Test results were to be used to "counsel" promising students to enter these career fields. Other titles of the act provided support for vastly expanded secondary school guidance programs and for university-sponsored institutes to train new counselors to staff these programs. Many of the graduate counselor education programs that are today training mental health counselors originated as a result of NDEA funding to train secondary school counselors.

The NDEA was renewed and amended in 1964, with new titles aimed at the support of counseling programs in elementary schools and in community colleges. Funds for counseling socially and economically disadvantaged students, especially at the elementary school level, were provided by the Elementary and Secondary Education Act (ESEA) of 1965. The Emergency School Assistance Act (ESAA) of 1971 funded additional school counselors to assist in the desegregation of school districts. Later in that decade the Education Amendments of 1976 (PL 94-482) strengthened the role of counseling in vocational education programs and authorized an administrative unit for counseling and guidance in the United States Office of Education. While a few more recent federal initiatives have provided funding for school counseling programs, none of these can be construed as having an impact on the development of mental health counseling.

The importance to mental health counseling of NDEA and subsequent federal education legislation lies in the impact of these laws on counselor education programs and on the economics of supply and demand as it affected counseling positions. By the late 1960s, nearly 400 colleges and universities offered at least master's degrees in counseling. Encouraged by federal funding and supplemented by other funding sources, schools of education were turning out counselors at rates that showed little regard for the demands of the marketplace. Birthrates were declining by the late sixties, a phenomenon that had the inevitable result of lower school enrollments. The drain on national resources created by the combination of federal spending on the Vietnam War and on the Great Society social initiatives (Lyndon Johnson's promise that the nation could afford both guns and butter) led to an economic recession in the early 1970s that took its toll on public school budgets. The combined effect of counselor oversupply and the reduced number of school counselor positions was predictable: those counselors entering the field increasingly found positions in nonschool settings. A quiet revolution was begun to which we shall return later.

Legislation Affecting the Delivery of Mental Health Services

The National Committee for Mental Hygiene (NCMH), founded by Clifford Beers during the Progressive Era, was quite active in improving mental hygiene education and patient treatment prior to and immediately following World War I. The National Mental Health Association, successor to NCMH, along with professional organizations representing a variety of mental health disciplines, has been a persuasive advocate for mental health legislation in the period since World War II. The National Mental Health Act was passed in 1946, authorizing the establishment of the National Institute of Mental Health (NIMH). The NIMH has in turn supported the training of psychiatrists, clinical and counseling psychologists, and psychiatric nurses.

The Joint Commission on Mental Illness was established by the National Mental Health Study Act of 1955. The findings of the commission provided the basis for Congressional passage of the Community Mental Health Centers Act of 1963. This act provided federal funds to states to plan, construct, and staff community mental health centers and to develop multidisciplinary treatment teams of professionals and paraprofessionals. Funding extensions were passed in 1965, 1970, and 1975, each of which expanded services to a broader population.

The Carter Administration's commitment to improvement of mental health services was first manifested in the 1978 report of the President's Commission on Mental Health, chaired by First Lady Rosalynn Carter. The report revealed problems and inadequacies in the mental health services delivery system and emphasized the need for community-based services, including long- and short-term care, access to continuity of care, changes to meet the needs of special populations, and adequate financing. Also addressed was the tension among the mental health professions. The Mental Health Systems Act of 1980 was based on the commission's recommendations and emphasized "balanced services" with appropriate attention to both preventive and remedial programs. This legislation mandated new services for children, youth, the elderly, minority populations, and the chronically mentally ill. The act was repealed almost before the ink was dry as the result of severe federal budget cuts for social programs during the first year of the Reagan Administration.

Federal mental health legislation since 1963 has been important to the development of mental health counseling for two reasons. First, the gradual evolution of models for community-based care of persons formerly housed in state hospitals has had profound effects on these individuals and their families as well as society at large. These effects will be dealt with in more detail in the next section. Second, the emergence of the community mental health center has provided a rich environment in which the counseling profession could develop and expand from its previous history in educational settings. The "quiet revolution," referred to earlier, continued as graduates of counselor education programs found that their skills were effective with populations and in settings other than those for which they had originally been trained. They gradually realized that they had been limiting themselves in the application of their skills, rather than the skills they possessed being the limiting factors.

These pioneer mental health counselors found, however, that there was much that they needed to know that was not covered by traditional counselor education curricula. They filled in the gaps in their knowledge base by additional coursework, by in-service training, by consultation with and supervision from other mental health professionals on the center staffs, and by their ongoing clinical experience. The presence of counselors in community mental health centers had an interactive effect as well, as they shared their expertise with their colleagues, especially in areas involving consultation and community education. Still missing in the early 1970s, however, was a coherent professional identity for counselors working in the centers and in other community settings. This deficit would not be remedied for a few more years.

OTHER OUTCOMES OF FEDERAL MENTAL HEALTH LEGISLATION

It is clear that federal mental health legislative initiatives have had a profound impact on the development of mental health counseling as a profession. The establishment of community mental health centers in particular provided the entree for counselors to move from primarily educational settings to community settings serving a much more varied population. It is also worthwhile to note several other outcomes of mental health legislation since World War II. Among these are the development of community-based delivery systems, the impact of the National Institute of Mental Health, and the organized efforts of community mental health centers through the National Council of Community Mental Health Centers (NCCMHC).

Community-Based Delivery Systems

Only in the last 35 years have mental health services begun to move toward community-based delivery systems on a large scale. The Joint Commission on Mental Illness established by the National Mental Health Study Act of 1955 realized that large state mental hospitals were becoming warehouses for the mentally ill, with little treatment taking place. It was as though the reforms instigated by Dix, Beers, and others had never happened.

After the passage of the Community Mental Health Centers Act of 1963, the state hospitals saw a dramatic decline in patient census. Halfway houses and group homes flourished as communities strained to find residences for the thousands of released patients. The bitter opposition to community-based treatment or residential facilities that is frequently seen today had not yet crystallized.

The mental health programs, with strong support from the Kennedy, Johnson, and Nixon Administrations, also improved services for the mentally retarded. The 1970 funding extension mandated programs for children and adolescents, drug and alcohol abuse, and for mental health consultation. Several additional programs were provided for by the 1975 amendments: follow-up care, transitional living arrangements, child and adolescent treatment and follow-up, screening, and additional programs in alcohol and drug abuse.

It is difficult to predict the effects of the Mental Health Systems Act of 1980 had it not been repealed in 1981. It is well accepted that community-based treatment is more cost effective than large-scale residential treatment and that "no treatment" eventually exacts a higher toll from the economy in general in terms of lost productivity and revenue than would be the case if public resources were committed to community care.

It is generally agreed that there are three optimal settings for primary prevention and treatment of mental and emotional disorders: the community, the schools, and the workplace. As has been shown, the future of publicly funded community-based care is somewhat in doubt in terms of necessary new initiatives to finish the process begun by the deinstitutionalization of the early 1960s. Unfortunately, the prospect is similar for mental health services in schools. One of the principal roles of the elementary school counselors who entered the field in the late 1960s was that of primary prevention of emotional difficulties in children. Many elementary counseling positions were funded by Title I of the Elementary and Secondary Education Act. When federal funds expired, the positions were funded by state and local authorities in some areas but by no means in all. The present situation is one of great variability. In some states, especially in the Sunbelt, elementary counseling programs are thriving, while in many others, elementary counselors are all but nonexistent. Regardless of the geographical location, secondary school counselors suffer from role confusion that is in part the legacy of the National Defense Education Act. Some secondary counselors have designed comprehensive, developmental guidance and counseling programs in which preventive mental health is a primary focus. Many others do little but process student schedules and seek appropriate post secondary educational placements for their clients. School-based counseling services may continue to drift or erode in many locales unless strong federal statements continue to be made, such as the Elementary School Counseling Demonstration Act, which was passed by Congress in 1995 (Paisley & Borders, 1995).

The outlook for mental health services in the workplace is fortunately much brighter. The employee assistance program (EAP) concept began when employers realized that it was more cost effective to treat and prevent alcoholism than to recruit and train new workers. The EAPs, while still dealing with alcoholism and alcohol-related problems, have expanded to include treatment of a wide range of drug abuse and personal problems. In many cases, EAPs provide (or make referrals) for marriage, family, and career issues as well. The *EAP Digest* is a source of information and innovative ideas for those interested in EAPs and provides advertising by the larger national corporations and inpatient centers who have entered the lucrative EAP field. With the privatization of services (as opposed to these services being available in tax-supported community agencies) which began with the Reagan Administration and which continues in the mid-1990s, EAPs and other private, for profit, community-based programs will likely continue to flourish. Those responsible for staffing EAPs are finding, as did administrators of community mental health centers nearly three decades earlier, that there is a pool of talented professionals trained as counselors at the master's degree level who can provide cost effective services and who can bring new dimensions of skills and services to the programs.

The National Institute of Mental Health (NIMH)

The National Institute of Mental Health is the oldest institute in the Alcohol, Drug Abuse and Mental Health Administration (ADAMHA), into which NIMH was incorporated by act of Congress in 1974. The NIMH, the National Institute on Alcohol Abuse and Alcoholism, and the National Institute on Drug Abuse are charged with advancing scientific knowledge in these fields.

Studies conducted by NIMH have shown that as many as one in five Americans suffer from mental or emotional problems. These range from anxiety and phobias to schizophrenia and other debilitating illnesses, with various types of depression accounting for the suffering of a significant portion of the population. The institute is devoted to the prevention and treatment of these illnesses through research, public education, and model treatment programs.

The NIMH supports a wide range of scientific studies in universities, hospitals, and other research centers to advance knowledge of the biological, genetic, and cognitive bases for behavior, and effective new ways to treat and prevent mental illness. Examples include fundamental studies of brain chemistry and the role of molecular and cellular mechanisms in triggering mental illness, as well as the normal processes of memory, learning, and cognition. Behavioral studies span mental, emotional, and behavioral development, and factors involved in dysfunctional behavior.

The NIMH also conducts and supports epidemiology research to collect national data on the incidence and prevalence of mental illnesses. These studies indicate the mental health status of various segments of the population.

In the area of prevention research, NIMH supports studies to promote healthy behaviors and coping skills, and studies of the most effective ways to help people who have undergone a life crisis such as death in the family, or a catastrophic event such as a flood, hurricane, or other natural disaster. A special focus of the institute's prevention studies are people considered at risk of developing mental and emotional problems, such as children of parents who are mentally ill or are separated or divorced. Studies are also supported in special areas, such as the mental health of minorities, antisocial and violent behavior, sexual assault, work and mental health, and the mental health of the elderly (DHHS Publication No. (ADM) 84-1320, 1984).

The National Council of Community Mental Health Centers (NCCMHC)

The National Council of Community Mental Health Centers is the national organization that represents community mental health centers in government relations efforts and serves a networking and clearinghouse function to enable its constituent members to better communicate among themselves. The NCCMHC is a nongovernmental body, but it is a direct result of federal legislative initiatives beginning with the Community Mental Health Centers Act of 1963.

Founded in 1970, NCCMHC represents more than 700 agencies comprising some 62,000 staff and board members nationwide. Through its sections and divisions, the organization also provides membership opportunities for individuals who share common interests in specialized areas of community mental health. The NCCMHC conducts an annual national convention that provides opportunities for professional development and renewal as well as consideration of policy and government relations initiatives.

MENTAL HEALTH COUNSELING: THE IDENTITY EMERGES

At the beginning of this chapter, the major historical antecedents of moral treatment and vocational guidance were presented. Antecedents in professional practice, including testing and assessment, nonmedical approaches to psychotherapy, theories of normal human development, group counseling and psychotherapy, and psychoeducational approaches to treatment were briefly sketched. These were followed by chronological accounts of legislative and public policy influences affecting the development of both the counseling profession and the delivery of mental health services. As important as all of these factors have been for the development of mental health counseling, none of them can be said to have been the causal factor of the dynamic profession that exists today. To be sure, all of them were necessary, but none is sufficient as an explanation. The heritage of mental health counseling cannot be traced so directly.

The "Quiet Revolution"

The date when the first counselor joined the staff of a community mental health center is not recorded. It is safe to say that the first cohort of counselors began working in the centers sometime in the mid-1960s. The decline in the number of school counselor openings coupled with the oversupply of counselor education graduates created a ready supply of personnel for the centers.

The staffing patterns of most community mental health centers recognized the established professions of psychiatry, clinical and counseling psychology, social work, and nursing. Most counselors were initially hired as paraprofessionals because their preparation was not in one of the recognized disciplines. Their status and pay were correspondingly lower than that of their colleagues. A wide variety of job titles, such as psych tech, mental health specialist II, and psychiatric aide, were applied to the counselors' positions.

As new community-based programs were inaugurated in the late 1960s, counselors found positions in these as well. Youth services bureaus, drug and alcohol rehabilitation centers, women's centers, and shelters for runaway youth were but a few of the agencies that provided career options for counselors. In these settings also, the recognized professions held the principal posts, with counselors often relegated to paraprofessional status.

By the early 1970s, professional counselors were becoming well entrenched in mental health centers and other community settings. Pay and status did not always improve commensurate with their skills, but counselors were becoming frontline providers of mental health services. Many doctoral graduates of counselor education programs, unable to secure licensure as psychologists as their forebears had done and finding positions as counselor educators increasingly difficult to obtain, began to set up private practices as professional counselors. They were gradually joined by more and more counselors with master's degree training, many of whom were veterans of community mental health centers. The "quiet revolution" was gathering momentum, but the identity of mental health counseling was yet to be affixed to its banners.

A New Professional Organization

The American Personnel and Guidance Association (APGA) had been founded in 1952 when four professional counseling and guidance organizations merged into a single association structure that permitted them to retain their separate identities while at the same time facilitating cooperative efforts. During the following 25 years, APGA grew to encompass 12 divisions accommodating counselors in school, college, rehabilitation, employment, and corrections settings. Divisions also represented special interests and skills, such as vocational counseling, measurement and evaluation, group work, religious and values issues, humanistic education, multicultural concerns, and counselor education and supervision.

Many counselors working in mental health and other community settings were APGA members, even though the association did not include a division that addressed their unique concerns. Calls for the formation of such a division began around 1975, setting in motion a series of events that led to the founding of the American Mental Health Counselors Association (AMHCA) as an independent organization in 1976 and its affiliation as APGA's 13th division in 1978 (Weikel, 1985). Chapter 2 contains a detailed account of AMHCA's history.

AMHCA: The Organization Becomes the Identity

From its founding in 1976 until around 1990, it was virtually impossible to separate the development of mental health counseling as a profession from its organizational expression. The new association seemed an idea whose time had come, attracting members from a variety of mental health and other community settings, from rehabilitation and corrections agencies, and from educational settings at all levels, elementary school through university. Growing to more than 10,000 in less than 10 years, AMHCA's membership was more diverse than any of its sister divisions, with the largest single group being private practitioners.

The association's agenda concentrated initially on issues related to professional identity and recognition. AMHCA's first major goal was to establish a national certification process for mental health counselors. The National Academy of Certified Clinical Mental Health Counselors was founded in 1979 to provide a vehicle through which the considerable skills of mental health counselors could be validated on a voluntary basis. Coupled with the national certification effort, AMHCA members threw their support behind the activities under way in a number of states to achieve passage of counselor licensure statutes.

During the 1980s, AMHCA leaders pressed NIMH officials and the Congress for full recognition of mental health counselors and for their involvement at all levels within NIMH. A priority still unrealized was to persuade NIMH to include mental health counselors in the national manpower studies to determine the extent to which direct client services were being provided by mental health and related counselors. Other early policy priorities included eligibility for clinical training funds and research into areas of concern to counselors. Professional counselors saw themselves as supporting the goals of NIMH without receiving any direct benefit from the institute. Mental health counselors were successful in negotiating a seat on the NIMH Advisory Council.

Concurrently, AMHCA sought a greater voice within the National Council of Community Mental Health Centers. The association was represented by its leaders at the NCCMHC conventions during most of the 1980s, but the relationship between the two groups has been less involved in recent years.

In the federal legislative arena, AMHCA supported legislation aimed at opening federally sponsored mental health programs to MHCs. Special targets during the 1980s were programs funded by Medicare and

Medicaid and by the Older Americans Act. These initiatives were unsuccessful in achieving their immediate goals, but mental health counselors learned a great deal about legislative advocacy during this period.

Following on the heels of efforts to secure state licensure and national certification was a cluster of priorities that focused on achieving parity with the older mental health disciplines. Labeled "recognition and reimbursement" by AMHCA President David Brooks (1986–87), these priorities encompassed third-party insurance reimbursement, recognition by federal benefit systems such as the Office of Civilian Health and Medical Programs of the Uniformed Services (OCHAMPUS) and the Federal Employees Health Benefits Program, official recognition in federal statutes as a core provider discipline of mental health services, and inclusion by title in state personnel classification systems, among others. Recognition by OCHAMPUS was accomplished in 1987 after an intensive three-year effort.

At the state level, mental health counselors achieved eligibility for health insurance reimbursement much more slowly. In some states, vendorship statutes were passed, while in others the insurance code was amended by rule. By the mid-1990s there was still considerable unevenness in patterns of reimbursement eligibility. The advent of managed care, even with the failure of the health care reforms of the Clinton Administration, raised the possibility that the decade-long effort to achieve reimbursement eligibility would become a moot point. At the time of this writing the situation was still too fluid and too diverse to be able to make general and definitive statements about the status of mental health counselors in a managed care environment.

AMHCA and ACA: Impact and Change

Mental health counselors and their professional organization have had substantial impact on the larger counseling profession as well. Immediately after affiliation in 1978, AMHCA leaders sought to change the name of APGA so that the word "counseling" was included in the name of the parent body. They achieved partial success in 1983 when APGA changed its name to the American Association for Counseling and Development (AACD). Following the disaffiliation of its college student development division in 1991, AACD, at AMHCA's urging, changed its name once more, this time to the American Counseling Association (ACA).

Tensions surrounding the name changes were mirrored in other policy differences among AMHCA, other units within APGA/AACD/ACA, and the parent body itself. Setting priorities for the government relations agenda was one flashpoint. ACA was comfortable lobbying for issues and funding affecting school counselors, but totally unfamiliar with mental health issues. AMHCA first hired its own lobbying firm, then in 1985 returned to a strategy of operating inside the ACA government relations apparatus. Other points of dispute have centered around internal governance, fiscal accountability, and ACA's general posture with respect to advocacy for mental health counselors.

Twice in the 1990s, relations between the elected leaders of AMHCA and the ACA governance structure reached the threshold of disaffiliation. In February, 1994, the AMHCA Board of Directors voted by a narrow margin to disaffiliate from ACA and to put the matter to an every-member referendum for ratification. They were opposed by a cadre of past presidents and other leaders who raised questions about the haste and wisdom of such an action. In April of that year, the membership voted by more than 70 percent to remain under the ACA umbrella (Smith & Robinson, 1995). In the summer of 1995, the AMHCA board took a similar action. At this writing, the outcome of the second referendum is unknown.

Counselor education programs have responded to the increasingly divergent career paths of their graduates by developing mental health counseling and community counseling training programs ranging in length from 48 to more than 60 semester credits. These programs, many of which are accredited by the Council for Accreditation of Counseling and Related Educational Programs (CACREP), are producing clinical mental health practitioners amply qualified to deliver services in a variety of public and private clinical settings. Forty-one states and the District of Columbia had responded to the professionalization of counseling by passing counselor licensure laws by the autumn of 1995.

SUMMARY

Descendants of a rich heritage extending back well before the 20th century, mental health counselors began their trek to professional identity and recognition in the late 1960s. Drawing from several historical and professional practice antecedents this new profession rose during the 1970s to the front line of service delivery in a variety of settings, but lacked a coherent identity until the American Mental Health Counselors Association was founded in 1976. During the last decade the AMHCA has experienced unprecedented growth and has emerged as an assertive and articulate voice for the identity and the advancement of mental health counseling. Its impact within and outside the counseling profession has been felt in areas of training and credentialing and of increased consumer access to mental health services.

REFERENCES

Alberti, R. E., & Emmons, M. I. (1970). *Your perfect right.* San Luis Obispo, CA: Impact Publishers.

Authier, J., Gustafson, K., Guerney, B., Jr., & Kasdorf, J. (1975). The psychological practitioner as a teacher: A theoretical-historical and practical review. *Counseling Psychologist, 5,* 31–50.

Beers, C. W. (1908). *A mind that found itself.* Garden City, NY: Longmans, Green.

Bernstein, D. A., & Borkovec, T. D. (1973). *Progressive relaxation training: A manual for the helping professions.* Champaign, IL: Research Press.

Brooks, D. K., Jr. (1984). *A life-skills taxonomy: Defining elements of effective functioning through the use of the Delphi technique.* Unpublished doctoral dissertation, University of Georgia.

Carkhuff, R. R. (1969a). *Helping and human relations. Vol. 1: Selection and training.* New York: Holt Rinehart & Winston.

Carkhuff, R. R. (1969b). *Helping and human relations. Vol. 2: Practice and research.* New York: Holt, Rinehart & Winston.

American Psychiatric Association. (1994). *Diagnostic and statistical manual of mental disorders* (4th ed.). Washington, DC: Author.

Egan, G. (1982). *The skilled helper: A model for systematic helping and interpersonal relating* (2nd ed.). Monterey, CA: Brooks/Cole.

Ellis, A., & Harper, R. A. (1975). *A new guide to rational living.* Hollywood, CA: Wilshire Books.

Freud, S. (1953). Three essays on the theory of sexuality. In J. Strachey (Ed.), *The standard edition of the complete psychological works of Sigmund Freud* (Vol. 7). London: Hogarth Press. (Original work published 1905).

Freud, S. (1961). The infantile genital organization: An interpolation into the theory of sexuality. In J. Strachey (Ed.), *The standard edition of the complete psychological works of Sigmund Freud* (Vol. 19). London: Hogarth Press. (Original work published 1923).

Galassi, M. D., & Galassi, J. P. (1977). *Assert yourself!* New York: Human Sciences Press.

Gazda, G. M. (1982). Group psychotherapy and group counseling: Definition and heritage. In G. M. Gazda (Ed.), *Basic approaches to group psychotherapy and group counseling* (3rd ed.) (pp. 5–36). Springfield, IL: Charles C Thomas.

Gazda, G. M., Asbury, F. R., Balzer, F. J., Childers, W. C., & Walters, R. P. (1984). *Human relations development: A manual for educators* (3rd ed.). Boston: Allyn & Bacon.

Gazda, G. M., & Brooks, D. K., Jr. (1985). The development of the social/life-skills training movement. *Journal of Group Psychotherapy, Psychodrama, & Sociometry, 38*(1), 1–10.

Green, T. F. (1985). The last forty years—The next forty years. *Nexus, 7*(2), 13–17.

Ivey, A. E., & Authier, J. (1978). *Microcounseling: Innovations in interviewing, counseling, psychotherapy, and psychoeducation* (2nd ed.). Springfield, IL: Charles C Thomas.

Kohlberg, L. (1973). Continuities in childhood and adult moral development revisited. In P. B. Baltes & K. W. Schaie (Eds.), *Life-span development psychology: Personality and socialization* (pp. 179–204). New York: Academic Press.

Lange, A. J., & Jakubowski, P. (1976). *Responsible assertive behavior: Cognitive/behavioral procedures for trainers.* Champaign, IL: Research Press.

Loevinger, J. (1976). *Ego development: Conceptions and theories.* San Francisco: Jossey-Bass.

McKinley, J. C., & Hathaway, S. R. (1940). A Multiphasic Personality Schedule (Minnesota): I. Construction of the schedule. *Journal of Psychology, 10,* 249–254.

Moreno, J. L., & Elefthery, D. G. (1982). An introduction to group psychodrama. In G. M. Gazda (Ed.), *Basic approaches to group psychotherapy and group counseling* (3rd ed.) (pp. 101–131). Springfield, IL: Charles C Thomas.

Murray, D. J. (1983). *A history of western psychology.* Englewood Cliffs, NJ: Prentice-Hall.

Paisley, P. O., & Borders, L. D. (1995). School counseling: An evolving specialty. *Journal of Counseling and Development, 74,* 150–153.

Parsons, F. (1909). *Choosing a vocation.* Boston: Houghton Mifflin.

Perry, W. G., Jr. (1970). *Forms of intellectual and ethical development in the college years: A scheme.* New York: Holt, Rinehart & Winston.

Rogers, C. R. (1942). *Counseling and psychotherapy.* Boston: Houghton Mifflin.

Rogers, C. R., Gendlin, E. T., Kiesler, D., & Truax, C. B. (1967). *The therapeutic relationship and its impact.* Madison: University of Wisconsin Press.

Rodgers, R. F. (1980). Theories underlying student development. In D. G. Creamer (Ed.), *Student development and higher education: Theories, practices, and future directions* (pp. 10–95). Cincinnati: American College Personnel Association.

Selman, R. L. (1976). Social-cognitive understanding. In T. Lickona (Ed.), *Moral development and behavior.* New York: Holt, Rinehart & Winston.

Selman, R. L. (1977). A structural-developmental model of social cognition: Implications for intervention research. *Counseling Psychologist, 6*(4), 3–6.

Smith, H. B., & Robinson, G. P. (1995). Mental health counseling: Past, present, and future. *Journal of Counseling and Development, 74,* 158–162.

Sprafkin, R. P. (1977). The rebirth of moral treatment. *Professional Psychology, 8*(2), 161–169.

Weikel, W. J. (1985). The American Mental Health Counselors Association. *Journal of Counseling and Development, 63,* 457–460.

Whiteley, J. M. (1984). A historical perspective on the development of counseling psychology as a profession. In S. D. Brown & R. W. Lent (Eds.), *Handbook of counseling psychology* (pp. 3–55). New York: Wiley.

Chapter 2

THE AMERICAN MENTAL HEALTH COUNSELORS ASSOCIATION

Wᴵᴸᴸᴵᴀᴹ J. Wᴇᴵᴋᴇʟ

This chapter traces the history and development of the American Mental Health Counselors Association (AMHCA), from its founding in 1976 to its present status as the leading voice for mental health counselors in the nation. It provides a rationale for AMHCA's rapid growth and rising influence in mental health care and examines issues of crucial concern for the future of the counseling profession. The chapter also addresses AMHCA's role in the establishment of professional identity for mental health counselors and credentialing and lobbying efforts. Finally, it discusses AMHCA's governance structure and its publications along with a list of the AMHCA presidents from 1976 to 1996.

By the mid 1970s, increasing numbers of counseling graduates were finding employment in a variety of community and nonschool settings. Yet, the American Counseling Association (ACA), then known as the American Personnel and Guidance Association (APGA), had no distinct division for community and agency counselors. Until the American Mental Health Counselors Association was founded, the thousands of professional counselors working in these settings had no organizational home. The American Psychological Association (APA) seemed to be emphasizing and supporting doctoral-level training, while APGA had a reputation as an association for school counselors, vocational counselors, college student development workers, and rehabilitation counselors.

AMHCA was born at just the right moment in time. People who were community counselors, agency counselors, and in private practice as counselors quickly latched onto the title "mental health counselor" and the idea that a unique professional group had been formed to meet their needs. AMHCA was born in May 1976, when James J. Messina and Nancy Spisso, then director and co-director, respectively, of the Escambia County (Florida) Mental Health Center, were discussing the issue of the lack of a professional organization for community counselors. Their discussion had been prompted by a letter to the *APGA Guidepost*, written by Edward Anderson and a group of his Wisconsin colleagues, calling for representation and recognition of nonschool counselors in APGA. About a year earlier, Gary Seiler of the University of Florida had written a similar letter.

Being action oriented, Messina decided to call APGA President Thelma Daley, who he knew from previous work with the American School Counselor Association. Daley promised to send the necessary information for establishing a new division. The process had begun. The name "American Mental Health Counselors Association" was chosen that first day "because we wanted to have counselors who worked in mental health settings identified and we wanted the name to have a good ring to it" (J. J. Messina, personal communication, November 14, 1983). Messina and Spisso contacted Gary Seiler and also James Hiett, also in Florida, for help, and AMHCA was off and running.

There was an excitement there in the early days that is hard to describe. I was invited to participate early on because I had been a University of Florida doctoral student with Spisso and Hiett. Messina and Seiler were at the Student Health Center as postdoctoral fellows and as adjunct faculty in the counseling program. Letters were sent to the *Guidepost* announcing the formation of a steering committee, and soon, Anderson and several Wisconsin counselors joined a growing nucleus of University of Florida graduates, faculty, and friends. The committee rapidly grew to 50 members. In July of 1976, the request to form a new division was presented to the new APGA President, George Gazda. However, at that July meeting, the APGA board had passed a resolution calling for a moratorium on the establishment of new divisions. Hence, the proposal was not acted upon. Undaunted, the steering committee decided to go ahead and establish an independent organization. By-laws were written and edited. They were approved by the members on November 7, 1976. AMHCA had become an official organization and was soon incorporated in the state of Florida.

The first annual AMHCA conference was scheduled concurrently with the APGA convention in Dallas, Texas on March 6, 1977. From November 1976 until March 1977, AMHCA had grown from the original 50 to almost 500 members. How exciting it was to be in Dallas and meet many of these pioneers face to face. For me it was an opportunity to develop friendships that continue today, twenty years later, with people who then and now are on the cutting edge of the profession. Dynamism and energy were abundant in Dallas. Most of the charter members were there, and several exciting new persons joined the movement. Programs and workshops were presented and the first board of directors was elected. Nancy Spisso was president; James Messina, president-elect; David Rouse Eastin from the Wisconsin group, treasurer; and Donald Didier as member-at-large. Committees were formed, and dedicated, motivated volunteers went to work. The official slogan, "AMHCA Works For You," was adopted, but at the late night parties and socials, the unofficial policy of "work hard, play hard" became the rule.

AMHCA's strong foundation was in place, cemented by competent, hardworking professionals in key positions. Norman Gysbers, APGA president-elect, attended the AMHCA meeting in Dallas, and by the close of the APGA convention, the moratorium on new divisions had been lifted. Because AMHCA was already incorporated, a membership vote regarding APGA affiliation was necessary. There were strong sentiments pro and con, but in a November 1977 referendum, the membership voted by a slim 51 percent to 49 percent margin to become a division of APGA. Also at this time, Steven Lindenberg was voted as the next AMHCA president-elect and James Messina began his term as president.

Throughout the remainder of 1977 and into 1978, the association continued to grow to almost 1500 strong. In March of 1978, prior to the APGA convention in Washington, D.C., another "First Annual AMHCA Conference" was held, this time in Columbia, Maryland. Twenty workshops and several membership and business meetings were conducted. However, the most important outcome of the Columbia gathering was the formation of AMHCA priorities such as licensure for MHCs, third-party payments, full parity with other mental health providers, private practice issues, and so forth. Many of these important issues continue to be association priorities at the present time.

Excitement at Columbia was high, because the APGA board was expected to act on AMHCA's proposal to become a division during their Washington meeting, a few days later. Dr. Gysbers delivered the good news to AMHCA leaders that, effective July 1, 1978, AMHCA would become APGA's 13th division. On that date, AMHCA President Messina took his seat on the APGA board, with Betty Knox presiding. There was not 100 percent crossover of members with the move to APGA, but

AMHCA quickly grew back to 1500 members and within the next few years to 12,000.

CERTIFICATION

Prior to the Columbia meeting, a special ad hoc committee within AMHCA composed the "Blueprint for the Mental Health Counseling Profession." This forward-thinking document added a sense of direction and continuity to the movement. Because counselor licensure was virtually nonexistent, except for Virginia (1976), AMHCA leaders proposed the founding of the National Academy of Certified Clinical Mental Health Counselors (NACCMHC). For legal purposes, the academy was established as a separate corporate entity. Its purpose was to certify counselors, via exam and competency assessment for the speciality of clinical mental health counseling. The first certification examination was given to a group of over 50 applicants on February 3, 1979, at the Johns Hopkins University Columbia, Maryland campus. Sitting next to me was early AMHCA leader, future AMHCA president and current (1995–1996) American Counseling Association President, Joyce M. Breasure. She still reminds me that I talked to myself throughout the entire difficult written examination. As I predicted in the 1986 writing of this text, the NACCMHC eventually affiliated with the National Board for Certified Counselors (NBCC) and is now administered as a speciality certification under the NBCC umbrella.

PUBLICATIONS

In April of 1978, Volume 1, Number 1, of the *AMHCA News* appeared replacing the mimeographed newsletters of the previous two years. Editor Colleen Haffner and Associate Editor Janet Asher Anderson, who later became editor, soon established the *AMHCA News* as a useful, high quality publication with a grassroots orientation. The News continued to expand and grow under a succession of future editors, including John Moracco, Charles Huber, William Weikel, and most recently, Carol Hacker. During Carol Hacker's tenure, the publication changed its name to the *Advocate.*

In 1978, I was selected to establish and edit the *AMHCA Journal.* Luckily, I was able to secure a top-notch editorial board of academics and practitioners. We sought a balance between theoretical manuscripts and practical articles that would be useful to AMHCA members. The charter issue appeared in January of 1979, carrying important articles about professional identity and certification and a warning to counselors about possible exclusion from the mental health care delivery system. The journal was published semi-annually until 1982, when James Wiggins became editor. By 1983, the budget allowed for the journal to become a quarterly. Under the successive editorial guidance of Linda Seligman, Lawrence Gerstein, and Earl Ginter, the *AMHCA Journal,* now known as the *Journal of Mental Health Counseling* has become a well-respected publication that disseminates research and applications to the international mental health community.

LEADERSHIP

AMHCA has been blessed and maybe sometimes cursed with strong and vocal leaders. Many in my opinion have been true visionaries while others have been content to nurture the seeds planted before them. All have given selflessly of their time and talents to promote the field of mental health counseling and to advance the profession. The presidents of AMHCA and their term in office follows:

Nancy Spisso	1976–1977	Nancy J. McCormick	1987–1988
James J. Messina	1977–1979	Howard B. Smith	1988–1989
Steven P. Lindenberg	1979–1980	Larry K. Hill	1989–1990
Joyce M. Breasure	1980–1981	Janet M. Herman	1990–1991
Gary D. Seiler	1981–1982	William Krieger	1991–1992
William J. Weikel	1982–1983	Gail Robinson	1992–1993
Edward S. Beck	1983–1984	Roberta M. Driscoll	1993–1994
Richard R. Wilmarth	1984–1985	John Nestor	1994–1995
Rory B. Madden	1985–1986	Glenda E. Isenhour	1995–1996
David K. Brooks, Jr.	1986–1987	Nancy Benz (elect)	1996–1997

These dedicated men and women guided the association through several stages of growth and not a small amount of controversy. In 1994, there was a major rift among past and present leaders over a decision by the 1994 board to attempt to disaffiliate from the American Counseling Association. By a vote of 76 percent, the rank and file members elected to stay in ACA. However, current leaders still feel it is best for the association to leave ACA and become a free-standing association and expect to put the question once again before the membership in early

1996. It is hoped that regardless of the outcome, the association will stay strong in its battle for the growth and advancement of the profession.

Perhaps the best overall view of the association is from the *1994 AMHCA Strategic Plan.* In summary, the plan advocates twelve goals for the association:

1. **Public Policy and Legislation** — Promote, support, and encourage the use of counseling professionals in all appropriate public policy and legislation, enhancing the profession and advocating for consumers.
2. **Professional Development** — Create comprehensive programs for continuing education, leadership development, counselor preparation, and professional recognition.
3. **Professionalization** — Implement a comprehensive plan for promoting the counseling profession that includes standards, credentialing, ethics, and advocacy.
4. **Public Awareness and Support** — Increase awareness and support for mental health counseling by educating and influencing the public, consumers, private and public decision-makers, the media, other mental health professionals, educators, and students.
5. **Membership** — Develop and implement a comprehensive membership recruitment and retention plan.
6. **Research and Knowledge** — Promote the development of research designs and paradigms to evaluate and enhance the practice of counseling, including efficacy research.
7. **Interprofessional-Interdisciplinary Collaboration** — Educate and involve the association and its members in interprofessional and interdisciplinary issues.
8. **Organizational Structure** — Provide an organizational structure that supports ongoing association activities and that is appropriate for the implementation of the strategic plan.
9. **Human Rights** — Develop, articulate, and implement a human rights agenda for the association.
10. **Resource Management** — Develop a resource management plan that supports ongoing association activities.
11. **Developmental Approach** — Collaborate with ACA on the development of an official statement regarding the developmental approach, particularly as to its application in mental health counseling.

12. **International Collaboration** — Promote international awareness of mental health counseling.

GOVERNANCE

In the 1980s, AMHCA abandoned the governance model of president, president-elect, past president, secretary, treasurer, and member-at-large in favor of a regional representation model. Now after various modes of experimentation, the board is comprised of: President, President-Elect, Past President, Four Regional Directors, a Director-at-Large/Secretary, and a Treasurer/Parliamentarian. AMHCA also has a full-time Executive Director, Mary Lyn Pike, who is an attorney and skilled association executive. The AMHCA central office is located in ACA headquarters at Alexandria, Virginia. The AMHCA toll-free number is 1-800-326-2642.

A RATIONALE FOR RAPID GROWTH

AMHCA grew rapidly for its first ten years of existence, then when they became the most expensive division of ACA, membership leveled off. It stays in the 10,000 to 12,000 range, even with significantly higher dues than most ACA divisions. AMHCA delivers. Its service to members, publications, and advocacy efforts are unsurpassed. One recent goal was to have 24,000 members by June 30, 1995. This goal was not reached as membership hovered at 10,000, yet AMHCA continued to provide a variety of first class services to members and to lobby for inclusion of MHCs in managed care programs. In my opinion, the AMHCA membership dollar has more often than not been well-stretched and well spent.

AMHCA has always welcomed all counselors to join and enjoy voting membership status. Usually about 70 percent of the members have a master's degree and about 20 percent the doctorate. Most are trained as counselors, but psychologists, psychiatrists, nurses, social workers, and paraprofessionals can also be found among the membership. Many work in full- or part-time private practices, private counseling centers, community mental health centers and clinics, while smaller numbers work for agencies, schools, and colleges. All members are invited to become involved in leadership and governance with constant calls for volunteers a regular feature of the AMHCA *Advocate.*

Future Direction

"AMHCA's Board of Directors has a vision and has adopted an agenda that will safeguard and enhance your ability to practice . . . " (Nestor, 1994). The association is strongly in favor of marketing mental health counselors to managed care companies; including MHCs in any reformation of the health care system; attaining core provider status for MHCs in all legislation; increasing membership; providing quality professional development opportunities; and developing state chapters. Current leaders are working to get AMHCA's financial situation turned around by increasing nondues revenue and adopting a sound investment policy (Isenhour, 1995). The priorities really aren't new. Many, in fact, follow AMHCA's twenty-year history, but they are vitally important to the future of the profession.

My greatest fear for the profession is that AMHCA will somehow leave ACA to become a freestanding association and that ACA will immediately institute another association for MHCs. This will dilute the power base of both associations and leave us with two groups of probably 5000–6000 each. Neither will have the membership dollars or lobbying clout to be an effective voice for the profession. In my opinion, AMHCA has a strong voice in determining ACA's agenda and can benefit from the power and resources of this 58,000 member group. Whether within ACA or without, whether there is one association or two, the mental health counseling revolution will continue thanks to dedicated professional women and men like you!

REFERENCES

American Mental Health Counselors Association. (1994). Strategic plan. Alexandria, VA. Author.

Isenhour, G. E. (1995 March/April). Setting priorities for 1995–1996. *Advocate*, p. 1.

Nestor, J. (1994 August). From the office of the AMHCA president . . . Alexandria, VA. Letter.

HIGHLIGHT SECTION

MENTAL HEALTH COUNSELING: PAST, PRESENT, AND FUTURE

HOWARD B. SMITH AND GAIL P. ROBINSON

This section examines the significant events in the history of mental health care that have contributed to the development of a specialty within the counseling profession referred to as mental health counseling. The development of credentials for the specialty and the issues currently facing mental health counseling are discussed, and a perspective on directions for the future is offered.

Mental health counseling brings a unique approach to the mental health care professions in that it offers a broader response to the definition of care than the traditional fields of psychiatry and clinical psychology. Historically, people who could benefit from mental health services were viewed as distinctly different from those who would be considered "healthy" (i.e., there is something "wrong" with them, or they are "ill" and therefore in need of treatment). If one considers mental health care to be a continuum based on needs of society with high-level wellness being on one end of the continuum and severe and persistent mental illness being on the other, virtually every person can improve their respective quality of life through the use of mental health services. Simply stated, mental health counseling believes that a person does not have to be sick to get better.

Seiler (1990) noted that mental health counseling emphasizes the developmental, preventive, and educational as well as the traditional remedial aspects of mental health care. Weikel and Palmo (1989) called mental health counseling a "hybrid" and suggested that it was "born from an uneasy relationship between psychology and educational counseling, but with family ties to all of the core mental health care disciplines" (p. 7). Hershenson and Power (1987) used words like "enabling," "asset oriented," and "skill based" (p. 18). They advocated assisting clients to help themselves by identifying and mobilizing the clients' strengths and developing the skills within the client that will carry them beyond the resolution of any immediate issue as opposed to simply "curing the patient" (p. 18). This article provides a brief outline of the history of

38

mental health counseling as a counseling specialty, a snapshot of the present, and some speculation about the future.

These statements appear to be fairly simple and straightforward; however, they are not as simple as they first appear. They set the stage for a profound effect on mental health care both philosophically and in the way it is delivered. Consider the mental health continuum mentioned earlier. Mental health counselors, with their definition, expand the range of treatment to include the concept of professionals delivering preventive services. This represents a fundamentally different concept of health care. It is truly health care rather than treatment of disorders, abnormalities, or disease amelioration. The health care industry of today is only beginning to consider the possibility of *health* care, having been obsessed with *illness* care since the beginning of time. With this as a backdrop, let us consider a brief history.

OVERVIEW OF HISTORICAL DEVELOPMENT

Brooks and Weikel (1986) traced the historical roots of mental health counseling back to the "moral treatment" of the mentally ill that was started by Philippe Pinel, director of the Bicetre (the largest mental hospital in Paris) in 1793. Pinel expanded the definition of mental health care to include the principles of "liberty, equality, and fraternity." Brooks and Weikel explained that Pinel forbade corporal punishment and demanded that the "inmates" be released from their chains. Pinel introduced the idea that individuals who were mentally ill had a level of competence and confidence that precluded the necessity of physical restraint unless, of course, they were a danger to themselves or others. He refused to assume that the "best" treatment was the most conservative, restrictive, and protective. Rather, he felt that a level of normalcy should be maintained or introduced into the clients' lives. About this same time, other reformers were beginning to introduce other more humane expansions to traditional forms of treatment (e.g., William Tuke of England and Dorthea Dix of the United States).

As history unfolded, there was not a straight-line development that led from the traditional, dichotomous thinking (i.e., healthy or sick) to where we are today. Instead, it followed a random and sporadic pattern through the late 1800s during which time there was a reversal from this gravitation toward humanitarian ideals back to a more conservative mentality. A decline in funding from both private and public sources undoubtedly played a role in this shift in that it is less costly to warehouse problematic individuals than to help them attain their potential.

As Brooks and Weikel (1986, p. 7) pointed out, the pendulum of change began to swing toward a broader, more humane position once again, with the publication in 1908 of Clifford W. Beers's autobiographical account of his experience as a patient in mental institutions. Public interest in the area of mental health care was heightened once again, and an organization which later became the National Mental Health Association was formed.

Other expansionist contributions led to the inclusion of occupational or vocational concerns to the definition of mental health, the development of the ability to estimate human abilities, and the measuring of differences between individuals through standardized tests. This was due in no small part to world events such as World Wars I and II, which created an interest in human aptitudes and abilities. This interest later was expanded to include personalities, for example, the publication of the Minnesota Multiphasic Personality Inventory by McKinley and Hathaway in 1940.

Again, Brooks and Weikel (1986, p. 10) pointed to the development of "nonmedical approaches" to psychotherapy being very significant in the continued evolution of this expanded definition of mental health care. Carl Rogers and Fritz Perls, for example, emphasized a client-centered theory, which had at its core the belief that the *client* is a partner in the healing process rather than a *patient* on which a cure is imposed by the professional.

Concurrent with this continuous refinement of the whole concept of mental health care and services were other significant events. Graduates of counselor education programs, who were primarily prepared to work in elementary and secondary education settings, were not able to find employment in those schools as the market was reaching a saturation point. Federal dollars for human services programs such as the Secondary Education Act of 1965 were being redirected into supporting the Vietnam war efforts. The effect of this was twofold. First, it meant less federal money for counseling services in school settings. Second, graduates from counselor education programs, especially those with doctorates, were beginning to find employment (often as licensed psychologists) in university counseling centers or in the Veterans Administration.

The latter was to be short-lived relief, however, as the psychology profession began to block the entrance of these mental health counselors into their "professional turf." The law of supply and demand dictated that the market for these educated and skilled professionals was drying up.

Brooks (1991) noted a number of other forces coming into focus at the same time. Some of these forces had positive effects on mental health counseling, such as the Community Mental Health Centers Act of 1963, which created employment opportunities. There were also increasing numbers of doctoral level counselors, which increased their viability as health care professionals.

STATEMENT OF NEED

According to Seiler (1990), mental health counselors "did not work exclusively with mental illness; we did not work solely through the social service system; nor was our clinical work mainly with marriages or families in trouble. Their roots had been influenced by developmental and prevention services and mental health education" (p. 7). In essence, by the 1970s, mental health counselors found themselves a loosely defined profession without a clear identity or a professional organization around which to rally or form the nucleus of an organizational structure for support or networking capabilities.

By the mid-1970s, it was clear that there was a critical mass of these individuals who (a) were educationally prepared at either master's or doctoral level; (b) worked in community agencies, community mental health, or private practice settings; (c) were delivering a wide variety of services very similar to the more established mental health care provider groups (psychiatry, psychology, social work, etc.); and (d) felt they had no professional home by virtue of their uniqueness (Seiler, Brooks, & Beck, 1987). Thus, the American Mental Health Counselors Association (AMHCA) was formed in 1976 around those things these individuals had in common. However, the central group of members soon discovered that they needed a larger identity or professional family to be able to move their agenda forward. They approached the American Personnel and Guidance Association, which is now the American Counseling Association (ACA), and eventually found, in 1976, a larger professional family with which to associate. By 1989, Ivey concluded, "it is clear that mental health counseling has reached the point at which it has become a heavyweight contender on the national scene" (p. 26).

RELATIONSHIPS WITH OTHER ASPECTS OF ACA

The early years of the relationship between AMHCA and ACA were often stormy and fraught with miscommunication and misunderstanding. It seemed that the AMHCA agenda (i.e., professional credentials, recognition, legislative activity, and third-party reimbursement) represented such a radical departure from the "business as usual" of pre-AMHCA days for ACA that the relationship would surely be strained beyond repair if not broken completely.

ACA had organizational maturity and strength of numbers and AMHCA had a youthful exuberance and had learned how to move swiftly and effectively in the public policy arena. Unfortunately, these respective descriptors occasionally led the two associations to be at cross-purposes. AMHCA sometimes perceived ACA as being too broadly focused and attempting to treat all divisions the same when AMHCA perceived its own needs to be very specific (e.g., ACA support in AMHCA's efforts to gain recognition as a mental health care provider). ACA sometimes perceived AMHCA as being too narrowly focused, and while they admired AMHCA's quest for quality through the development of credentials (e.g., the National Academy of Certified Clinical Mental Health Counselors in 1979), ACA's support and encouragement was somewhat less than impressive in AMHCA's eyes. However, 3 years after the Academy was established, ACA established its own credential, the National Board for Certified Counselors (NBCC). AMHCA continues to be more clearly focused than ACA on legislative activities that affect mental health counselors' right to practice, such as licensure, vendorship, freedom of choice, core-provider status, and third-party reimbursement. ACA, by definition and function, must respond to the legislative needs of the other 15 divisions that represent counselors in other work settings in addition to AMHCA.

AMHCA's relationship with the other divisions of ACA has been cordial and cooperative for the most part. Rarely has it been adversarial, even when the agenda of mental health counseling and other ACA divisions has been at cross-purposes. Over the years, the clear movement has been one of assuming an increasing leadership role within the ACA family. AMHCA, as a division of ACA, has moved from being the "new kid on the block" to being one of the largest divisions whose counsel is sought by other divisions and ACA itself. The emphasis of all of the divisions within ACA has shifted away from emphasizing their uniqueness and professional diversity toward emphasizing cooperation and professional unity. However, from time to time, the unique needs of ACA division members have resulted in dissatisfaction with the overall organization as not responsive and helpful. In a rare instance, this resulted in disaffiliation based on divergent goals. In most instances, the commonalities among counselors have led to problem resolution and a continued desire to maintain ACA's common professional identity, as is the case of the 1993 referendum initiated by the AMHCA Board of Directors.

SPECIALTY TRAINING STANDARDS

AMHCA and the Association for Counselor Education and Supervision (ACES) formed a Joint Committee on Education and Training for Mental Health Counselors in 1978. This was followed shortly in 1979 by the National Academy of Certified Clinical Mental Health Counselors appointing a task force to develop a system of counselor preparation that was competency based. The outcome of this effort came in 1981 when Messina and Seiler (1981) published the *Ideal Training Standards for Mental Health Counselors.*

By the mid-1980s, it had become obvious that if mental health counselors were to work in the health care system, new and more rigorous standards were going to have to be established. The marketplace demanded proof of clinical skills if mental health counselors were to be taken seriously as qualified providers. This meant including issues such as the nomenclature of psychopathology, diagnosis, and treatment planning if mental health counselors were to be viable vendors of quality care as defined in the marketplace.

The 1986–1987 AMHCA Board of Directors adopted a set of comprehensive training standards for mental health counselors. These training standards required at least 60 semester credit hours and a minimum of 1,000 clock hours of clinical supervision. These standards were finally adopted, with some modifications, by the Council for Accreditation of Counseling and Related Educational Programs (CACREP) in July 1988.

SPECIALTY ACCREDITATION

Also in the mid-1980s, AMHCA began to promote specialty accreditation for certain areas within the broader mental health counseling area, such as marriage/couples and family counseling. In keeping with the strong emphasis on competency-based programs, it was the considered opinion of AMHCA that programs preparing mental health counselors to enter certain areas of specialty in practice should also guarantee skill and provide for supervised clinical instruction for these specialty designations. These special competencies were to be added to the common core and the environmental curriculum as specialized studies designed to "give the trainee a foundation and overview of this field of study," which would "provide an adequate basis for the mental health counselor to begin to utilize the knowledge and skills in practice" (Seiler, 1990, p. 85).

AMHCA's efforts to promote these subspecialty standards within the mental health counseling area (e.g., marriage/couples and family counseling) met with resistance partially from other ACA entities with differing agendas (i.e., the International Association for Marriage and Family Counselors and CACREP) and from other internal circumstances such as not having the energy and resources to address AMHCA's full agenda. CACREP now has adopted specialty standards for marriage and family counselors that are quite similar to those initially proposed by AMHCA.

SPECIALTY LICENSURE

A major focus for mental health counselors has been to gain licensure. Licensure laws differ from state to state. For example, counselor licensure laws have resulted in the use of at least 16 different titles and a different definition of counseling in virtually every state. In most cases, licensure laws were written to cover a broad spectrum of counseling services. Several states have chosen to license counselors only at the clinical level. These laws specify that diagnosis and treatment of mental and emotional disorders are appropriate practices for qualified counselors. Still other states have provisions for recognizing clinical and other counselor specialties within their laws.

Licensure laws may be either *title* acts, which protect the use of particular titles such as Licensed Professional Counselor, or *practice* acts, which require the practitioner to hold a license in order to practice. In cases in which a generic counselor license provides the right to practice but does not provide a clear scope of practice, the counselor may be able to establish competence through specialty certification or by meeting national standards for clinical mental health counseling.

NATIONAL STANDARDS

By the late 1980s, it had become obvious that mental health counselors would not be recognized for reimbursement by third-party payors without standards of preparation and practice. Preparation standards for the specialty of mental health counseling were established by CACREP in 1988. ACA had adopted a policy statement on advocacy for counselors. In 1993, using the CACREP standards and ACA policy as starting points, AMHCA adopted a comprehensive set of national standards for mental health counselors who deliver clinical services.

These national standards were designed to enable the mental health counselor to satisfy requirements of third-party payors, particularly multistate insurance companies, and to pave the way for greater reciprocity among state regulatory bodies. A mental health counselor can achieve a Certified Clinical Mental Health Counselor (CCMHC) credential or meet the categories of criteria of the AMHCA National Standards for Mental Health Counselors, which include the following:

1. Education: completion of a CACREP-approved program in Mental Health Counseling or the equivalent (see Appendix A);
2. Experience: completion of at least 3,000 hours of clinical experience;
3. Supervision: completion of at least 100 hours of face-to-face supervision by a qualified supervisor;
4. Standards of practice: adherence to the AMHCA Standards of Clinical Practice;
5. Ethical standards: adherence to appropriate statutory or certifying body or professional association code of ethics;
6. National clinical examination: achievement of a passing score on clinical exam;
7. Competency-based criterion (work sample): submission of a satisfactory sample of counseling session on audio or video tape; and
8. Statutory regulation: appropriately licensed where available.

Many practicing mental health counselors received their training long before these standards were in place. They have wanted to establish their professional viability as providers but have not been able to return to school full time, or perhaps enter a new degree program, in order to keep up with current education and training requirements. Now the mental health counselor may attain national standards by taking one of several paths that have been designed to guide them toward meeting the standards (see Table 1). Again, one of the paths (often referred to as the "path of choice"), is to become a Certified Clinical Mental Health Counselor (CCMHC) through the NBCC.

The CCMHC was created by AMHCA in 1979 when it established the National Academy of Certified Clinical Mental Health Counselors. Soon after, the NBCC was founded. In 1993, the National Academy and NBCC merged to provide a unified certification program.

The most critical piece of the comprehensive national standards that was missing was the standards of clinical practice. Mental health counseling is practiced all along the continuum of mental health as mentioned above, and the diagnosis and treatment of mental and emotional disorders are necessary practices on part of that continuum. Consequently, AMHCA adopted national standards to serve as guidelines for the "best practice" of clinical mental health counseling. The standards of clinical practice will help ensure the delivery of high-quality clinical services to clients.

FUTURE TRENDS AND ISSUES

On the basis of changes in the health care marketplace, we believe that the term *mental health counseling* will come to mean the delivery of counseling services along the full continuum of mental health services. If the reimbursement climate remains as it is today, a specialty in the clinical practice of mental health counseling may continue to be necessary. We also believe that all counselors will find it necessary to have at least entry-level education and experience along the full continuum of services. The identification of mental and emotional disorder is essential to proper treatment, referral, or both.

At the same time, mental health counselors will be articulating a diagnostic system based on developmental theories and determining appropriate intervention or treatment (D'Andrea, 1994). We hope that, through these efforts, preventive counseling will become respected as cost saving and effective as the practice of preventive medicine.

National standards for counselor preparation will continue to evolve to acknowledge a profession truly worthy of the status afforded other mental health care providers. We anticipate that all practicing mental health counselors will have basic knowledge and skills in the diagnosis and treatment of mental disorders as a part of their core coursework. This, in addition to the preventive, developmental, holistic, and multi-

TABLE 1.

Uniform National Clinical Standards for Mental Health Counselors

Component	CCMHC	Board Eligible	CACREP-Approved Program in Mental Health Counseling	Equivalent Education
Education	60 semester hours	60 semester hours	60 semester hours	60 semester hours
Experience	3,000 hours of clinical experience	3,000 hours of clinical experience	3,000 hours of clinical experience	3,000 hours of clinical experience
Supervision	100 hours of face-to-face	100 hours of face-to-face	100 hours of face-to-face	100 hours of face-to-face
Standards of practice	Clinical standards of practice	Clinical standards of practice	Clinical standards of practice	Clinical standards of practice
Ethics	NBCC Code of Ethics AMHCA Code of Ethics	NBCC Code of Ethics AMHCA Code of Ethics	NBCC Code of Ethics AMHCA Code of Ethics	NBCC Code of Ethics AMHCA Code of Ethics
Examination	National Clinical Mental Health Counselor Exam	National Clinical Mental Health Counselor Exam	National Clinical Mental Health Counselor Exam	National Clinical Mental Health Counselor Exam
Competency-based work sample	Work product sample	Work product sample	Work product sample	Work product sample
Statutory regulation	1. Clinical license 2. Clinical license beyond general license 3. Clinical designation	1. Clinical license 2. Clinical license beyond general license 3. Clinical designation	1. Clinical license 2. Clinical license beyond general license 3. Clinical designation	1. Clinical license 2. Clinical license beyond general license 3. Clinical designation

Note. CCMHC = Certified Clinical Mental Health Counselor; CACREP = Council for Accreditation of Counseling and Related Educational Programs; NBCC = National Board for Certified Counselors; AMHCA = American Mental Health Counselors Association.

disciplinary emphasis, will remain unchanged as mental health counselors continue to broaden the continuum of care.

We hold out much hope for the counseling profession to seek unity to maximize its impact on the field of mental health. The concepts of "continuum of care," "continuum of mental health services," and "multidisciplinary" will take precedence over special interests that cordon off specific parts of the continuum. The uniqueness that counselors offer is the application of counseling processes all along the continuum.

We anticipate that specific techniques, special populations, or work settings will become subsumed under the identity of being mental health practitioners. If counselors really want to be viewed as members of a mental health profession, then they must truly become mental health counselors qualified to practice on the continuum of mental health services.

REFERENCES

American Psychiatric Association. (1994). *Diagnostic and statistical manual of mental disorders* (4th ed.). Washington, DC: Author.

Beers, C. W. (1908). *A mind that found itself.* Garden City, NY: Longmans, Green.

Brooks, D. K. (1991). Mental health counseling. In D. Capuzzi & D. R. Gross (Eds.), *Introduction to counseling: Perspectives for the 1990s* (pp. 250–270). Boston: Allyn & Bacon.

Brooks, D. K., & Weikel, W. J. (1986). Mental health counseling in an historical perspective. In W. J. Weikel & A. J. Palmo (Eds.), *Foundations of mental health counseling* (pp. 5–28). Springfield, IL: Charles C Thomas.

Council for Accreditation of Counseling and Related Educational Programs. (1994). *CACREP accreditation standards and procedures manual.* Alexandria, VA: Author.

D'Andrea, M. (1994, April). *Creating a vision for our future: The challenges and promise of the counseling profession.* Paper presented at the American Counseling Association convention, Minneapolis, MN.

Hershenson, D. B., & Power, P. W. (1987). *Mental health counseling: Theory and practice.* New York: Pergamon.

Ivey, A. E. (1989). Mental health counseling: A developmental process and profession. *Journal of Mental Health Counseling, 11,* 26–35.

Messina, J. J., & Seiler, G. (1981). *Ideal training standards for mental health counselors.* Tampa, FL: Advanced Development Systems.

Seiler, G. (1990). Shaping the destiny of the new profession: Recollections and reflections on the evolution of mental health counseling. In G. Seiler (Ed.), *The mental health counselor's sourcebook* (p. 85). New York: Human Sciences Press.

Seiler, G., Brooks, D. K., & Beck, E. S. (1987). Training standards of the American

Mental Health Counselors Association: History, rationale and implications. *Journal of Mental Health Counseling, 9,* 199–210.

Weikel, W. J., & Palmo, A. J. (1989). The evolution and practice of mental health counseling. *Journal of Mental Health Counseling, 11,* 7–25.

APPENDIX A
CURRICULAR EXPERIENCES FOR MENTAL HEALTH COUNSELING PROGRAMS

In addition to the common core curricular experiences found in Section II.J of the *CACREP Accreditation Standards and Procedures Manual* (Council for Accreditation of Counseling and Related Educational Programs, 1994, pp. 73–74), curricular experiences and demonstrated knowledge and skill in each of the following areas are required of all students in the program.

A. Foundations of Mental Health Counseling

Studies in this area include, but are not limited to, the following:
1. Historical, philosophical, societal, cultural, economic, and political dimensions of mental health counseling;
2. Roles, functions, and professional identity of mental health counselors;
3. Structures and operations of professional organizations, training standards credentialing bodies, and ethical codes pertaining to the practice of mental health counseling;
4. Implications of professional issues unique to mental health counseling, but not limited to recognition, reimbursement, right to practice, core provider status, access to and practice privileges with managed-care systems, and expert witness status; and
5. Implications of sociocultural, demographic, and lifestyle diversity relevant to mental health counseling.

B. Contextual Dimensions of Mental Health Counseling

Studies in this area include, but are not limited to, the following:
1. Assumptions and roles of mental health counseling within the context of the health and human services systems, including functions and relationships among interdisciplinary treatment teams, and the historical, organizational, legal, and fiscal dimensions of the public and private mental health care systems;
2. Theories and techniques of community needs assessment to design, implement, and evaluate mental health care programs and systems;
3. Principles, theories, and practices of community intervention, including programs and facilities for inpatient, outpatient, partial treatment, and aftercare, and the human services network in local communities; and
4. Theoretical and applied approaches to administration, finance, and budgeting; management of mental health services and programs in the public and private sectors; principles and practices for establishing and maintaining both solo and

group private practice; and concepts and procedures for determining accountability and cost containment.

C. Knowledge and Skills for the Practice of Mental Health Counseling

Studies in this area include, but are not limited to, the following:

1. General principles of etiology, diagnosis, treatment, and prevention of mental and emotional disorders and dysfunctional behavior, and general principles and practices for the promotion of optimal mental health;
2. Specific models and methods for assessing mental status; identification of abnormal, deviant, or psychopathological behavior; and the interpretation of findings in current diagnostic categories (e.g., *Diagnostic and Statistical Manual of Mental Disorders* [4th ed., DSM–IV; American Psychiatric Association, 1994]);
3. Application of modalities for maintaining and terminating counseling and psychotherapy with mentally and emotionally impaired clients, including crisis intervention, brief, intermediate, and long-term approaches;
4. Basic classifications, indications, and contraindications of commonly prescribed psychopharmacological medications for the purpose of identifying effects and side effects of such medications;
5. Principles of conducting an intake interview and mental health history for planning and managing client caseload;
6. Specialized consultation skills for effecting living and work environments to improve relationships, communications, and productivity and for working with counselors of different specializations and with other mental health professionals in areas related to collaborative treatment strategies;
7. The application of concepts of mental health education, consultation, outreach, and prevention strategies, and of community health promotion and advocacy; and
8. Effective strategies for influencing public policy and government relations on local, state, and national levels to enhance funding and programs affecting mental health services in general and the practice of mental health counseling in particular.

D. Clinical Instruction

For the Mental Health Counseling program, the following standard should be applied in addition to Section III, Standard I of the *CACREP Accreditation Standards* (Council for Accreditation of Counseling and Related Educational Programs, 1994):

A minimum of 300 clock hours of supervised experience must be completed in an appropriate setting under the direct supervision of a qualified mental health professional (e.g., CCMHC). The total internship experience will, therefore, consist of a minimum of 900 clock hours.

Chapter 3

PROFESSIONAL IDENTITY OF THE MENTAL HEALTH COUNSELOR

ARTIS J. PALMO

In order to understand the complexities of the problem of professional identity for the Mental Health Counselor (MHC), one must examine the historical roots of the counseling movement over the past 100 years. As Aubrey (1983) pointed out, the beginning of the counseling movement stems from the many social reform activities surrounding the Industrial Revolution of the late 1800s to the early 1900s. According to Aubrey, " . . . the early pioneers of guidance and counseling (Jesse Davis, Frank Parsons, Eli Weaver) were quite adamant in wishing to prepare people to successfully cope with and master the social environment" (pp. 78–79). At this early time, guidance was the only function, with counseling being mentioned in the literature for the first time in 1931. From a historical standpoint, counseling as a professional function has been discussed for only the past 64 years!

Probably the most important professional change for counseling occurred during the 1940s and 1950s. During this time, there was a dramatic shift from the "mechanistic-deterministic" philosophy of behaviorism and psychoanalysis to "self-determinism" of the humanistic philosophy espoused by Carl Rogers (Aubrey, 1983, p. 79; Aubrey, 1977). Rogers' overall impact upon the field of counseling, both philosophically and pragmatically, was tremendous. The birth of the field of counseling as a separate entity from guidance, psychology, and psychiatry can be traced directly to the work of Rogers. Although many varied techniques and theories of counseling exist today, the philosophical groundwork for the profession of counseling rests on the humanistic work of Rogers and his contemporaries. With Rogers' work, the guidance role has expanded to include a wide range of counseling functions as well.

Two other important historical events need to be mentioned in relation to the professional identity of the MHC. First, the training of counselors took a giant step forward in 1958 (Aubrey, 1983) with the establishment of the National Defense Education Act (NDEA). This legislation was in direct response to Russia initiating the space race with the launching of Sputnik. Along with the emphasis on math and science education in the schools, the NDEA legislation resulted "... in the preparation of thousands of counselors ... " (p. 79). The legislation promoted the rapid growth of counselor education programs throughout the country, which leads to the second point.

Following the decline of the NDEA programs in the 1960s, counselor education programs began a slow transition from the training of guidance counselors for the schools to the training of counselors who could function in a variety of mental health settings besides the schools. This shift in the professional direction of counseling was a tremendous divergence from the early roots of the guidance and counseling movement. Counselors began to function effectively in settings that were traditionally the exclusive propriety of the fields of psychology and medicine. By the late 1970s and early 1980s, the counseling professional could be found in such varied roles as "... developing career education programs; ... working to help chronic schizophrenics attain optimal vocational adjustment, and ... dealing with adolescent developmental crises" (Goodyear, 1976, p. 513). The roles performed and work settings occupied by the professional counselor are numerous, as noted in a recent article by Zimpfer and DeTrude (1990).

In summary, the broadbased, developmental nature of professional counseling can be traced from the early vocational exploration of the 1900s, Rogers' self-theory of meeting individual needs in the 1940s and 1950s, the development of professionalism in the 1960s, and the use of counseling methodologies with all types of clientele in the 1970s and 1980s (Bradley, 1978). Having such a broad base, however, does cause the profession to have a severe identity crisis, as Aubrey noted in 1977 and Sherrard and Fong noted again in 1991. Important questions arise as a result of the identity crisis. What type of clientele should be served? What counseling methodologies should be employed by the counselor? What is the goal of the profession of counseling?

The intent of this chapter is to answer the questions posed above as well as to provide the reader with a framework for mental health counseling. Although counseling as a profession has a general identity problem, the field of mental health counseling has some very specific issues that it faces. The struggle for an accepted identity for the MHC within the overall field of mental health has been a relatively recent phenomena spanning the '70s, '80s, and '90s. Although the roots of mental health counseling can be found in the guidance movement explained here, and in Chapter 1, the true identity of the MHC has been defined only recently in the practice and the professional literature of mental health counselors. With this in mind, the chapter will explore the basic philosophical and theoretical premises that underlie the profession of mental health counseling which make the MHC a distinct entity in the helping professions.

Mental Health Providers

Development of AMHCA

The identified field of the professional MHC can be traced directly to the development of the American Mental Health Counselors Association (AMHCA) during the late 1970s within the American Personnel and Guidance Association (later named the American Association for Counseling and Development and presently the American Counseling Association). AMHCA's development was the direct result of the dissatisfaction of many counselors with the existing professional groups and associations primarily oriented toward clinical and counseling psychology, psychiatry, social work, marriage and family counseling, and guidance counseling. These early counseling professionals felt that their training and orientation did not fit the traditional, contemporary styles of existing professionals in the field of mental health. Rather than attempt to fit within the existing organizational structures, a group of counseling professionals initiated AMHCA with the expressed purpose of providing counselors working in the field of mental health a vehicle for the exchange of ideas, methods, and research.

The development of AMHCA parallels the development of the professional title, Mental Health Counselor. Through the efforts of the early AMHCA leaders, the title Mental Health Counselor has become the accepted designation for those counseling professionals whose primary affiliation and theoretical basis is counseling and not psychology, psychiatry, or social work. Through the work of the founding AMHCA professionals, such as Steve Lindenberg, James Messina, Nancy Spisso, Joyce Breasure, Gary Seiler, and Bill Weikel, tremendous strides were made in developing the concept of Mental Health Counselor.

It is very important to note the development of AMHCA as a professional association, since the contemporary title of Mental Health Counselor is a direct result of that group's founding. Although the roots of the MHC, and the resultant identity problems, can be traced to the beginnings of the guidance movement, the title MHC is a recent happening. Therefore, the professional identity of the MHC is founded in the beliefs and philosophies of counseling's past as well as the very recent developments of the '70s, '80s, and '90s. The primary purpose for MHCs during the past 25 years has been to establish themselves as one of the core providers of mental health services along with psychiatrists, psychologists, social workers, and psychiatric nurses. In order to do this, MHCs have had to demonstrate why they belong as well as how they differ from existing professionals in the field of mental health.

MHC Defined

Prior to 1980, if one were to review the professional literature, the titles most frequently used to distinguish the professionals associated with community mental health are the community counselor, community psychologist, psychologist, psychiatrist, or social worker. Other than an article by Seiler and Messina (1979), it was unlikely that the reader could find literature that related directly to the issue of the professional identity of the MHC and the role of the MHC within community mental health (Lewis & Lewis, 1977). Not until the 1980s and 1990s does the literature regularly begin to discuss the issues surrounding the identity crisis being faced by MHCs within the community mental health movement.

In 1981, Palmo developed a manuscript for the AMHCA Board of Directors which described the role and function of the MHC. This manuscript was developed and approved for the purpose of ultimate inclusion in the *Dictionary of Occupational Titles and the Occupational Outlook Handbook.* Eventually, in 1984, segments of the description were placed in the OOH establishing, for the first time, mental health counseling as one of the core providers of mental health services.

Previously, four groups of helping professionals had been recognized and identified legislatively as being the core providers of mental health services. They included psychiatrists, psychologists, psychiatric nurses, and clinical social workers (Asher, 1979; Lindenberg, 1983; Randolph, Sturgis, & Alcorn, 1979). With the advent of licensure and certification throughout the United States, the core providers today primarily include psychiatrists, psychologists, clinical social workers, licensed professional counselors and marriage and family counselors. Although there are significant overlaps between and among the roles and functions of the identified core providers and the MHC, there are several important differences that must be presented and discussed. First, the definition of an MHC:

> Performs counseling/therapy with individuals, groups, couples, and families; collects, organizes, and analyzes data concerning client's mental, emotional, and/or behavioral problems or disorders; aids clients and their families to effectively adapt to the personal concerns presented; develops procedures to assist clients to adjust to possible environmental barriers that may impede self-understanding and personal growth (Palmo, 1981).

This early definition of the MHC provided the necessary distinctions between MHCs and the other core providers. Primarily, the MHC has a concern for the environment surrounding the client (Hershenson & Strein, 1991). Although there is an emphasis upon the identified client, the MHC has a more global view of the client concern that includes family and other personal associations. As Hershenson and Strein relate, "Clients rarely spend more than a few hours each week in counseling; the bulk of their time is spent in other settings, such as home, work, and community" (p. 248). The concern for the environmental factors is a major aspect of the MHCs' approach to treating clients.

Another primary goal of counseling is the development of the client's self-understanding and promotion of his/her personal growth. Self-understanding and personal growth on the part of the client means continued self-direction and effective mental health for the individual. The definition of MHC also includes the following:

> Utilizes community agencies and institutions to develop mental health programs that are developmental and preventive in nature. Trained to provide a wide variety of therapeutic approaches to assist clients, which may include therapy, milieu therapy, and behavioral therapy. Employed in clinics, hospitals, drug centers, colleges, private agencies, related mental health programs, or private practice. Required to have knowledge and skills in client management, assessment, and diagnosis through a post-graduate program in mental health or community mental health counseling (Palmo, 1981, p. 1).

The second aspect of the definition expresses more clearly the major distinguishing characteristics for the MHC. A key characteristic is the emphasis on a developmental model of counseling and therapy within an overall prevention scheme, with a "... focus on promoting healthy development of coping capacities and on using environmental forces to contribute to the goal of wellness . . . " (Hershenson & Strein, 1991, pp. 250–251). What this means is that the MHC examines clients' concerns as a part of the normal developmental issues and crises faced by most people as they progress through daily living experiences. The client is not viewed as "sick," but rather, as an individual who must learn more effective coping mechanisms in order to function appropriately and gainfully within society (Lindenberg, 1983; Hershenson & Strein, 1991; Weikel & Palmo, 1989). It is important to stress the developmental/ preventive model does not deny that client concerns vary in severity, and at times, the client suffering from more severe distress may be referred to the services of other professionals in the helping fields.

Prevention, as discussed in another section of the text, is a very important role that is stressed by the professional MHC. Prevention has been a defining characteristic to mental health counseling from the beginning of the movement (Kiselica & Look, 1993). As outlined by Goodyear (1976), prevention counselors " . . . build on clients' strengths and teach clients the life skills necessary for problem mastery" (p. 513). This does not mean that the client may never face the need for direct counseling intervention, but rather the role for the MHC is one of mental health educator (Heller, 1993; Lange, 1983; McCollum, 1981; Myers, 1992; Shaw, 1986; Sperry, Carlson, & Lewis, 1993; Westbrook, Kandell, Kirkland, Phillips, Regan, Medvene, & Oslin, 1993). Mental health education means instructing the public regarding various methodologies that can be utilized to handle the everyday stressors of life.

In summary, an examination of the MHC definition shows several important distinctive qualities for the counseling professional. First, there is an environmental/milieu approach to the client which stresses the client's adjustment to societal pressures, whether it be at home, school, work, or in the community. Second, there is a developmental/ preventive model that underlies the orientation the MHC utilizes in his/her work with individuals, groups, and families.

Before continuing the discussion of the MHC's role definition, it is useful to define the role and function of the other major core providers— psychiatrists, psychologists, and social workers. In order to fully understand the role and function of the MHC, it is important to be familiar with the definitions of the other mental health care professionals.

Mental Health Providers

Psychiatry

A professional psychiatrist, according to the *Dictionary of Occupational Titles* (1991), is defined as follows:

Diagnoses and treats patients with mental, emotional, and behavioral disorders: Organizes data concerning patient's family, medical history, and onset of symptoms obtained from patient, relatives, and other sources, such as **NURSE, GENERAL DUTY** (Medical ser.) 075.364-010 and **SOCIAL WORKER, PSYCHIATRIC** (profess. & kin.) 195.107-034. Examines patient to determine general physical condition, following standard medical procedures. Orders laboratory and other special diagnostic tests and evaluates data obtained. Determines nature and extent of mental disorder, and formulates treatment program. Treats or directs treatment of patient, utilizing a variety of psychotherapeutic methods and medications (Volume I, p. 57).

There are several key aspects to the role of the psychiatrist that differ from all other mental health professionals. First, the psychiatrist utilizes the medical model in his/her interventions with a client, or as the model dictates, patient. The medical model assumes there is an illness or sickness, with the best intervention for the patient being medicinal. Second, since the psychiatrist is a physician, he/she is the only mental health professional who can prescribe psychopharmocological drugs. Because many serious mental illnesses involve some form of organic problem (Lindenberg, 1983), the use of drugs as a treatment of choice has become more and more popular.

A third important role most often assumed by the psychiatrist is the director of a team of professionals working with patients. This means the psychiatrist is usually the most powerful professional in determining the direction of the therapy to be completed with the patient. Most frequently, in hospitals and other agencies, the psychiatrist has the final say regarding the methods to be utilized by the mental health care team.

As with other mental health professions, the field of psychiatry has had to make significant changes in its role and function. Because of the proliferation of mental health providers from other fields, psychiatry has taken a more consultative role in working with the other core providers of mental health services. MHCs have taken effective and active roles in the private and public sector of community mental health, forcing the other professional groups to adapt their treatment approaches to better treat the clientele seeking assistance.

A brief case example will demonstrate the consultative relationship than can exist between an MHC and a psychiatrist:

> Bill was an MHC working in private practice and treating Warren, a 17-year-old high school junior who was having severe socialization problems at home, school, and community. In addition to individual counseling with Warren, Bill did family counseling as well as maintaining a consultative relationship with Warren's school counselor. Warren's primary problems had subsided as a result of counseling, but he continued to have severe behavioral outbursts whenever he was faced with stressful situations. For example, one Saturday, Warren's girlfriend broke-up with him, creating a situation where Warren became angry and abusive with her and the family. This was just one example of his behavioral outbursts that had occurred recently. Since Bill was no longer sure that the problem was environmental/social, he referred Warren to the psychiatrist who headed the local hospital's adolescent psychiatric unit. The psychiatrist determined some organic abnormalities with Warren, and placed him on medication. Warren was told to remain in counseling in addition to the medication. In the consultative role, the psychiatrist was able to assist Bill in treating this young boy and his family.

This case is a good example of how the professional fields can come together to treat someone, rather than to make arbitrary distinctions between mental health groups. As the world of community mental health changes, there are more and more collaborative efforts in the field. MHCs have contributed a great deal to this collaborative effort over the past 15 years through their active involvement with all professional groups in the field.

Psychology

Utilizing the DOT (1991) description, clinical psychologist is defined as follows:

> Diagnoses or evaluates mental and emotional disorders of individuals, and administers programs of treatment: Interviews patients in clinics, hospitals, prisons, and other institutions, and studies medical and social case histories. Observes patients in play or other situations, and selects, administers, and interprets intelligence, achievement, interest, personality, and other psychological tests to diagnose disorders and formulate plans of treatment. Treats psychological disorders to effect improved adjustments utilizing various psychological techniques, such as milieu therapy, psychodrama, play therapy and hypnosis. Selects approach to use in individual therapy, such as directive, nondirective, and supportive therapy and plans frequency, intensity, and duration of therapy (Volume I, p. 51).

There are several other aspects to the role and function of the clinical psychologist mentioned in the DOT that are important. The clinical psychologist usually collaborates with a psychiatrist in diagnosis and treatment; frequently is responsible for the research that is conducted with patients; develops mental health programs for social, educational, and welfare agencies; and generally has a specialty such as the severely disturbed, criminals, delinquents, or other special group.

The field of psychology has many varied specialties, as can be noted by reading the list of professional divisions of the American Psychological Association. According to the OOH, the listing of titles includes: Experimental, Developmental, Personality, Social, Comparative, Physiological, Counseling, Psychometrician, Educational, School, Industrial, Community, and Health. There is much confusion surrounding the title of psychologist, with the academics and training requirements varying from state to state (Brown & Srebalus, 1988; Wayne, 1982). Each state psychology licensure board has been left to define the title and function of psychologist on its own; however, through a coordinated effort on the part of state psychological associations, there is a more consistent set of national standards defining the field of psychology.

For the purposes of the discussion in this chapter, the term psychologist will refer to clinical and counseling psychologists, since those are the two most frequently used titles related to the treatment of clients in the mental health field. In addition, the professional definition most closely related to mental health counseling is either clinical or counseling psychology.

As noted in Brown and Srebalus (1988), many of the doctoral programs in counseling that once existed have become counseling psychology programs. Many colleges of education that once offered Doctorates in Education in Counseling, now offer Doctorate of Philosophy in Counseling Psychology. This trend toward PhD's in Psychology has been to meet the demands of the field of community psychology, which in most instances means a license as a psychologist. Although there has been an attempt to have more doctoral level MHCs, the terminal degree seems to be the master's degree or specialist's degree.

There are many similarities between the role definitions for psychologists and MHCs. The most important distinctions include the psychologist's emphasis on psychometrics and various forms of assessment. Generally speaking, projective and intellectual assessments are almost always done by the psychologist. The clinical psychologist frequently works with institutionalized persons or those with more severe problems, in conjunction with the psychiatrist. Evaluations and assessments by the psychologist are very important to the diagnostic evaluation ultimately completed by the psychiatrist. Many therapeutic interventions are based upon the assessments done by the psychologist, but psychopharmocological treatments are always assigned by the psychiatrist.

As with psychiatry, the field of psychology has made some drastic professional changes over the past 30 years. Private practice (Davis, 1981; Snow, 1981) was originally the domain of the psychiatrist, but with modern society came many social changes demanding treatments beyond the psychopharmocological treatment of the psychiatrist. Many mental health professionals, including MHCs and psychologists, began to offer the general community some alternative treatments, such as family counseling, school interventions, marriage counseling, and other forms of proactive counseling. In fact, many of the early participants in the MHC movement were psychologists, social workers, and psychiatrists who believed in a community mental health model that was based on wellness and not illness, in proactive treatments not reactive treatments, and in collaboration and not separatism.

Since there has been a broadening of the roles performed by psychologists, many are presently providing services in private practice settings. Being a licensed professional makes the private practice setting a viable alternative to the traditional role of assessment and treatment within an institutional setting. The key issue is licensure, along with acceptance by insurance carriers who often pay for part of the treatment through major medical insurance. For the MHCs in many states, licensure has become a reality but acceptance by insurance carriers is often another issue of discussion. In this area of practice, psychologists have become widely accepted, along with psychiatrists, by the insurance industry while MHCs are continuing to work in this important area.

In summary, utilizing various forms of assessments, the clinical psychologist is the primary nonmedical diagnostician of the mental health care professionals. In addition, the broadening of the roles performed by psychologists have lead them into all areas of psychology and counseling practice, including private practice. Historically, psychologists have worked closely with psychiatrists in the management of cases as well as being direct providers of service. Although they have made many changes in their approach to counseling and therapy, psychologists remain directed by the medical model because of the need for diagnosis and illness identification.

Social Work

The third core provider with legislative recognition (Randolph et al., 1979) is the field of social work. No professional field has had the major growth in all areas of mental health care as social workers. From advancements in licensure to expanded roles in institutions to private practice, social workers have made great professional strides to reach acceptance in the community. Two titles are most frequently used when discussing social work—Clinical or Psychiatric Social Worker. Like the MHC, both titles usually require two years of graduate study leading to a Master's degree in social work with specialties in psychiatry or clinical practice (Kyes & Hofling, 1974).

The DOT (1991) defines social worker as follows:

> Provides psychiatric social work assistance to mentally or emotionally disturbed patients of hospitals, clinics, and other medical centers, and to their families, collaborating with psychiatric and allied team in diagnosis and treatment plan: Investigate case situations and presents information to **PSYCHIATRIST**... and **PSYCHOLOGIST, CLINICAL**... and other members of health team, on patient's family and social background pertinent to diagnosis and treatment. Helps patients to respond constructively to treatment and assists in adjustment leading to and following discharge. Interprets psychiatric treatment to patient's family and helps to reduce fear and other attitudes obstructing acceptance of psychiatric care and continuation of treatment. Serves as link between patient, psychiatric agency, and community. May work directly in treatment relationship with patients, individually or in groups... (Volume I, p. 161).

Historically, the role of the social worker has remained somewhat defined and stable through the 1970s and early 1980s. The professional social worker was generally the link between the client and the community, providing adjustment counseling and support for the client and his/her family. More recently, however, the role has been expanded to include long-term individual and family counseling through community agencies and institutions. In addition, as noted above, social workers have expanded their role by becoming involved in private practice.

The important distinction to make with social work is between bachelor's level and master's level. Bachelor's level social workers are generally involved with an agency, institution, or hospital, assisting patients and their families in readjusting to the community from which they came. The master's level social worker may be involved in these functions but is also trained to provide counseling services.

Psychiatric social workers generally serve several distinct functions according to Kyes and Hofling (1974), including: (1) helping the individual utilize the social environment; (2) helping the individual find work, housing, and monetary support; (3) family planning; (4) explaining the various aspects of the hospital services; (5) utilizing community agencies; and (6) being a member of the mental health care team planning treatment for the individual. The psychiatric social worker generally has distinct functions that relate directly to the treatment of hospitalized patients.

Psychiatric Nursing

Generally, the professional nurse associated with mental health care is usually employed in a hospital or institution for the chronically ill. In this medical position, the professional nurse is a critical part of the mental health team headed by the psychiatrist or other medical staff. Once again, besides the psychiatrist, the psychiatric nurse is the only mental health professional with a medical background in addition to mental health training.

The psychiatric nurse has intensive training in working with the severely emotionally disturbed individuals. They are the medically trained assistant to the psychiatrist entrusted with the responsibility for medical care, distribution of drugs, and offering some therapeutic interventions with individuals and groups of patients in institutional settings or community readjustment programs.

Because of the shift from the hospitalization of severe, long-term disturbed patients to less restricted community-based programs, psychiatric nurses are performing more of their functions in outpatient settings. As a core provider, psychiatric nurses have been accepted by insurance carriers for quite some time because of their advanced training and the necessity for a license to practice. However, nurses do not usually open private practices or compete in the open community mental health market; therefore, they are not often compared to MHCs because of their specific functions within treatment.

Summary

The four previously defined core providers have some distinct individual characteristics, but also many overlapping functions. Also, the MHC has different, as well as similar functions to the other core providers. The overlapping role for all five professional groups (Psychiatry, Psychology, Social Work, Nurse, and MHC) is counseling or therapy. Each professional group is involved in some level of counseling/therapy, although the orientation or model utilized may differ as well as the content and style of advanced training. For the reader's purpose, the following general definitions for each profession should be kept in mind for the remainder of the chapter:

1. **Psychiatrists** are the only mental health professionals who can **administer drugs** (although the Veterans Administration Hospitals are beginning a project to teach psychologists the use of psychopharmocological treatments;

2. **Clinical Psychologists** are the professionals generally entrusted with the **assessment** of intellectual and personality functioning, in addition to providing counseling/therapy;

3. **Psychiatrist** and **Psychologist** are usually the mental health professionals **directing mental health care teams** in agencies, hospitals, and institutions;

4. **Social Workers** usually provide the **link** between the institutional services for clients/patients and the integration of the individual back into the social milieu; and

5. **Psychiatric Nurses** provide the **medical linkage** between the agency or institution and the client/patient after hospitalization.

The key to this chapter is to examine the role, function, and identity of the MHC in comparison to the other mental health care providers. Hopefully, the previous discussion has clarified the roles performed by each of the core providers which will permit an in-depth discussion of the specific professional characteristics of the MHC that makes mental health counseling a profession unto itself.

MHC as a Profession

Back in 1979, Seiler and Messina stated that "Although mental health counselors have existed for many years, they have labored under the burden of being professionals without a distinct identity" (p. 3). This identity crisis for the MHC remains, with trained counselors being labeled as psychologist in some instances or case worker in other instances. The overlap between and among the MHC, psychologist, and social worker has negated a separate identity for the MHC. However, there are distinctions that make mental health counseling a separate profession

(Hershenson & Strein, 1991; Sherrard & Fong, 1991; Weikel & Palmo, 1989).

One of the important questions that arises from this discussion is, "What is a profession?" Messina (1979) presents Peterson's long accepted criteria for a profession: (1) defined objectives for the professional work; (2) techniques of the profession that can be taught to attain the objectives; (3) techniques are basically intellectual operations and the techniques are applied according to the individual problems; (4) techniques are founded in principles of science, theology, or law and not readily accessible to the novice; (5) professionals are members of an organized society; and (6) the professional organization has altruistic goals, is not totally self-serving, and has a statement of professional ethics.

The field of mental health counseling has all the necessary characteristics to be noted as a profession along with the other four core providers of mental health care. An examination of the most recent standards published by the Council for Accreditation of Counseling and Related Educational Programs (CACREP, 1994) for the profession of Mental Health Counseling demonstrates that MHCs have to meet the academic and professional training qualifications that make it a profession. The professional techniques are founded upon a sound body of knowledge, the goals of the profession have been clearly stated, training programs have an established set of standards, and the MHC is associated with two primary professional groups (American Counseling Association and AMHCA). ACA and AMHCA have existing professional groups who are responsible for the development of training standards (CACREP) as well as standards for professional certification (National Board of Certified Counselors, NBCC).

The true test of the distinctiveness of mental health counseling as profession was the historic legal case of John I. Weldon vs. Virginia State Board of Psychologist Examiners in 1972. Lindenberg (1976) reported at that time that the decision of the court was that the profession of counseling was a distinct and separate entity. This court decision provided the foundation and framework for finally establishing counseling as a true profession.

The discussion that follows will provide some specific philosophical and theoretical orientations that make mental health counseling distinct from the other core mental health providers.

The Distinctiveness of the MHC

Counselor Use of Self

Probably, the most important aspect of the theoretical and philosophical foundations of mental health counseling is the MHC's therapeutic use of his/her own experiences, reactions, and information in the counseling relationship. Although there are many variations and styles of counseling used by today's MHC, historically, the field of counseling is founded in the works of Carl Rogers (Aubrey, 1977). Rogers' approach was based on field theory and founded in the client's present rather than the past, as previously emphasized by Freudian psychology (Hershenson & Strein, 1991; Meador & Rogers, 1973). Rogers' strong belief in the " . . . dignity of the individual . . . " (p. 121) permeates the philosophy and theory underlying mental health counseling.

The counseling relationship provides a permissive environment where a client can explore his/her own needs, desires, and goals (Weikel & Palmo, 1989; Hershenson & Strein, 1991). More importantly for the professional MHC, Rogers advocated that the counselor also be free in the counseling relationship to use his/her experiences in the sessions as feedback for the client. Thus, the concept of the active "use of self" on the part of the counselor became a critical part of the professional counselor's role and function. This aspect of the MHC's role makes the MHC a distinctly different professional from other mental health care providers.

Traditionally, other mental health providers have followed a more analytic therapeutic approach. The psychiatric/medical model has permeated the helping profession since the time of Freud. Using the work of Rogers as a foundation, professional counseling became the first helping profession that advocated the "use of self" as a necessary aspect of therapy that provides the groundwork for client improvement. The "use of self" is one professional characteristic that sets the MHC apart from all other helping professionals.

Positive Approach to Mental Health

A second differentiating factor for the MHC is the belief that the individual has the capability to correct whatever problems he/she faces (Weikel & Palmo, 1989). As Seiler and Messina (1979) stated in one of the original articles on mental health counseling, the MHC model is based " . . . on the client's strengths and on helping develop skills necessary for successfully dealing with life" (p. 5). The medical model is based on the premise someone is sick, while the developmental and preventive model emphasizes the need to focus upon normality and wellness.

This leads to the second aspect of the positive approach to mental health—prevention. As noted earlier in the chapter and in the Highlight Section on prevention, the MHC's primary professional responsibility and energy is placed in the prevention of mental illness as well as assisting individuals and groups in crisis. The MHC has to be " . . . prepared . . . to work more on preventing onset (primary prevention) and less on the overwhelming task of working with already affected individual clients (secondary prevention)" (Hershenson & Strein, 1991, p. 250). Mental health counseling remains dedicated to primary prevention within the total model.

The concept of prevention does not deny the existence of crises in each person's life. Rather, it is expected that everyone goes through a variety of crises, large and small, throughout a lifetime. Crises are a part of every individual's normal development. The community at large is frequently "turned off" by the terms therapist, therapy, psychotherapy and psychotherapist (SERCO, 1984), and refuse to seek assistance, even when needed. However, the community at large is more comfortable with the concepts of prevention, which views people in positive ways, and not labeling them as mentally ill. Therefore, the MHC philosophy of prevention as a major aspect of the model helps alleviate the stigma usually associated with mental health services.

Self-Development as a Continued Process

Normal development for any individual is fraught with many crises and problems. The problem for most individuals is not *how to avoid a crisis*, but rather, *how to deal with a crisis* once it is upon them. The MHC's basic philosophy is founded in the belief that a person has the capability to handle the problems he/she faces and to continue to develop personally while attempting to "fix" the problem. Therefore, not all individuals should be labeled "sick" when they are having difficulty facing a certain problem situation. A person who is temporarily nonfunctional because of a problem may not be necessarily "sick", but in need of assistance in order to overcome his/her difficulties.

Although a certain percentage of the individuals seeking mental health services may need consistent and continual care, a majority of the population needs help to get through crisis situations only. The effects of the crisis may last one month or one year, but eventually the person can function on his/her own. The MHC believes that an individual, who may be nonfunctional for a period of time, will more than likely return to functional in the future. Self-development is a process of personal "ups and downs" that continues throughout a person's life, with dysfunctional not necessarily meaning abnormal.

Counseling Relationship

As Boy and Pine (1979) so masterfully wrote, "Counselors may be the last professionals in our society who are committed to meeting the needs of clients through the process of counseling" (p. 527). Although this statement is 16 years old, it remains true for MHCs today! The MHC's role and function in prevention is quite important, but *mental health counseling is founded in the counseling process.* Of all the core providers, the MHC remains the helping professional who is committed to the counseling relationship. Although the MHC may function in a variety of settings and roles, his/her primary function is counseling (Bubenzer, Zimpfer, & Mahrle, 1990; Seligman & Whitely, 1983; Weikel & Taylor, 1979; Wilcoxon & Puleo, 1992; Zimpfer & DeTrude, 1990).

Summary

Although mental health counseling is a relatively new profession when compared to the other core providers of mental health services, it has now emerged and been recognized as an important part of the total health care system. The field of mental health counseling is seen as growing in the future (Weikel & Palmo, 1989) because of the needs of the community at-large.

The need for MHCs has been demonstrated, but the road ahead to full acceptance by the national health care system is not likely a smooth highway. The recent recognition by the Civilian Health and Medical Program of the Uniformed Services (CHAMPUS) has been a crucial breakthrough for MHCs. Not only have MHCs been recognized, but an agreed upon definition of a reimbursable MHC was developed (Weikel & Palmo, 1989). The consistent work of the professional MHCs over the past 20 years has assured a bright future for the newest group of the mental health care providers.

REFERENCES

Asher, J. K. (1979). The coming exclusion of counselors from the mental health care system. *American Mental Health Counselors Association Journal, 1*(1), 53–60.

Aubrey, R. F. (1983). The odyssey of counseling and images of the future. *Personnel and Guidance Journal, 62*(2), 78–82.

Aubrey, R. F. (1977). Historical development of guidance and counseling and implications for the future. *Personnel and Guidance Journal, 55*(6), 288–295.

Bradley, M. K. (1978). Counseling past and present: Is there a future? *Personnel and Guidance Journal, 57*(1), 42–45.

Boy, A. V., & Pine, G. J. (1979). Needed: A rededication to the counselor's primary commitment. *Personnel and Guidance Journal, 57*(10), 527–528.

Brown, D., & Srebalus, D. J. (1988). *An introduction to the counseling profession.* Englewood Cliffs, NJ: Prentice-Hall.

Bubenzer, D. L., Zimpfer, D. G., & Mahrle, C. L. (1990). Standardized individual appraisal in agency and private practice: A survey. *Journal of Mental Health Counseling, 12*, 51–66.

Council for Accreditation of Counseling and Related Educational Programs. (1994). *CACREP accreditation standards and procedures manual.* Alexandria, VA: Author.

Davis, J. W. (1981). Counselor licensure: Overkill? *Personnel and Guidance Journal, 60*(2), 83–85.

Dictionary of occupational titles (1991, 4th Ed.). Indianapolis, IN: JIST, Inc.

Goodyear, R. K. (1976). Counselors as community psychologists. *Personnel and Guidance Journal, 54*(10), 512–516.

Heller, K. (1993). Prevention activities for older adults: Social structures and personal competencies that maintain useful social roles. *Journal of Counseling and Development, 72*, 124–130.

Hershenson, D. B., & Strein, W. (1991). Toward a mentally healthy curriculum for mental health counselor education. *Journal of Mental Health Counseling, 13*, 247–252.

Kiselica, M. S., & Look, C. T. (1993). Mental health counseling and prevention: Disparity between philosophy and practice? *Journal of Mental Health Counseling, 15*, 3–14.

Kyes, J., & Hofling, C. (1974). *Basic psychiatric concepts in nursing.* Philadelphia, PA: J. B. Lippincott.

Lange, S. (1983). The ten commandments for community mental health education. *Personnel and Guidance Journal, 62*(1), 41–42.

Lewis, J. A., & Lewis, M. D. (1977). *Community Counseling: A Human Services Approach.* New York: John Wiley & Sons.

Lindenberg, S. P. (1976). Attention students: Be advised . . . *Personnel and Guidance Journal, 55*(1), 34–36.

Lindenberg, S. P. (1983). Professional renewal: Counseling at the crossroads. *Pennsylvania Journal of Counseling, 2*(1), 1–10.

McCollum, M. G. (1981). Recasting a role for mental health educators. *American Mental Health Counselors Association Journal, 3*(1), 37–47.

Meador, B. D., & Rogers, C. R. (1973). Client-centered therapy. In R. Corsini (Ed.), *Current psychotherapies* (pp. 119–165). Itasca, IL: Peacock.

Messina, J. J. (1979). Why establish a certification system for professional counselors?: A rationale. *American Mental Health Counselors Association Journal, 1*(1), 9–22.

Myers, J. E. (1992). Wellness, prevention, development: The Cornerstone of the profession. *Journal of Counseling and Development, 71,* 136–139.

Occupational outlook handbook. (April, 1984). U.S. Department of Labor, Bulletin #2205, Washington, D.C.

Palmo, A. J. (1981). Mental Health Counselor. Unpublished manuscript developed for the American Mental Health Counselors Association Board of Directors, Washington, D.C.

Randolph, D. L., Sturgis, D. K., & Alcorn, J. D. (1979). A counseling community psychology master's program. *American Mental Health Counselors Association Journal, 1*(2), 69–72.

Seiler, G., & Messina, J. J. (1979). Toward professional identity: The dimensions of mental health counseling in perspective. *American Mental Health Counselors Association Journal, 1*(1), 3–8.

Seligman, L., & Whitely, N. (1983). AMHCA and VMHCA members in private practice in Virginia. *American Mental Health Counselors Association Journal, 5*(4), 179–183.

SERCO. (1984). *Fighting the stigma: An up-to-date pilot promoting mental health care.* SERCO Marketing: Dayton, OH.

Shaw, M. C. (1986). The prevention of learning and interpersonal problems. *Journal of Counseling and Development, 64,* 624–627.

Sherrard, P. A. D., & Fong, M. L. (1991). Mental health counselor training: Which model shall prevail? *Journal of Mental Health Counseling, 13,* 204–210.

Snow, B. M. (1981). Counselor licensure as perceived by counselors and psychologists. *Personnel and Guidance Journal, 60*(2), 80–83.

Sperry, L., Carlson, J., & Lewis, J. (1993). Health counseling strategies and interventions. *Journal of Mental Health Counseling, 15,* 15–25.

Wayne, G. (1982). An examination of selected statutory licensing requirements for psychologists in the United States. *Personnel and Guidance Journal, 60*(7), 420–425.

Weikel, W. J., & Palmo, A. J. (1989). The evolution and practice of mental health counseling. *Journal of Mental Health Counseling, 11,* 7–25.

Weikel, W. J., & Taylor, S. S. (1979). AMHCA: Membership profile and journal preferences. *American Mental Health Counselors Association Journal, 1*(2), 89–94.

Westbrook, F. D., Kandell, J. J., Kirkland, S. E., Phillips, P. E., Regan, A. M., Medvene, A., & Oslin, Y. D. (1993). University campus consultation: Opportunities and limitations. *Journal of Counseling and Development, 71,* 684–688.

Wilcoxon, S. A., & Puleo, S. G. (1992). Professional-developmental needs of mental health counselors: Results of a national survey. *Journal of Mental Health Counseling, 14,* 187–195.

Zimpfer, D. G., & DeTrude, J. C. (1990). Follow-up of doctoral graduates in counseling. *Journal of Counseling and Development, 69,* 51–56.

SECTION II
THEORY AND PRACTICE
OF MENTAL HEALTH COUNSELING

Chapter 4

THE ROLE OF THEORY IN THE PRACTICE OF MENTAL HEALTH COUNSELING: HISTORY AND DEVELOPMENT

Thomas A. Seay and Mary B. Seay

"The growth of mental health counseling as a viable discipline has been phenomenal" (Seay, 1986, p. 59). The preceding statement is as true today as it was in 1986 with the first edition publication of Palmo and Weikel's *Foundations of Mental Health Counseling*. Much of what the first author had to say concerning the historical role of theory in the practice of mental health counseling also is as true today as ten years ago. Particularly important is the current significance of the **PHILOSOPHY → THEORY → PRACTICE** paradigm (Seay, 1980a) in an age where over 60 percent of practitioners consider themselves eclectic in their approaches to the conduct of counseling (Mahoney, 1991; Lazarus, Beutler, & Norcross, 1992; Lazarus, 1993; Norcross, 1993). However, problems associated with eclecticism abound.

The underlying paradigm for therapeutic intervention **PHILOSOPHY → THEORY → PRACTICE** has contributed in many important ways to the development of counseling as a vibrant profession. This philosophy to practice paradigm is the foundation for advancements in therapeutic intervention. Furthermore, it has provided the cushion necessary for deviations from tradition to occur. Revolutionary changes are occurring in the field of mental health, and they portend further changes. As teachers and practitioners, we must be able to understand the meaning and significance of the field's history in relation to future directions if we are to continue to provide quality services. The present chapter will explore the history and development of this paradigm, and more specifically the role of theory, as an influential force on the directions taken by mental health counselors (MHCs) as core providers of mental health services.

To fully understand the role of therapy in contemporary mental

73

health, we must first look at its philosophical and historical roots. Only then does the phenomenon of mental health counseling make some sense. This chapter will examine historical antecedents, and current trends and developments to determine the role played by contemporary mental health counseling theory. What is required is an understanding of what brought about these changes, what the changes mean for the profession, and what impact they are likely to have on the future of counseling. However, first it is necessary to examine the legitimacy of the mental health counselor's role and skills.

Role Legitimacy

MHCs have joined the ranks of psychiatrists, psychologists, social workers, and psychiatric nurses as primary mental health care providers. But are we legitimate primary care givers? Acceptance has not been easy; nor have we fully won over significant power brokers in the mental health field. The primary reason can be found in the developmental history of the practice of mental health care.

While the origins of mental health counseling are multifarious, three major trends have played a more immediate and potent role in mental health counseling. Each deserves special attention. The first trend refers to the numerous changes in the methodology of psychotherapy used to treat society's mental health casualties. Such changes are tied directly to the history and evolution of psychotherapy. The history of the field shows movement from model dependency with a restricted range of strategies and techniques to an attitude of eclecticism where almost any strategy or technique is acceptable. This trend will receive detailed attention throughout the remainder of the chapter.

The second development is of more recent origins, and can be found in the community mental health movement of the 1960s and 1970s. Returning society's casualties to the community for treatment was a revolutionary step toward recognizing the relationship among intrapsychic, interpersonal, and environmental sources of etiology and between etiology and treatment. This trend has provided an organizational model for mental health counseling.

The third trend grew from the guidance movement of the 1950s, and, while it resulted in the production of counselors who worked primarily in educational settings, the methodology used by these counselors was drawn almost entirely from models of psychotherapy. Consequently, it should come as no great surprise that this body of counselors would eventually turn their knowledge and skills toward a larger population of people in need. These three developments, changes in psychotherapy delivery, ecological psychology, and production of psychologically-trained and educationally-trained counselors, have come together to create a fifth core mental health provider, who has the knowledge and skills necessary to work with society's casualties. Yes, we are legitimate.

Counseling and Psychotherapy: What's In A Name?

One of the perennial controversies within the health care professions is whether counseling can be considered the same as psychotherapy, or does the counseling profession represent different roles, skills, and methods. Many leading authorities believe that the two represent distinctive approaches to helping people, and that they differ in essential, identifiable ways. Other professionals hold that such a controversy is meaningless, and that any distinction serves the sole purpose of creating professional elitism.

It is indeed difficult to distinguish between the two on the basis of the type of client served, the theoretical underpinnings, the therapeutic processes, and the major strategies and techniques. Practitioners of counseling and psychotherapy work with the same people, use the same methodology, and work towards the same goals.

In the past, factors such as the type of therapy delivered, the degree of disturbance, the clinical work setting, and the type of training received (Patterson, 1974) have been employed to distinguish between counseling and psychotherapy. Differentiation based on type of therapy delivered follows the argument that counseling is emotionally expressive, supportive, and educative, while psychotherapy is depth-oriented, uncovering, and remediative.

Such a distinction creates problems. Persons employed as counselors encounter clients who begin to disclose deep levels of self. Thus, counselors are either moved or "shoved" into an uncovering process. Furthermore, uncovering is the first step in any therapeutic encounter. It is impossible to remain at a superficial level for any length of time. Also, remediation is the desired outcome whether one is attempting vocational counseling or attempting to therapeutically intervene into the private world of a schizophrenic. To create such a distinction is unrealistic.

At one time the work setting served as an adequate means of differentiating between counseling and psychotherapy. Historically, counselors were employed primarily in educational settings while psychotherapists worked in clinics, mental health agencies, hospitals, and private practice. This is no longer true, as can be easily verified by examining current employment practices across the nation. Today, practitioners whose primary identification is with counseling and those who identify with psychotherapy are employed in all major work settings, and work side by side for the betterment of their common clientele.

Traditionally, the medical degree and the Ph.D. in clinical psychology represented the necessary training to function as psychotherapists. Persons who held the Ed.D. or Ph.D. in counseling psychology were labeled counselors, and were expected to work with clients other than mentally disturbed patients. Not only have these practitioners earned the right to practice psychotherapy, but over the past 15 years, people trained at the master's level (M.A., M.S., M.S.W., and M. Div.) have moved toward, and in some instances, won recognition as legitimate practitioners in mental health. As the demand for services continues to increase and the supply of practitioners continues to be at inadequate levels to meet current mental health needs, the line of differentiation based on professional degree will continue to diminish. It can also be anticipated that the master's level practitioner will continue to gain recognition as a mental health provider. Licensure for the master's level counselor is already a reality in over forty-one states, and promises to become a reality in the remainder within the foreseeable future. In part, the impetus toward licensure is being assisted by the Managed Health Care movement, with its emphasis on reimbursement of licensed practitioners.

None of the above arguments suffice to distinguish between counseling and psychotherapy. The professional community of mental health providers must now recognize at least five core providers in the treatment of society's casualties. The tasks of the future will be to recognize that these practitioners share common theoretical nets and a core of therapeutic intervention skills, and to then actually identify the unique contribution that each practitioner can make. For example, psychiatry is unique in that the practitioner can dispense medication, and not that he/she can deliver psychotherapy that differs from that of the psychologist. Each core provider should and can provide something unique. The professional community must seek both that uniqueness and the core skills shared in common, rather than mire itself in inane debates over whose credentials are best or which practitioner is the rightful heir of therapeutic intervention.

Historical Perspective

Counseling is an artistic endeavor which uses scientific methodology to help people lead more effective lives. Counseling, growing as it has from the practice of psychotherapy, is now over ninety years old. Much time and effort has been expended in developing the philosophies, theories, and practices of therapy. For such a young endeavor, compared to other sciences, it has been relatively successful (Smith, Glass, & Miller, 1980).

Counseling is still a vibrant profession. Practitioners, over the last fifteen to twenty years, have witnessed phenomenal changes. The plethora of strategies and techniques available today were either absent or enjoyed only restricted use in the 1960s. Research has grown into a more sophisticated endeavor, moving from questions such as "which approach is best" to "what are the components of effective therapy." The next ten to twenty years will witness even more changes. The rapidity and the magnitude with which these changes are occurring present difficulties for the novice and the experienced counselor alike in gaining a firm grasp of the field.

To understand what is currently happening in the field of mental health counseling, it is necessary to understand how the field evolved into its present status. Numerous changes in the philosophical and theoretical foundations for intervention have led to innovations in processes and strategies. These, in turn, have resulted in major breakthroughs in the treatment of society's casualties.

Philosophical Foundation

One of the major strengths of counseling/psychotherapy has been the internal consistency which binds a set of practices to a theoretical net and a philosophical foundation. That is, the foundations for various counseling models are composed of a set of philosophical beliefs about human beings, which in turn guides the formation of theoretical propositions about human functioning. Based on these theoretical propositions, a set of practices for the conduct of counseling has evolved. To be a viable force, however, the movement from philosophical beliefs to counseling practices must be internally consistent. Such consistency has enabled counseling to make its impact on society. Figure 4.1 represents how this internal consistency may be achieved.

PHILOSOPHY → THEORY → PRACTICE

Figure 4.1. Internal consistency as a foundation for counseling.

The philosophy to practice consistency enables practitioners to evaluate how well their theory predicts actual behavior in counseling, provides an explanation for how change occurs, and establishes expectations for what should be done to help clients. The theory builder develops certain philosophical assumptions about the nature of "humanness," and about the source of knowledge (epistemology) or how change occurs. These assumptions should lead directly to a set of theoretical propositions about human functioning. The theory of human functioning would dictate the nature of the counseling process and the intrasessional behavior that is necessary to create change.

Following this paradigm, some concepts would be appropriate within a given model, while others would not. If a primary assumption concerning the source of knowledge is that the human mind is essentially a blank paper "written on" by environmental forces, then "wired-in" or inherited cognitive configurations for learning and such notions as memory traces and insight would not be postulated.

Seay (1980b; Braswell & Seay, 1984) traced the development of various counseling (psychotherapy) models from their philosophical foundations. As can be seen by examination of Figure 4.2, the lines of influence have not been clearcut. Current philosophical beliefs have developed from the Greek traditions. Plato's world of representations of ideals has resulted in contemporary phenomenology; Aristolean thought is expressed in modern empirical philosophy.

Contemporary phenomenology is best expressed through the work of Leibnitz in philosophy and by the humanistic or "third-force" movement in psychology. Leibnitz provided the defining characteristics of phenomenology, when he proposed that the subjective world of the mind was the source of knowledge. The basic datum for phenomenologists is experience. Thus, knowledge or the source for client change resides in the perceptual awareness of the individual. Considerations of an external reality are useless, since the only source of knowledge about reality is created through the subjective, interpretive system inherent to

them through insight—oriented techniques. The model had a high degree of internal consistency from its foundational philosophy to its set of prescribed practices. The underlying theme that held the model together was that knowledge (psychological change) came from cognitive activity (subjective) of natural events (objective).

The first of Rychlak's (1965) motives, the scholarly motive, corresponds to the purpose of psychotherapy best represented by Freud. By examining intrapsychic dynamics using the psychoanalytic method, the analyst could learn about human nature and human motives. The therapist was essentially a scientific scholar. In fact, the technique of free association was analogous to the scientist's microscope. The fact that Freud had no difficulty in seeing the applicability of the natural sciences to the study of mental activity is a direct demonstration of the power of Kantian philosophy—an external reality examined from the internal world of perceiver. Freud's emphasis influenced Seay's (1980b) designation of psychoanalysis as a cognitive paradigm.

The second original paradigm was created by Carl Rogers. Rogers focused on the subjective experiencing of people and on how change was created within these subjective experiences. Rogers' approach corresponded to Rychlak's second motive. "Felt" levels of experiencing come from interpersonal relationships, relationships that either did or did not provide the necessary elements of growth. Rogers' model focused on the interpersonal difficulties of clients. Thus, Rogers' Person-Centered therapy represented an affective, interpersonal model.

Rychlak's second motive emphasized the ethical consideration of helping people to grow, and was primarily the focal point of Rogers. The basic reason for conducting psychotherapy was to help people grow. This task was accomplished through a subjective encounter with the patient. Rogers (1964) labeled this type of epistemology "interpersonal knowing or phenomenological knowledge." The primary analogy is experience. The therapist comes to know the patient's attitudes and emotions (the 'felt' level of experiencing). Rychlak (1965) refers to this emphasis on felt experiencing as "the ethics of self-determination through congruent interpersonal relations" (p. 115).

Locke's philosophy gave rise to modern scientific inquiry. A scientific model of counseling and psychotherapy was a natural extension of the Lockean tradition. Behavior Therapy, the application of learning theory to human suffering, represents the third motive—the curative purpose. The therapeutic emphasis is to help people change their ineffective behaviors. This orientation is epitomized by the work of Wolpe (1973). The purpose for conducting therapy is to cure the patient. The appropriate analogy for therapy is the experimental design (Rychlak, 1965). Treatment is established as an experiment in the modification of behavior. Behavior is the focal point because it is an observable event. The experimental design calls for observation as the method used to derive basic data. In this sense, Behavior Therapy is consistent with the Lockean tradition (British Empiricism) with its emphasis on the observable, external reality. Human suffering is explained as learned associations. What was once learned could be unlearned or relearned. True to Lockean philosophy, Behavior therapists see little need to postulate internal processes to account for mental dysfunctions. Thus, Behavioral Counseling completes the therapeutic triad corresponding to the triad of human modalities—cognition (Psychoanalysis), affect (Person-Centered Therapy) and behavior (Behavior Therapy).

Each of these three basic models form the tradition (cognitive, affective, and behavioral modalities) from which numerous other models were derived. Each of the three models represents a major shift of focus in both theory and practice. Each represented a paradigm shift from what was tradition at that time.

Beyond the Original Paradigm

The human mind thrives on inquiry. Not long after the development of each of these three paradigms, members of the professional community began to modify the original paradigms, thus ushering in the second stage of development—the Modification Stage. Stage two developments occurred when proponents of the original paradigm discovered a lack or an unfulfilled need in the original theory. For example, Jung tempered Freud's biosexual theory with a philosophical perspective, and Adler provided a social perspective. Both theorists gave psychoanalysis depth and breadth, but neither changed the basic structure of the paradigm.

The third stage was classified by Seay as the Specificity Stage. During this stage, proponents of a particular paradigm adapted aspects of the original paradigm to their needs. Thus, while leaving intact the basic structure of the parent paradigm (e.g., Berne's use of parent, child, and adult for Freud's superego, id and ego), they developed approaches to counseling based on some aspect of the original. Within stage three adaptations, the integrity of the original paradigm suffered few violations to its parameters.

Current Developments: Stage Four Experimentation

Current Status

Counseling has undergone radical changes over the past thirty years. Also, the rules used to signify appropriate conduct in counseling have changed. As a result, it is difficult for practitioners to fathom the multitude of innovations and current practices as organized and following a specific path of development.

Seay (1980b) indicated that a fourth stage, which he labeled the Experimentation Stage, could account for these changes. This stage reflects the current status of the profession. Theoreticians have violated the parameters of the original paradigm by experimenting with theoretical structures, processes, and paradigm-linked techniques. The counseling profession has just entered stage four experimentation, but the resulting changes and innovations to emerge thus far have already profoundly impacted the practice of counseling (Lazarus, Beutler, & Norcross, 1992; Mahoney, 1991; Ellis & Dryden, 1987). For example, once behaviorists accepted internal processing, such as cognitions, they violated the parameters of their basic paradigm. However, in doing so, they, as a group, have moved closer to the humanists. Also, some practitioners having a primary identification with psychoanalysis sound more like behaviorists than many current behaviorists. In addition, with the growing acceptance of family therapy, itself a stage four development, as a viable methodology for treatment, the panorama of therapy has been explicitedly altered.

Stage four, however, has yet to run its course. The experimental manipulation of paradigm parameters has only just begun. Also, researchers are only beginning to emphasize the scientific validation of strategies and techniques. Once paradigm parameters have been breached, the philosophy to practice internal consistency that gave counseling its foundation falls apart. For example, the Lockean philosophy cannot provide a firm foundation for cognitive-behavior therapy. A cognitive-behavioral view implies an interactive involvement with the environment and inherent structures of cognitive organization. Also, an affective-behavioral approach such as Carkhuff's (1969) model is a reinterpretation of Rogers' Person-

Centered Therapy, and as such, can no longer claim a Leibnitzian base. Thus, stage four is a stage of models without foundational supports. This is Lazarus' (1976; Lazarus, Beutler, & Norcross, 1992) "technical eclecticism" in action.

At some point in the future, this problem, for it is a problem, must be reconciled. The profession must have a means of anchoring its practices. Perhaps a new philosophy will evolve. Perhaps a combinatory alternative to current philosophical positions will be found (Seay, 1978). While the future does not lend itself easily to accurate predictions, sufficient evidence is accruing that points to a fifth stage. As previously mentioned, practitioners are becoming more and more alike in their actual intrasessional behaviors. In addition, theoretical efforts are assuming a combinatory flavor by adapting concepts drawn from diverse models. It is no longer unusual to talk of cognitive-behavioral, or affective-behavioral approaches. Speculation on the outcome of these changes leads to what Seay called the Consolidation Stage. Stage five represents the evolution of a single paradigm for the conduct of counseling. Such a paradigm would be based on scientifically validated processes, strategies, and techniques. Once such a model is established, it becomes possible to build an appropriate theoretical net. From a well-defined theory, philosophical propositions can be ascertained, thereby reconstituting the philosophy to practice internal consistency. Finally, counseling and psychotherapy can enter Kuhn's (1970) scientific era.

As previously mentioned, stage four developments are having a significant impact on counseling. Part of this impact can be seen in the restraint exercised by theoreticians on further theoretical developments. None have expressed this better than Lazarus (1976), who called for a "technical eclecticism" until the field could grow into its own. Kuhn (1970) proposed that a true scientific discipline is one where only a single paradigm existed as the guiding model for the discipline. Counseling currently has no fewer than 250 such competing paradigms (Herink, 1980). Lazarus' call for a moratorium on theorizing was appropriate and timely. The effect of deemphasizing theory building has been the granting of freedom from the shackles of model dependency. The price, however, is the desperate need for a scrupulously delimited research mosaic.

By deemphasizing theoretical dependency, the diminution of model dependency occurs and model boundaries are crossed. Counselors are free to create a mixture of models or what some have identified as eclecticism (Norcross, 1986; Seay, 1978). Such mixture is easily demonstrated and more clearly conceptualized if the various models are loosely classified into one of three categories (Seay, 1978; 1980b). All approaches, where the primary focus for change is on thinking (cognition) such as Freud's insight-oriented psychoanalysis and Beck's Cognitive Theory, can be grouped together as Cognitive approaches. Other approaches focus almost entirely on the "felt" level of experiencing such as Rogers' Person-Centered Therapy. Rogers (1964) refers to this felt level of experiencing as phenomenological knowledge. These approaches can be classified as Affective. Finally, the behavioral approaches such as Wolpe's Behavior Therapy and the behavior modification movement (Meichenbaum, 1985) will be classified as Behavior because of the primary emphasis on changing current maladaptive behaviors. Using such a classification system, it becomes easy to diagram the changes that are occurring.

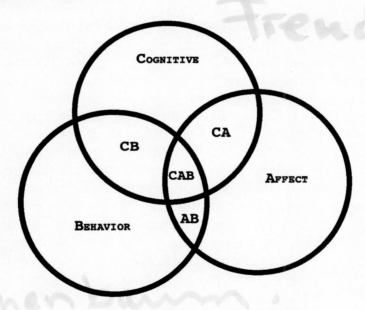

Figure 4.4. Mixing models of counseling.

With areas of uncrossed lines pure models are represented. These are models emphasizing only a single modality such as cognition. Where the lines do cross, two or more human modalities become the point of focus for client change, where the first term (e.g., cognitive in the cognitive-behavior therapy model) is the modifier of the second term (e.g., behavior in the cognitive-behavior therapy model). Thus, counselors are crossing model lines to combine theoretical components, strategies, and processes from different models. The **CB** component refers to practices which combine the cognitive and behavioral modalities. Thus, the cognitive-behavior therapy movement of recent years (e.g., Meichenbaum, 1977; 1985) can be understood and explained from this perspective. This **CB** group emphasizes a modification of behavior, but they may accomplish the modification by enabling the client to restructure or otherwise change thinking first. The **CA** refers to those theorists and practitioners who combine information processing models of thinking with affective models to form a cognitive-affective approach to counseling (Wexler & Rice, 1974). The **AB** designation accounts for approaches that combine the affective modality with the behavioral, such as Krumboltz & Thoresen (1969) and Carkhuff (1969). Few approaches, at this point, emphasize equally all three modalities (**CAB**). Lazarus' (1981) Multimodal therapy approach stands as an exception. As research continues to identify appropriate tools and processes for counseling, all three modalities (**CAB**) can be expected to play a more prominent role. Perhaps, new strategies will be developed that are designed to address all three modalities simultaneously. Perhaps, a new model will emerge.

　　Practitioners, in crossing the boundaries of models, are forcing paradigm shifts to occur. As paradigm shifts occur theoretically, divergent practitioners are finding common ground in their practices. What the outcome of this movement will be is difficult to determine, but the profession may be moving towards a consolidation of paradigms (Seay, 1980b). If so, Kuhn's (1970) criterion for a scientific discipline may be achieved in the not-so-distant future. Once the scientific component of counseling has achieved a strengthening of practice, the remaining task becomes one of integrating the artistic encounter of counseling with its scientifically-established practices.

　　Due to the crossing of paradigm boundaries, counselors can identify a multitude of strategies and techniques currently available for their use. In the past, counselors rigidly adhered to a particular model for knowledge concerning appropriate conduct for their counseling practices. Such adherence brought a measure of security and the ability to communicate with other professionals of an alike mind. However, within these models, practitioners were limited in their ability to utilize strategies and techniques (Seay, 1980b). In fact, they typically were limited to only techniques identified for their model as being appropriate methods of accomplishing the goals of the model. The effect was to force all clients who walked through the door to conform to the model parameters. Model dependency appears to have ended. Counselors are more free to use a wide variety of techniques drawn for diverse models. A counselor who claims allegiance to one of the humanistic models of counseling may be found using systematic desensitization or cognitive restructuring (Raimy, 1975). By the same token, it is not at all unusual to find Behavior therapists engaging in cognitive restructuring or affective focusing (Lazarus, 1976; 1981; Mahoney, 1991).

Paradigm shifts and multidimensional strategies are not the only changes growing from stage four experimentation. Practitioners are decidedly more eclectic in their approach to helping people. They seem more willing to use whatever they deem necessary to help their clients without fear of paradigm violations. Obviously, problems result from a haphazard application of techniques. Eclecticism, to be a viable force in counseling, must be systematic, integrative, and process-oriented (Seay, 1978). In lieu of philosophy and/or theory, practitioners must evolve some method of case conceptualization to anchor their practices. Examples of case conceptual methods can be found in Lazarus (1976), and Seay (1978).

Additional Stage Four Developments

Another major development that has occurred recently may eventually change the face of applied psychology. Community psychology, a relatively recent entry in the field of psychology, has already had a significant impact on professional practices (Seay, 1983). Community psychology, as the words imply, is the application of psychological principles to community elements, structures and dynamics. The origins of community psychology are diverse, but its primary impact can be traced to the conditions within the mental health field in the early 1960s. Because of the recognition that major changes must occur in mental health delivery, John F. Kennedy, then president of the United States, signed into law a bill calling for the establishment of community mental health centers. These centers shifted the responsibility for providing mental health services from state-maintained hospitals to the community itself. Psychiatrists, psychologists, and social workers were quick to become involved in this new movement, but it has taken the counseling profession somewhat longer to move from a primary emphasis on school settings to the community.

In many areas of the country, counselors have now earned the right to take their place alongside other practitioners in community mental health delivery. In fact, in the authors' geographical area, counselors represent one of the largest, if not the largest, professional group. Thus, the community mental health movement has opened a new arena for professional employment. In so doing, however, the impetus has fallen back to colleges and universities to upgrade and update their training programs. Counselors whose training was geared toward schools have found themselves inadequately trained for the majority of a community's mental health needs. Counselors have found that working in the community necessitates using counseling skills more similar to those of psychiatrists, psychologists, and social workers than those skills derived from the old guidance movement of the 1950s, and the early 1960s. However, the outcome of the community mental health movement has been to demonstrate the degree of importance of environment in the remediation of mental health problems.

Developments in Nontraditional Directions

Delivery Systems

There are many different ways to deliver counseling. However, only three basic types of therapy are readily identifiable. The types are: (1) individual, (2) group, and (3) family therapy. The distinguishing features of each type are their theoretical nets and their delivery rather than the processes or methodologies involved.

Individual Therapy: The individual form of psychotherapy refers to the processes and techniques for encountering the client in a one-to-one relationship. The focus of this relationship is on the client and the client's modes of experiencing. The methodology of individual psychotherapy is designed to identify and modify specific aspects of the client's intrapsychic (internal), interpersonal, behavioral, and/or environmental dysfunctions.

Group Therapy: The group approach still focuses on the individual, but uses the natural force of group interaction as part of the therapeutic process. Group members become the primary ingredient of change as each person discloses "self." Each member contributes to the process by supporting and uncovering "self" with other members. The methodologies (e.g., psychoanalytic techniques) used in group therapy may not differ greatly from those used in individual therapy, but the mutual support and the direction that psychological change takes through the group effort will differ extensively.

Family Therapy: Family therapy is the newest form of therapy to appear on the professional scene. It differs from the other two types in that family, as an interlocking, interacting system, is the focal point for treatment rather than an individual who may be identified as the patient. The systemic interaction of the family provides the avenue for intervention and change.

The dynamics of the therapeutic interaction differs extensively among the three types of delivery. The dynamics of family therapy acknowledge that the family comprises a powerful social institution, and that it has internal supports and motivational systems for change not found in other types of therapy. Family therapy utilizes such forces to impact the family structures and the family members' patterns of interaction.

Also as subclassifications of family therapy, marital therapy, divorce therapy, and sex therapy have gained recognition as legitimate approaches to specific dysfunctions within the family unit. Each of these approaches can be expected to continue to have an impact on the way mental health counseling is practiced.

Innovative Models

Counseling models cross paradigm boundaries by focusing on more than one modality. The three modalities are Cognition (C), Affect (A), and Behavior (B). Models or approaches classified as nontraditional are those models based on more than one of the basic three human modalities-cognition, affect, and behavior. Several additional nontraditional systems are described.

Humanistic Behaviorism (A)

Robert Carkhuff (1969) developed a model that follows three process stages: (1) the facilitation or relationship stage; (2) the self-development, self-understanding stage; and (3) the action stage. Carkhuff combined aspects of client-centered and behavior therapy to form the elements of this model.

[handwritten margin note: I would like to learn more here]

Personal Science (CB)

Michael Mahoney (1977; 1991) developed a cognitive-behavioral approach to therapy. Personal Science, the title he used, indicates that the client performs his/her own scientific investigation into the nature of personal coping skills, and monitors his/her own behavior. Mahoney employs an acronym, **SCIENCE,** to describe the therapy process involved. Specifically, Mahoney's stages are: (1) specify problem area (**S**); (2) collect data (**C**); (3) identify patterns or sources (**I**); (4) examine options (**E**); (5) narrow options and experiment (**N**); (6) compare data (**C**); (7) extend, revise, or replace (**E**). This therapy process is a basic problem-solving sequence in which the therapist serves as a consultant and trains the client to use his/her own resources as a problem-solver. By 1991, Mahoney had expanded his approach to resemble more of a CAB model of eclecticism.

Rational Behavior Therapy (CB)

Maultsby's (1977) RBT approach is derived from Ellis' (1973) Rational Emotive therapy. Unlike Ellis, however, Maultsby employs concerted and direct effort toward working with the client's emotionality. The context is still cognitive, but the techniques that he uses tend to follow a more affectively-oriented and behaviorally-oriented therapy. Maultsby employs a five-step process (Emotional Re-education): (1) intellectual insight (created through rational self-analysis); (2) converting practice (behaving consistently with the newly gained insight); (3) cognitive emotive dissonance (focusing on the gap between what the client thinks and what he/she may feel that is caused by converting practice); (4) emotional insight (feeling right or being consistent in feelings that correspond to the newly acquired rational thinking); and (5) new personality trait (causing the new way of thinking and feeling to become as much a habitual and natural way of living as was the old, more irrational way).

Psychobehavioral Therapy (CB)

Woody (1971) has attempted to combine technique and theory from the psychoanalytic and behavioral approaches. To some extent, Woody is eclectic in that he is willing to use many of the insight techniques, while relying on behavior modification techniques to enhance transfer of learning.

Cognitive-Client-Centered Therapy (CA)

David Wexler (1974) outlined a theoretical modification in Client-Centered thinking that reemphasized the role of cognition in affective experiencing. Wexler draws extensively from Information Processing

Theory as the basis for his position on the role of cognition. He, like the cognitive-behaviorists, places emphasis on cognitive control. Emotional experiencing cannot occur without thought occurring first.

Multimodal Behavior Therapy (CAB)

Arnold Lazarus (1976; 1981) has proposed what is probably one of the most comprehensive methods of combining client-conceptualization and therapy procedures developed to date. Lazarus proposed that a client utilizes many human modalities in everyday living. Effective therapy capitalizes on this fact. Traditional approaches to therapy are usually modality limited (i.e., Psychoanalysis focuses on cognition, Rogerian therapists on affect, and Behavior therapists on behavior), while no approach fully utilizes all of the human modalities. Lazarus identified seven modalities, which are summarized by the acronym **BASIC ID.** The corresponding modalities are behavior, affect, sensory, imagery, cognition, interpersonal, and drugs. Lazarus' method of therapy was one of the first to identify and use essential problem themes. These themes were classified according to the **BASIC ID** category that best represented the item. Thus far, there is no theoretical base to guide the therapist in choosing useful techniques. Lazarus has emphasized that there is no therapy process involved in multimodal therapy. A theme is identified and a technique is applied.

Brief Counseling

With few exceptions, the various approaches to counseling had their origins in methodologies developed for individual treatment. However, in recent years a dire need for brief, crisis intervention methodologies, requiring short periods of time to produce meaningful results, has come to the notice of the professional community.

Several reasons exist to explain why this development has occurred. One of the primary social changes supporting brief intervention is the growing public demand for mental health services and the corresponding shortage of professionals available to deliver services. More people require services than there are services available.

Also, technological and institutional changes are occurring at such a rapid pace that the human condition is one of accelerating difficulty in adequately coping (Toffler, 1980). These technological changes are out pacing social-value changes to the extent that a gap now exists between the values produced by technology (e.g., the meaning in one's life is brought about through the creative use of leisure time) and the values attributable to social conformance and social convention (e.g., the meaning in one's life is gained by the quality of one's life work). The times in which we live are difficult because they create mental health coping problems. The briefer methodologies offer a less costly process of remediation because of the limited time involved.

An additional, but seldom mentioned, reason is that psychotherapy is a short-term process for most clients. A review of the current literature (Garfield, 1978) on the average number of therapy sessions revealed that the typical client remains in therapy for only three to eight sessions. It would seem that therapy in general is not the long-term venture that professionals have been led to believe. If the typical client is to benefit, the benefit must come in a relatively short period of time.

Another impetus is worth mentioning. The Managed Health Care movement (Wooley, 1993; Berman, 1992; Austad & Hoyt, 1992), with its primary emphasis on containing excessively escalating mental health costs, is gaining ground. The movement may result in a complete change in the conduct of psychotherapy, or it may not last, losing ground to some other cost containment method.

Butcher and Koss (1978) have listed several characteristics which seem common to most brief approaches. These characteristics include: (1) the time factor (25 sessions or less); (2) limited goal setting; (3) focused interviewing (problem-centered); (4) present-centeredness; (5) active and directive intervention; (6) quick assessment (diagnostics); (7) flexibility (eclecticism) in the use of therapeutic tools; (8) prompt intervention; (9) inclusion of a ventilation process; (10) the therapeutic relationship (positive transference); and (11) careful selection of clients.

Of the several approaches to brief crisis intervention, Small (1979) has developed a six-step model that seems to offer promise as a methodology for conducting therapy. The first step is to identify and continually focus on the presenting problem. Next (Step 2), a personal history should be taken to assist in determining essential characteristics of the client's situation. The third step is to establish a therapeutic relationship with the client. This relationship is essentially the same as establishing positive transference. The fourth step is to devise a plan for intervention which includes strategies (and a wide variety of techniques) specific to the client and the client's situation. The fifth step in Small's model is to resolve or otherwise work through the problem. This step includes reinforcing the client for transferring learning outside the specific therapy context. The final step is successful termination of therapy. Success includes leaving the client with positive transference feelings and positive attitudes toward returning if the need arises. This last step recognizes that therapy is not forever, that people's life situations change as they change and develop, and as their milieu changes.

A more recent development, but still within the framework of Small's model, is Solution Focused Therapy. The goal of Solution Focused Therapy (SFT) is to construct an atmosphere in which clients can generate specific solutions to their presenting problems (Lipchik, 1990; de Shazer, 1988). The fundamental assumptions of this approach holds that clients, in an atmosphere of acceptance and support, will generate possible positive solutions to their problems. The therapist functions as a cofacilitator, providing support and a non-defensive climate. The therapist assists the client through guided and scaled questions to clarify the problem and to examine situations when the problem is "better" or less intense. The therapist reinforces the existing strengths of clients and the positive and useful ways clients are currently reacting. Therapy focuses on clients' assessment of the problem. Clients are entreated to define clear, and specific goals which lead to the generation of client-specific solutions. There is little focus of the roots of the problem or the past in the therapy session, and Solution Focus Therapy does not use diagnostic categories as a guide to strategies or treatment. While originally Solution Focused Therapy dealt primarily with client's cognitions and behaviors, recent authors (e.g., Kiser, Piercy, & Figley, 1993) have focused more on the role of emotion in the therapeutic process.

Diagnostic and Assessment Procedures

When drastic changes in theory occur, the way becomes open for difficulties in the use of old methods and for the development of new methodologies. As shifts in theory occur, the focus centers more on the practices of counseling than was true of the past. Nowhere is this more apparent than with diagnosis and assessment. Psychological testing and assessment appears to have fallen into disfavor. In some circles an antitesting attitude seems to prevail. Alternative methods are being explored, and new techniques are being developed. Traditional techniques of diagnosis include a medical exam, life history questionnaire, projective tests, and paper and pencil tests. Recent trends indicate that therapists are less inclined to use these measures, and they are less inclined to use the corresponding restrictive nomenclature, preferring instead to engage in alternative methods of diagnosis and assessment. Three such alternatives are present. These methods are derivations from current theoretical developments, and each is forcing a rethinking of current theoretical propositions.

Neuropsychological Assessment

One such alternative that has gained in popularity in recent years is neuropsychological assessment. Neuropsychology is the study of the relationship between brain and behavior. Neuropsychology acknowledges that human psychology is related to a physiological/neurological base (Diamond, 1978). Every human action is caused by some finite physiological or neurological change, or causes some physiological/neurological change. Neuropsychology has three primary purposes: (1) diagnosis; (2) patient care; and (3) research (Lezak, 1976).

Behavioral Assessment

Behavioral assessment differs from traditional assessment procedures in two essential ways: (1) what is examined and (2) what is done with the findings. The behavioral assessor looks at observable biological, physiological, and social behaviors, to determine how each impacts adaptive functioning. The behavior assessor attempts to assess the degree to which a particular behavior (e.g., social relations skills) is present or absent. These behaviors are then related directly to desired outcomes.

Thematic Assessment

Assessment of major themes that occur in a person's life offers another way of understanding the client (Braswell & Seay, 1984; Seay, 1978). Usually assessment occurs as a natural part of the therapeutic process. Major themes emerge as clients talk about their problems. Thematic assessment attempts to translate findings into concrete statements about the various interrelated themes that tie together the client's life. These themes are usually interdependent, and assessment should be oriented toward understanding their interrelatedness. Actual assessment procedures can range anywhere from paper-pencil tests such as the Minnesota Multiphasic Personality Inventory (MMPI) to behavioral charting (e.g., frequency of disruptive anger) to process assessment techniques (e.g., cognitive imagery) to clinical interview techniques.

Methodological Innovations

While counseling methodology per se is not of concern in this chapter, how it relates to theoretical developments is. The major thesis of this chapter is that theory has and is undergoing radical changes. These changes are resulting in numerous innovative strategies and techniques. The methodology used by practitioners is no longer dependent on theoretical orientation for legitimacy. In short, the base for conducting counseling has expanded considerably. Methodology refers to the processes, strategies, and techniques used in therapy to create client change (epistemological change). Although there are numerous methodological advances available, only a few will be presented here, along with several general references. In addition, since one of the major themes has been the examination of therapy in terms of three human modalities, consistency will be maintained by subdividing the presentation of methodological innovations according to their use in the cognitive, affective, and behavioral modalities.

Cognitive Techniques

Of the three modalities, the greatest development in technique usage seems to have occurred in relation to cognition. All of these techniques are used to modify faulty thinking (irrational ideas, misconceptions, and automatic thoughts), instill decision-making, and engage in reality testing (Seay, 1980c). Cognitive strategies include such techniques as advanced therapy organizers, bibliotherapy, blow-up, cognitive imagery, cognitive rehearsal, cognitive restructuring, cognitive self-talk, covert reinforcement, free association, graded task assignments, mastery and pleasuring, paradoxical intention, rational self-analysis, reality testing, distancing and centering, and repeated review. Several general references for cognitive techniques are available: Beck (1976); Foreyt and Rathjen (1978); and Lazarus (1981).

Affective Techniques

Affective strategies and techniques are designed to bring a 'felt' experience into full awareness so that it can be fully experienced, understood, and diffused. The techniques in the affective domain include affective focusing, body awareness, catharsis, emotional reeducation, empathic responding, empty chair, evocative reflections, here and now focus, iconification of feeling, psychodrama, stress inoculation, ventilation, and

plus other kinds
of expressive arts therapy

warmth and acceptance. References for affective techniques include Gendlin (1978), Hart and Tomlinson (1970), Seay (1980c), and Wexler and Rice (1974).

Behavioral Techniques

Various behavioral techniques are designed to focus directly on the observable behaviors of the client and on the environmental contingencies supporting those behaviors. The behavioral techniques include assertiveness training, audiovisual feedback, aversive control, behavioral rehearsal, contracting, decision-making, escalation, extinction, feedback, fixed role therapy, homework, hypnosis, minimal effective response, modeling, pain control, reinforcement, relaxation training, role reversal, self-control procedures, time out, systematic desensitization, and contingency management. Several general references for behavioral techniques include Foreyt and Rathjen (1978), Lazarus (1971), and Masters et al. (1987).

Future Directions

A Physiological Basis for Psychotherapy

Of increasing importance is the biopsychological approach to therapy, which assumes that psychological disorders are related to physiological, primarily brain dysfunctions. The assumptions underlying much of the current biopsychological research is that all human behavior can be accounted for by knowledge of the biological mechanisms involved (Uttal, 1978). By understanding these mechanisms, it is possible to understand human behavior.

Treatments altering brain chemistry, drug therapies, have been used since the 1950s and remain an important treatment approach today. However, alternate means of altering psychology, such as the use of exercise with depressed clients, increasingly demonstrate the intricate relationship of physiological and psychological processes. Future research can be counted on to further elaborate the role of biology in psychological processes.

Community Psychology as an
Organizational Model for Intervention

All societies experience psychological casualties. Casualties create a severe drain on a nation's economy and they represent a terrible waste of human resources. Numerous intervention strategies and programs have been developed to provide therapeutic relief for psychological suffering and to counteract the losses suffered by society. These efforts, while producing limited successes, have proved to be expensive and are less effective than originally expected (Rappaport, 1977; Sarason, 1974).

Traditional approaches treat the psychological casualty as victimizer-victim; that is, the victim is to blame for his/her own difficulties. Professional thinking has centered on intrapsychic conflicts, interpersonal (affective) deficits, or maladaptive behaviors (Seay, 1978; 1980b) as the sources for mental illness. Regardless of the external or interpersonal events, clients now carry these internalized processes as their own. Person-created difficulties such as internal conflicts, lack of love and caring, or inappropriate behaviors have resulted in the victim status. Since these conditions are internal they must be treated by changing or otherwise modifying the person. Experience, however, has taught us that while theories that focus on human dynamics do result in change, the change may be short-lived, lasting only until the return of the person to the original environment where conditions and natural support systems work against previously acquired changes.

Alternatives to the human dynamics theories have been proposed and include the social reform/social action movement. Such reflections have led to attempts to change major structures within society. These efforts also have been less effective than desired. In many instances, they have been resisted by the very people for whom they were intended.

An alternative to traditional treatment models is emerging in the literature (Rappaport, 1977; Sarason, 1976). Rappaport (1977) refers to this alternative as the psychoecological perspective (theory). From this perspective, mental health, mental illness, and a host of psychosocial problems such as crime and delinquency are better understood by looking at the person-environment interactions. This theory provides a basis for incorporating and solidifying mental health practitioners and practices. Psychoecology, as applied to the community, refers to the psychological effects of the interaction between people and their environment.

The major premise presented here is that historically either the person or the society has been labeled as sick. Such views place severe limits on the type of treatment that can be provided. Professionals are encouraged instead to view the fit between person and community as being in accord, thereby representing healthy living, or being in relative discord and representing mental and/or social illness (Rappaport, 1977).

Effective treatment, then, must impinge on the interaction between person and environment. To accomplish the necessary changes, psycho-ecological treatment requires the use of strategies designed to modify aspects of the person that contribute to the overall problem, strategies designed to modify aspects of the environment which provides stress and otherwise hinder growth, and strategies designed for problems resulting from the interaction between person and environment.

Seay (1983) has indicated that almost everything in a client's environment, including the intrapsychic and interpersonal interactions, can become therapeutic. In fact, intervention should occur on a number of levels simultaneously. Psychotherapy (individual, group, and marriage/family) should be considered only one strategy among numerous possibilities when attempting to help a client modify his/her life functioning. What is necessary for the professional community at this time is an organizational model that brings together all of the different therapeutic intervention methodologies and community resources for comprehensive intervention. The professional community can no longer afford the limited intervention approaches so characteristic of our past history, where agencies and professionals isolated themselves away from each other and provided services from only their limited perspective, thereby effectively ignoring the contributions that could be made from other resources.

Seay (1983) presented an example of a theoretical and an organizational model for psychoecological delivery based on targets of delivery, sources of psychoecological effects, and services to be delivered. Seay's model identified the target areas for mental health delivery as Primary (direct preventive interventions), Secondary (remediative), and Tertiary (aftercare) Prevention. These areas are consistent with the recommendations of Caplan (1964).

The psychoecological environments or sources of intervention were: (1) residential; (2) community/society; (3) educational; (4) business and political; and (5) the private sector. Together, these five areas constitute most of the major environments of clients.

Identified services required for the model were: (1) psychotherapy (including individual, group, and family); (2) consulting; (3) educational programming; (4) coordinating the various systems in operation; (5) environmental structuring/restructuring; (6) community networking; (7) advocacy; (8) referral; (9) professional training; (10) psychodiagnostics; (11) research and evaluation; and (12) funding.

The intent of this tripartite model is to bring all therapeutic intervention methods under one theoretical and organizational model. Thus, counseling/psychotherapy, marital and family therapy, drug and alcohol therapy, environmental restructuring, funding, community health centers, and the host of other strategies are simply strategies in the larger intervention system of community mental health. Whether this model or some other similar model can accomplish its intended goal remains to be demonstrated. However, the idea offers great potential for organizing the mental health field. The model also provides the opportunity to bring the five core providers under one roof and on an equal status basis, since each would provide unique aspects of the model.

Perhaps psychoecology can provide the necessary organization that is currently so lacking in the field. Certainly, the field needs a theoretical net that will allow all of the various practices and practitioners to function in concert.

Unified Paradigm for Mental Health Counseling

As practitioners used mixed models of therapy to guide their practices, the face of mental health counseling is forced to change. What are the short-term and long-term effects of these changes? One such effort is the movement away from the **Philosophy** $\rightarrow$ **Theory** $\rightarrow$ **Practice** paradigm in favor of a "technical eclecticism" that, to some extent, ignores philosophical and theoretical foundations. Abstinence from theory and philosophy frees the practitioner to use a wide variety of strategies and techniques. In examining the use of mixed models, it would seem that the diversity of therapeutic views are slowly becoming more similar. A single paradigm for therapeutic intervention may eventually emerge. Arguments against an emerging unified paradigm are based on the idea that existing models are drawn from irreconcilable philosophical positions. While therapists may agree on practical theory procedures, they may never agree on a unified philosophical or theoretical base for those procedures. Using existing philosophies (Seay, 1980b), this argument is undoubtedly valid. Traditional philosophies are, in many instances, in direct opposition to one another. Nothing short of developing a new philosophy, one that can reconcile the different views of human behavior, increasingly has distinct possibilities. In the past, philosophical beliefs have evolved from day-to-day living and practices. Philosophy is the explanation of the abstract human being. Thus, by developing a scientific approach to conducting therapy, it may become possible to build a theory of human functioning around those practices. From theory, a philosophy becomes possible.

REFERENCES

Allport, G. (1955). *Becoming.* New Haven: Yale University Press.

Austad, C. S., & Hoyt, M. F. (1992). The managed care movement and the future of psychotherapy. *Psychotherapy, 29,* 109–118.

Beck, A. (1976). *Cognitive therapy and emotional disorders.* New York: International Universities Press.

Berman, W.H. (1992). The practice of psychotherapy in managed health care. *Psychotherapy in Private Practice, 11,* 39–45.

Braswell, M., & Seay, T. A. (1984). *Approaches to counseling and psychotherapy.* Waveland Press.

Butcher, J. N., & Koss, M. P. (1978). Research on brief and crisis-oriented psychotherapies. In S. L. Garfield & A. E. Bergin (Eds.). *Handbook of psychotherapy and behavior change (2nd ed.).* New York, Wiley.

Caplan, G. (1964). *Principles of preventive psychiatry.* New York: Basic Books.

Carkhuff, R. R. (1969). *Helping and human relations* (Vol. 1). New York: Holt, Rinehart & Winston.

Corsini, R. J. (1989). Introduction. In Corsini, R. J., & Wedding, D. (Eds.) *Current psychotherapies (4th Ed.).* Itasca, Ill.: F.E. Peacock.

de Shazer, S. (1988). *Clues: Investigating solutions in brief therapy.* New York: Norton.

Dimond, S. J. (1978). *Introducing neuropsychology.* Springfield, IL: Charles C Thomas.

Ellis, A., & Dryden, W. (1987). *The practice of rational emotive therapy.* New York: Springer.

Ellis, A. (1973). *Humanistic psychotherapy: The rational-emotive approach.* New York: Julian Press.

Foreyt, J., & Rathjen, D. (1978). *Cognitive behavior therapy.* New York: Plenum.

Garfield, S. L. (1978). Research on client variables in psychotherapy. In S. L. Garfield & A. E. Bergin (Eds.), *Handbook of psychotherapy and behavior change (2nd ed.).* New York: Wiley.

Gendlin, E. (1978). *Focusing.* New York: Everest House.

Hart, J., & Tomlinson, T. (1970). *New directions in client-centered therapy.* Boston: Houghton-Mifflin.

Herink, R. (1980). *The psychotherapy handbook.* New York: New American Library.

Kiser, D.J., Piercy, F.P., & Figley, E. (1993). The integration of emotion in solution-focused therapy. *Journal of Marital and Family Therapy, 19*, 233–242.

Krumboltz, J., & Thoresen, C. (1969). *Behavioral counseling.* New York: Holt, Rinehart & Winston.

Kuhn, T. (1970). *The structure of scientific revolutions.* Chicago: The University of Chicago Press.

Lazarus, A. A. (1993). Tailoring the therapeutic relationship, or being an authentic chameleon. *Psychotherapy, 30*, 403–407.

Lazarus, A. A. (1976). *Multimodal behavior therapy.* New York: Springer.

Lazarus, A. A., Beutler, L.E., & Norcross, J.C. (1992). The future of technical eclecticism. *Psychotherapy, 29*, 11–20.

Lezak, M. D. (1976). *Neuropsychological assessment.* New York: Oxford University Press.

Lipchik, E. (1990). Brief solution-focused psychotherapy. In Zeig, J.K., & Munion, W.M. (Eds.). *What is psychotherapy.* San Francisco: Jossey-Bass.

Mahoney, M. J. (1991). *Human change processes.* New York: Basic Books.

Mahoney, M. J. (1977). Personal science: A cognitive learning therapy. In A. Ellis & R. Grieger (Eds.), *Handbook of rational-emotive therapy.* New York: Springer.

Masters, J.C., Burish, T. G., Hollon, S.D., & Rimm, D.C. (1987). *Behavior therapy.* Fort Worth: Harcourt, Brace, Jovanovich.

Maultsby, M. C. (1977). Emotional re-education. In A. Ellis & R. Grieger (Eds.). *Handbook of rational-emotive therapy.* New York: Springer.

Meichenbaum, D. (1985). *Stress-inoculation training.* New York: Pergamon.

Meichenbaum, D. (1977). *Cognitive behavior modification.* New York: Plenum.

Norcross, J.C. (1993). Tailoring relationship stances to client needs: An introduction. *Psychotherapy, 30*, 402–403.

Norcross, J.C. (Ed.). (1986). *Handbook of eclectic psychotherapy.* New York: Brunner/Mazel.

Patterson, C. H. (1974). *Relationship counseling and psychotherapy.* New York: Harper & Row.

Raimy, V. (1975). *Misunderstandings of the self.* San Francisco: Jossey-Bass.

Rappaport, J. (1977). *Community psychology.* New York: Holt, Rinehart & Winston.

Rogers, C. R. (1964). Toward a science of the person. In T. W. Wann (Ed.), *Behaviorism and phenomenology.* Chicago: The University of Chicago Press.

Rychlak, J. F. (1969). Lockean vs. Kantian theoretical models and the "cause" of therapeutic change. *Psychotherapy: Theory, Research and Practice, 6*(4), 214–223.

Rychlak, J. F. (1965). The motives of psychotherapy. *Psychotherapy, 2*, 151–157.

Sarason, S. B. (1976). Community psychology, networks, and Mr. Everyman. *American Psychologist, 31*(5), 317–328.

Sarason, S. B. (1974). *The psychological sense of community.* San Francisco: Jossey-Bass.

Seay, T. A. (1983). Psychoecological treatment as a model for community psychology. *Journal of Counseling and Psychotherapy, 5*(1), 1–12.

Seay, T. A. (1980a). Nontraditional psychotherapy. *Journal of Counseling and Psychotherapy, 3*, 1–5.

Seay, T. A. (1980b). Toward a single paradigm. *Journal of Counseling and Psychotherapy, 3*, 47–60.

Seay, T. A. (1980c). Recent innovations in counseling. *Pennsylvania Personnel and Guidance Journal, 7,* 29–39.

Seay, T. A. (1978). *Systematic eclectic therapy.* Jonesboro, TN: Pilgrimage Press.

Shlien, J. (1970). Phenomenology and personality. In J. Hart & T. Tomlinson (Eds.), *New directions in client-centered therapy.* Boston: Houghton-Mifflin.

Small, L. (1979). *The brief psychotherapies (rev. ed.).* New York: Brunner/Mazel.

Smith, M. L., Glass, G., & Miller, T. I. (1980). *The benefits of psychotherapy.* Baltimore: The Johns Hopkins University Press.

Toffler, A. (1980). *The third wave.* New York: William Morrow.

Uttal, W. R. (1978). *Psychobiology of the mind.* Hillsdale, NJ: Lawrence Erlbaum.

Wexler, D. A., & Rice, L. N. (1974). *Innovations in client-centered therapy.* New York: Wiley.

Wolpe, J. (1973). *The practice of behavior therapy.* New York: Pergamon Press.

Woody, R. H. (1971). *Psychobehavioral counseling and psychotherapy.* New York: Appleton-Century-Crofts.

Wooley, S. C. (1993). Managed care and mental health: The silencing of a profession. *International Journal of Eating Disorders, 14,* 387–401.

HIGHLIGHT SECTION

SEX POSITIVISM FOR
MENTAL HEALTH COUNSELORS

Robert H. Rencken

S-E-X. The word almost leaps off the page. In our society, it is a study in paradox. Sexuality is both hidden and glaringly before us. It is seen as a gift of God and the tool of the devil. An intimate way of unifying people, it is a powerful weapon in the hands of others.

Why do mental health counselors have to deal with sex? Aren't there specialists for that kind of thing?

Perhaps the most comprehensive "why" is that sexuality is such a major part of our client's lives, regardless of activity level, preferences, or attitudes. Sexuality is a potent dynamic force that must be acknowledged by the counselor as an integral part of the whole person. It includes our whole identity as male and female.

It is clear, then, that even if we could leave sex problems to the specialists, we are always confronted with **sexuality** issues, feelings, and concerns. For some of us, that presents a difficult challenge.

One helpful way of meeting this challenge is by adopting a "sex-positive" perspective. Essentially, this means viewing our sexuality in a positive way regardless of our behavior, identification, or values. One can be sex-positive whether he/she is celibate or active, gay or straight, liberal or conservative.

There are three components to sex-positivism: knowledge, consensus, and lack of harm.

Knowledge

As counselors, our sexual knowledge unfortunately reflects that of society as a whole—it is not good enough. There are few formal training programs in sexology and sex counseling and equally few sexuality components in counselor training programs. We simply haven't received the information.

Most mental health counselors have to rely on two sources of information: books and seminars/workshops. How do we evaluate that information?

The information needs to be nonjudgemental with an extra measure of objectivity because of the strong attitudes and values associated with sexuality. It should also be consistent (different theories can still reflect consistency). Finally, there should be cautions against simple solutions. Sexuality is a complex composite of physiology, psychology, spirituality, and cultural issues.

Another component of knowledge is the counselor's awareness of his/her attitudes and values regarding sexuality. What are the messages that I've received about sex? What did my parents think? What seems strange? What seems normal? Why? There is no "right" attitude, but we have to be aware of those attitudes and their potential effect on our clients.

Consensus

The concept of consensus or agreement is often misinterpreted as "whatever turns you on," an extension of the "permissiveness of the sexual revolution." The true issue is equality between partners. When there is an equitable relationship, informed choices can be discussed and acted upon. When there is a power discrepancy or role dominance, there is a limited chance of consensus.

Not only does a lack of consensus open the door to exploitation, but it also tends to put pressure for performance on the partner in the "power" position; a classic "no-win" situation. The expectation of a certain performance (intensity, frequency, or duration) has certainly had a crippling effect on sexuality.

While we usually think of consensus between or among partners, sexuality is, also, importantly, an individual issue. While we may readily ask a couple about their sexual relationship, how often do we ask an individual about sexuality. Intrapersonal consensus is a significant issue. Am I okay with my masturbation? Do I feel settled about my body image? Is my masculinity and femininity in balance?

Lack of Harm

Too often, sex has been associated with harm. In the 1960s, we heard about "sex and drugs" and now certain groups deride "sex and violence" as if those dyads really go together. We've been prone to blame the demise of horrible relationships on a sexual affair or lack of sexual performance. And, of course, we have attempted to link sexual issues with the tragic violence of rape.

A lack of harm is both a cause and effect of healthy sexuality. Our sexuality provides a conduit for the expression of love, for ourselves and others. It is only harmful if we make it that way.

As counselors, we are committed to preventing harm to our clients. Sexuality, like any powerful force, involves some risks—sexually transmitted disease, compulsive behaviors, pathological relationships. We are particularly obliged to protect our children. Hundreds of thousands of children are victimized by sexual abuse, abuse that could well be prevented by better education, gender equity, and a more positive attitude towards sexuality.

Mental health counselors, regardless of setting or clientele, will be dealing with powerful sexuality issues. A sex-positive approach to those issues provides a functional and comfortable way of assisting our clients to effectively channel that power in a healthy and pleasurable way.

Chapter 5

CAREER COUNSELING FOR ADULTS: IMPLICATIONS FOR MENTAL HEALTH COUNSELORS

Linda Brooks and Duane Brown

The relative importance of work to human existence has been argued at length in the professional literature. What is not arguable is that, for most people, work occupies a major portion of the waking hours and that the quality of the occupational experience impinges upon other life roles. Conversely, the influence of family, leisure, and other life roles can attenuate or exacerbate the negative psychological impact of work (Billings & Moos, 1982; Holahan & Moos, 1982). Given the dynamic interaction between work and other life roles and their cumulative impact upon mental health, it is regrettable that mental health counselors (MHC) and career counselors alike have failed to recognize the interrelationship between personal and occupational functioning. The result of this view has been that career and personal counseling are viewed as distinct enterprises. The authors' view is that the goal of both of those forms of counseling includes facilitating personal adjustment. Similarly, Blocher and Biggs (1983) assert that the dichotomization of career and personal counseling represents a "muddle headed" view of human needs. A more charitable interpretation is that career counseling is frequently misunderstood. For example, it is the author's impression that career counseling is viewed by many as nonpsychological in nature and limited to helping youth with occupational choice using "test and tell" approaches (Crites, 1981). If this stereotyped view of career counseling is indeed prevalent, then, career counseling is an underutilized intervention.

One purpose of this chapter is to present a definition of career counseling that captures its true complexity and expands the purview of its applicability. Additional purposes are to offer a model of the career counseling process and to raise the awareness of MHCs regarding when career counseling should be selected as the treatment of choice. The authors challenge the view of Crites (1981) that career counseling should follow psychotherapy and offer an alternate viewpoint that career counseling is sometimes the first, only and most appropriate mental health intervention, even when the client has what appears to be debilitating psychological concerns. The chapter is concluded with a discussion of some issues in the field.

What Is Career Counseling?

Before presenting a definition of career counseling, it is useful to take a brief historical excursion. Parsons (1909), who began the Guidance Bureau in Boston to help youth, is credited with one of the earliest definitions of vocational guidance. According to him, the process involved three steps: (a) gaining an understanding of self, including aptitudes, abilities, and interests; (b) collecting information about the requirements, conditions for success, and rewards of various occupations; and (c) "true reasoning" on the relation between the individual's attributes and job requirements. In Parson's view, the **goal** of vocational guidance was choosing an occupation and the **process** was rational, highly dependent on information, and focused solely on the occupational aspects of one's life. Moreover, an underlying assumption of Parson's model was that occupational choice is a one-time event.

Another early definition of vocational guidance was that adopted by the National Vocational Guidance Association (NVGA) in 1920:

> Vocational guidance should be a continuous process designed to help the individual choose, to plan his preparation for, to enter upon, and make progress in an occupation. (cited in Miller, 1973, p. 9)

The above definition expands the **goal** from occupational choice to preparing, entering, and progressing in an occupation. As Miller (1973) observed, this early definition contains the "germ of a concept of developmental guidance" (p. 9). Much like Parson's definition, however, the above statement seems to assume that occupational choice is a one time event.

Parson's view of vocational guidance was the foundation for the trait-and-factor approach to career guidance. What the trait-and-factor model added to Parson's approach was precision of person-assessment through the use of vocational, personality, and aptitude inventories. These psychometric devices could presumably help the counselor predict which occupations might be most satisfying for the client.

The view of vocational guidance as primarily a rational process that involved matching occupational requirements to individual traits dominated the scene until 1951 when Super offered a substitute definition of vocational guidance that was adopted by NVGA. According to Super, vocational counseling was:

> The process of helping a person to develop and accept an integrated and adequate picture of himself and of his role in the world of work, to test this concept against reality, and to convert it into a reality, with satisfaction to himself and to society. (Super, 1951, p. 92)

Super's definition represented a significant shift in the focus and purpose of vocational guidance. The emphasis on the integral relationship between self-concept and occupational roles introduced the psychological nature of career choice. Furthermore, the definition reflected Super's view of career choice and adjustment as an ongoing developmental process that required accurate self-understanding. A careful reading of Super's article reveals that he formulated his definition, in part, as a reaction against the rational, information centered approach that was associated with trait-and-factor counseling. For Super, "Good vocational counseling deals with both the emotional and the rational" (Super, 1951, p. 90).

Over the years, others have urged counselors to reject early trait-and-factor assumptions. Tyler (1961), for example, stated that the underlying "square-pegs-in-square-holes" philosophy was obsolete. "Vocational choice is a **process,** not an **event**" (pp. 60–61). Crites (1974) proclaimed that the trait and factor approach was atomistic. Following Super, most researchers and theorists today view choice as a developmental and psychological process. Moreover, occupational choice is seen as only one of many career issues faced by individuals.

Clearly, understanding of vocational behavior has increased considerably since the days of Parsons and the original formulations of the trait-and-factor approach. These new understandings are reflected in the growing trend to substitute the term career counseling for vocational guidance (Crites, 1981). The authors applaud this trend and believe that an adequate definition of career counseling should reflect the following ideas:

1. Career development is a psychological process that occurs throughout the life span. This means that career problems may occur at

any age and are not limited to indecision about occupational choice, but also include concerns related to work adjustment, work performance and satisfaction, career change, and integration of career with other life roles.

2. Career development and personal development are reciprocally related. This means, among other things, that psychological symptoms may have their roots in career and work related problems (e.g., an incongruent or unhealthy work environment). Adjustment in one's career, then, may enhance personal adjustment.

3. Counseling is an interpersonal process.

The authors propose that an adequate definition, which would include all of the above features, is the following:

> Career counseling is an interpersonal process designed to assist individuals with career development problems. Career development is that process of choosing, entering, adjusting to and advancing in an occupation or occupations. It is a lifelong psychological process that interacts dynamically with other life roles. Career development problems include but are not limited to career indecision and undecidedness; work performance, stress and adjustment; incongruence of the person and the work environment; and inadequate or unsatisfactory integration of work roles with other life roles (e.g., parent, friend, citizen).

When Is Career Counseling Needed?

The above definition of career counseling implies that it is an appropriate intervention in a variety of situations — many of which are not often recognized. For example, since many psychological symptoms are due to job stress (c.f. Caplan et al., 1975; Kohn & Schooler, 1973; Van Dijkhuidzen & Reiche, 1980), career counseling for occupational change or work adjustment may be more appropriate than stress management interventions. The latter may erroneously assume that the problem lies within the person or that the only choice open to the individual is to adapt to the work situation. Similarly, psychotherapy generally assumes an intrapsychic problem.

Consider the following case. Jean is in a middle management position with a large corporation. She is extremely depressed, cries at the "drop of a hat," and has frequent bouts with insomnia for no apparent reason. At first glance, she appears to be a classic case of a depressive disorder. Further inquiry reveals, however, that none of these symptoms existed before she assumed her current position. Furthermore, she is in an all-male department, is new in the city, and describes her work environment as cold and rejecting, in contrast to the supportive atmosphere she experienced in her last position.

Two career problems are evident in this case: work adjustment and an unhealthy work environment. No amount of psychotherapy purely focused on intrapsychic phenomenon will change the reality of her situation. In fact to focus on the depressive symptoms betrays a lack of recognition that the roots of many psychological problems are career related. According to Blocher and Biggs (1983), "Most major life crises have a heavy vocational component" (p. 263). Maccoby (1980) has criticized mental health workers for assuming that certain symptoms such as acute anxiety and feelings of persecution indicate psychopathology or are due to intrapsychic difficulties. He urges that before a conclusion be drawn, the counselor explore the goals and strivings of the person and the reality of the work situation. "The worker might be extremely neurotic, but the symptoms might result from his (sic) efforts to adapt to, or struggle with humanly destructive conditions" (1980, pp. 509–510). Additionally, the work situation need not be unhealthy to produce such symptoms, but may simply be the result of a poor person-environment fit, for example, the activities that are rewarded are not those valued by the worker or the work requires different abilities than those possessed by the worker.

In light of the above, the authors disagree with Crites (1981) that career counseling should follow psychotherapy in the presence of psychological symptoms. In some circumstances career counseling should be offered first and may render psychotherapy unnecessary. In other situations, career counseling may follow psychotherapy or be offered concurrently. In essence, this discussion points to the need to complete an accurate diagnosis before choosing the appropriate intervention. The next section deals with this issue in some detail.

The Process of Career Counseling

Probably no one has given more thought to the process of career counseling than Crites (1974; 1976; 1981). In his writings he has examined the fundamental characteristics of trait-and-factor, client-centered, psychodynamic, developmental, and behavioral approaches to career counseling (1974; 1981), and presented his own comprehensive approach to career counseling (1976; 1981). What is most obvious from the analyses presented by Crites is that the theoretical orientation of the counselor impinges upon the process. A client-centered career counselor will approach each phase of the career counseling process somewhat differently from a career counselor who subscribes to a trait-and-factor point of view. Persons interested in a full elaboration of the different theoretical approaches to career counseling should consult either the work of Crites (1981) or Brown and Brooks (1984). Because these discussions are available elsewhere, the presentation here will be a generic look at the process of career counseling. An attempt is made in this discussion to present a model for the process of career counseling that transcends theoretical orientation.

When looking at the process of career counseling one major arbitrary decision must be made: what should be included in the process? In his discussions, Crites (1974; 1976; 1981) chose to look at diagnosis and outcomes as separate from the process. The authors have chosen what is probably a more conventional approach and have incorporated diagnosis (here termed assessment) and outcomes into the process. Accordingly, the process of career counseling is made up of a series of dynamic stages: (1) relationship development; (2) assessment and problem identification; (3) goal setting; (4) intervention; and (5) evaluation. This type of listing makes these stages appear to have a definite temporal and linear relationship but nothing could be further from reality. The major assumptions are that the career counseling process begins with relationship building, the sine quo non of counseling, and that appropriate interventions cannot be initiated without first conducting assessment. No other assumptions are made about the order of or nature of the process. It is quite likely that relationship building will have to reoccur from time to time throughout the process; similarly, while assessment begins with relationship development and continues as the exact nature of the client's concerns unfold, it may have to be reconducted after interventions are attempted and either fail or succeed. Career counselors have erred by conducting career counseling by the numbers: (1) test, (2) interpret, (3) provide occupations. This approach is so foreign to the authors' conceptualization of career counseling as not to warrant the label at all.

Relationship

Brammer and Shostrom (1982) assert that "vocational psychology cannot be singled out as a special branch of counseling and psychotherapy, largely because career counseling must be accomplished in the context of the individual's total life style and in relationship to his or her subculture" (p. 390). It can be taken from this statement that career counseling requires the same depth of understanding as does personal counseling and thus must be predicated upon the same relationship if open, genuine communication is to occur. In other words, the same careful attention should be given to the development of the relationship in career counseling as it is in any other form of counseling. The practices of some agencies that dictate that a battery of tests and inventories must be taken prior to seeing a career counselor, is deplorable, because one of the early agenda items becomes test interpretation. Relationship development must be the number one priority. The model proposed by Carkhuff (1969) can serve as the basis of this phase of the counseling process.

Assessment Phase I

Assessment is that aspect of the counseling process in which the counselor and the client develop a full and mutually agreed upon understanding of the client's concerns. Initially, the primary assessment device is the interview. Later other more formal assessment strategies may be used ranging from interest inventories to role playing. The first question that must be answered during the assessment (phase I) is "what is the appropriate intervention; personal counseling or career counseling?". This conclusion should not be drawn until the client and counselor have had an opportunity to develop a relationship and the counselor has developed a high degree of understanding of the client's intrapersonal state and environmental circumstances. To put this point differently and bluntly, just because clients ask for career counseling does not mean that they should receive it, and vice versa. What then are the factors that dictate the type of intervention to be employed?

Brown (in press) has identified a number of key variables that should be considered in making a determination regarding personal vs. career counseling, including the client's perceptual clarity, chronicity of the problem, psychological symptoms, sources of environmental support (nonoccupational), the occupational environment, the match between worker and job, demographic characteristics of the client, motivation, and situational factors such as having a working spouse. Each of these will be discussed separately.

Perceptual Clarity: Perceptual clarity is the ability to accurately perceive one's self, one's environment, and the relationship of the two.

Lack of perceptual clarity has long been viewed as an indication of poor mental health, and more recently theories have pinpointed it as one of the bases of occupational maladjustment (Caplan, 1972; Caplan, Cobb, French, Harrison & Pinneau, 1975). Assessing perceptual clarity requires that the counselor collect data from the person and to some degree from extrapersonal sources so that an objective standard can be set. For example, if the client perceives his or her work supervisor to be cold and nonsupportive, some data may need to be collected regarding the accuracy of the client's observation. Similarly, a client who claims to have been passed over repeatedly for promotions and raises because of "office politics" or discrimination may be quite accurate in that perception. On the other hand, the real reason the individual may not have received the rewards expected is because of job performance.

One of the difficulties involved in assessing perceptual clarity is determining whether or not distortions are the result of psychological or informational deficits. It is quite possible for an individual to draw conclusions based upon insufficient data and be relatively healthy psychologically. Therefore, one of the tasks to be accomplished in assessing perceptual clarity is to identify situations where the individual has the facts and determine whether or not distortions are still present. For example, if promotion to sargeant in the police department is contingent upon scoring at the seventy-fifth percentile on a qualifying examination, and a client who has consistently failed to achieve that score still claims that his or her failure is the result of politics or discrimination, a tentative hypothesis regarding that individual's perceptual clarity can be established. Other similar data would lead to the conclusion that perceptual clarity is absent.

Chronicity: If perceptual clarity is not present, career counseling should not be provided until the condition is remediated. Personal counseling is the intervention of choice. Evidence of chronicity would also lead to a similar conclusion. Individuals who have experienced repeated failures in various aspects of their lives, particularly in their work, often seek career counseling. An investigation may reveal that the person has a high absentee rate, fails to get along with co-workers or supervisors, or has other personal deficiencies that preclude them from being successful workers. In these instances personal counseling will be the initial intervention. Career counseling may, and probably should, follow after the deficiencies have been addressed.

Psychological Symptoms: The presence of psychological symptoms such as depression and psychosomatic illnesses have often led counselors and psychologists to provide personal counseling or stress management training (Abush & Burkhead, 1984). In some instances, at least, the intervention probably should have been career counseling. There is abundant evidence that certain characteristics (or lack of them) in the work environment (e.g., social support, autonomy, clarity of job definition) can produce not only severe psychological symptoms but debilitating physical problems as well (Ivancevich & Donnelly, 1974; Johnson & Stinson, 1975; Keenan & McBain, 1979; Moos, 1981; Moos & Insel, 1974). Assessment of noncompatibility between workers and environments requires thorough person assessment and the ability to assist clients in making an analysis of their work environment and its congruence with their aptitudes, values, and interests. While lack of social support may be debilitating for some workers, others may not find this situation problematic. Some workers may thrive in an atmosphere that requires high levels of productivity while others may suffer. The questions that must be answered are: (1) How well is the worker able to perform the tasks required by the job (aptitudes and skills)?; (2) How interested is the person in the job?; (3) Are the persons' basic values accommodated by the job environment?; and (4) Is the job environment manipulable?

Mismatches between the person and the work environment can produce stress and other mental health problems. Career counseling focused upon identifying alternate careers may be the intervention of choice, as may career counseling focusing upon adjustment within the current job setting (e.g., developing new job skills, negotiating a job redefinition). In certain instances adjustment within an occupation is not possible because of the rigid structure of the work environment. While career counseling for career change would appear to be the intervention of choice in these situations, other data must be collected prior to arriving at this conclusion.

Other Factors: Perceptual clarity and/or chronicity of problems dictates that personal counseling be the first intervention. The presence of psychological symptoms does not result in a similar conclusion because they may be related to an occupational concern—the work environment. Before making a final decision regarding the course of counseling, a number of other factors must be considered. Foremost among these is the possibility of making a job shift. Some workers are precluded from making a job change by interpersonal situations (e.g., a working spouse who cannot move), economic commitments, age, health problems, and skills deficits. These persons will clearly not benefit from career counseling. Counseling aimed at generating additional support from the family or other social groups may be useful in offsetting the negative impact of the work environment (Billings & Moos, 1982; Eaton, 1978; Gore, 1978; Holahan & Moos, 1982), as may stress management programs (Fields & Olsen, 1980). Other workers are not motivated to make a job shift because of some of the factors already mentioned. Career counseling would not be indicated for these workers either.

When then is career counseling the intervention of choice? When the client has perceptual clarity, does not present a history of chronic mental health problems, has both the opportunity and the motivation to make a change in the job situation, and, of course, when the job is problematic. In all other instances some form of personal counseling, psychotherapy, or perhaps stress management intervention is indicated (Brown & Brooks, in press).

Assessment: Phase II

Phase one of the assessment process ends with a decision either to pursue career counseling or some other form of intervention. This is, of course, a mutually agreed upon conclusion. Once this conclusion has been reached, phase two of the assessment process begins which may be comprised of both informal and formal assessment procedures. If the client is currently employed, a decision must be reached as to whether to attempt to restructure the current work environment in order to bring it in line with the client's needs or to make a job shift. If the client decides that a viable course of action is to restructure the present work environment, an assessment of the problematic aspects of the occupation must be conducted along with the client's ability to alter those situations. If a job change appears to be the most appropriate course, some of the traditional assessment procedures may be used to look at interests, aptitudes, and values. In adults, interests and values may be well crystallized and aptitudes fairly evident on the basis of life experiences; thus inventories and tests may not be required. That will of course be a decision left to the counselor and client. It will also be necessary at some point to assess employability skills (e.g., job hunting, interviewing, resume preparation, etc.) with young workers and with adults who have never worked or who have been absent from work for an extended period of time. Practically speaking, it is probably wise to postpone assessment of employability skills until after some closure is reached on the types of jobs to be sought by the worker.

Problem Identification and Goal Setting

In a sense, problem identification and goal setting began when a decision to pursue career counseling was reached. However, formal goal setting within career counseling is the process of establishing an agenda aimed at addressing the problem(s) identified by the counselor and client. The first step is to agree upon the precise nature of the client's concern. Some typical problems might be:

1. A salesperson has unrealistically high expectations for her performance which cause undue stress.
2. Office automation has taken much of the contact with people out of a secretary's work and she has a growing dissatisfaction with the job.
3. A corporate reorganization has resulted in a middle manager receiving notice that he will be terminated in 90 days.
4. The local factory has announced that it will close permanently in six months and layoffs will begin immediately. A worker with 15 years seniority realizes that she will need to relocate.

Counseling goals growing out of these respective problems might be:

1.a To consider realistic earnings expectations based upon the opportunities provided by the current job situation.
1.b To explore new job opportunities that will enable the client to meet current earnings expectations with less effort.
2.a To gain employment that affords more opportunity to work with people in a new setting.
3.a To identify management placement services that might be useful in acquiring a similar position with another company.
3.b To identify alternative careers to management.
3.c To develop the personal skills needed to seek employment as a manager.
4.a To identify jobs that require skills similar to those utilized in the current job and geographic regions where those jobs are available.
4.b To identify potential problems related to relocation and to establish plans for coping with them as they arise.

4.c To identify resources that can be tapped to assist with the job search (agencies, family members, friends, etc.).

4.d To develop employability skills.

Goals focus the counseling effort. However, they must be flexible. As career counseling progresses new information surfaces and goals may change. If the counselor senses even the slightest resistance to pursuing a particular goal, the goals should be rediscussed and reconfirmed.

Selecting Interventions

Interventions are strategies, employed to assist the client in achieving the objectives that have been established. As one would suspect, there are numerous potential strategies and space will not permit a full exploration of all of them. Instead the focus here will be upon identifying the major types of interventions used by career counselors and discussing them briefly.

Probably the most common tool used by career counselors can be classified as informational interventions. For the most part these are designed to assist individuals to cope with career problems by providing them with data about themselves and the world of work. The most commonly used information sources are tests and inventories and various forms of occupational information including simulations, interviews, and job shadowing. These interventions were first employed by trait-and-factor counselors and their use is predicated upon the assumption that human beings are totally rational and only require the right data to make appropriate decisions. While all career counselors use information interventions, the assumption of rationality is not necessarily made by all.

A second set of interventions which have developed over the past 20 or so years are decision making process interventions. These interventions are designed either to enhance the client's decision-making capabilities or, in those cases where faulty decision making styles are discerned, remediate those styles. Typical decision making interventions range from teaching systematic problem solving skills to clients who simply have not developed a good decision making model, to cognitive restructuring for individuals who have developed faulty decision-making styles (e.g., impulsive or dependent). Simulation and modeling (Mitchell & Krumboltz, 1984) can also be employed in this area. Horan's (1979) book, *Counseling for Effective Decision Making* (pp. 201–216), should be contacted for a more complete discussion of this topic.

A third type of intervention can be classified as behavior development interventions. These interventions are designed primarily to assist clients in developing new behaviors or to overcome behavioral deficiencies that either impede their functioning on the job or their ability to get a new job. Role playing or behavioral rehearsal strategies are often used in assisting clients to develop employability skills (e.g., interviewing). Bibliotherapy can also be viewed as a behavioral development intervention (although it is obviously informational as well) if the readings are focused in a manner that stimulates the development of a set of behaviors. The dozens of books that tell people how to search for, acquire, and be successful in jobs are an example of this type of intervention.

To reiterate, the purpose of the intervention is to assist the client in achieving the goals that have been established. The final step in the process, evaluation, provides the data necessary to draw conclusions about whether or not the tasks have been accomplished.

Evaluation

Evaluation, like assessment, can be formal or informal. Informal evaluation consists of gaining casual opinions from the client, perhaps others associated with the process, and counselor judgments regarding the success or failure of the career counseling process. Formal evaluation, of course, involves systematically collecting data relative to the goals that have been established. Needless to say, most evaluation is informal if it is conducted at all. The authors do want to make a place for at least some informal evaluation of the career counseling process at the time the process is terminated and, if possible, some weeks and months after the process. Questions that need to be answered are:

  a. Did the client achieve his/her goals?
  b. How satisfied is he/she with both the process and outcomes?
  c. Were the interventions used helpful in achieving the goals?
  d. What suggestions would the client make for improving the career counseling process?

Formal evaluations of career counseling also need to be conducted and inserted into the professional literature. *The Vocational Guidance Quarterly** has an In-The-Field section that provides an ideal forum for publishing these evaluations.

---

*Now *The Career Development Quarterly*.

Some Additional Issues

One issue repeatedly addressed in this chapter is when career counseling should be the treatment of choice. It would be remiss to fail to discuss additional issues of importance to the practice of career counseling. Thus, the remainder of this chapter will discuss the following: self-directed procedures versus career counseling, sex bias, the role of career development theory, and the status of career counseling.

Self-Directed Approaches Versus Career Counseling

Holland (1974, 1978) has been a strong advocate of self-directed approaches to helping clients with career choice problems. He chastises counselors for doggedly offering individual counseling when less expensive, more efficient forms of assistance are available, such as Holland's Self-Directed Search (SDS, 1977). Some support for Holland's positions is found in a limited number of studies showing that counselors are not better than interest inventories (Holland, Magoon & Spokane, 1981). As Brown (1984) and Spokane and Oliver (1983) have observed, however, the available research has methodological problems and no final conclusions are possible regarding the effectiveness of do-it-yourself approaches as compared with individual counseling. Furthermore, it is important to point out that the self-directed materials developed by Holland thus far are potentially useful for only one type of career problem; namely, indecision about occupational choice. As previously discussed, career indecision is only one of many vocational problems that may warrant career counseling.

Even in those cases where the primary problem is career indecision, self-help approaches may be effective only for certain subgroups of clients. Power, Holland, Daiger, and Takai (1979), for example, found that students with low vocational identity and high decision-making difficulty rated the SDS lower than students with high vocational identity and low decision-making difficulty. They concluded that the more vocationally confused student may need something more than self-help. Insofar as Holland's assertions are motivated by a concern for offering more efficient and less expensive forms of career assistance, self-directed approaches certainly deserve continued attention and research. Any blanket offering of self-help devices for assistance in career choice must be tempered, however, by the need to complete an accurate diagnosis of the client's situation. Holland apparently concurs with this viewpoint for he recently provided an assessment device, *My Vocational Situation* (Holland, Daiger, & Power, 1980), designed to distinguish the low from the high vocationally confused client. For the former, the SDS may be adequate. For the latter, Holland developed another self-help instrument, *The Vocational Exploration and Insight Kit* (VEIK) (Holland et al., 1980). Whether the VEIK will prove effective for the client with more complex career decision problems is a question that needs further research. In the meantime, there is some doubt about whether or not self directed approaches can meet the needs of more than a limited number of clients.

Sex Bias in Career Counseling

A variety of factors enhance or deter career choice and advancement, for example, individual abilities and interests, socioeconomic status, family background, and cultural norms. In regard to women, more attention in recent years has been devoted to variables that deter rather than facilitate career development. One such environmental factor of concern is counselor bias. Fitzgerald and Crites (1980) have summarized the research documenting various forms of counselor bias (e.g., counselors disapprove of women entering nontraditional careers and roles).

So much emphasis has been placed on counselor bias and sexist attitudes since the middle 1970s, that many assume that counselor consciousness has been raised to the point where counselor bias has vanished. A recent study suggests it has not, however (Haring, Beyard-Tyler, & Gray, 1983). Moreover, some charge that only blatant forms of bias have been eliminated; subtle bias is still pervasive. Sheridan (1982) asserts, for example, that passive bias may still operate since sexism is as much a function of what is not done as well as what is. "A therapist need not actively discourage a female client from going to engineering school when the same effect may be obtained by simply not raising the possibility" (p. 82). Similarly, Fitzgerald and Betz (1983) warn that even a neutral stance contributes to the existence of a "null" environment (Freeman, 1975) (i.e., support or encouragement is lacking). Failure to challenge "women's socialized expectations serves . . . to reinforce and perpetuate traditional sex-role stereotypes." (Fitzgerald & Betz, 1983, p. 108).

Whether counselor sex bias in either blatant or subtle forms is a widespread problem is an empirical question that has not yet been answered satisfactorily. Few would disagree, however, with the position that counselors should avoid blatant and subtle bias in their work with women. Such an avoidance requires both a thorough awareness of one's own and society's sexist assumptions and the special career development issues faced by women. Among the latter are both internal variables (e.g., fear of success, home-career conflict) and external or environmental obstacles (e.g., job discrimination, family attitudes) (Farmer, 1976). Fitzgerald and Betz's (1983) commendable and comprehensive review of these issues is highly recommended reading in this regard.

Sex bias is not confined to women, however, as Fitzgerald (1980) and Skovholt and Morgan (1981) have discussed. Men, too, are restricted by sex-typed expectations. Counselors are thus advised to examine their assumptions about both sexes.

The Role of Career Development Theory

Thus far, little mention has been made of the role of theory in career counseling. Few would question the need for counseling in general and career counseling in particular to be guided by some theoretical framework. Without theory, counselors will wander aimlessly through all phases of career counseling, from diagnosis and assessment to goal setting, and evaluation. The specific implications of the various career development theories for career counseling is beyond the scope of this chapter but have been addressed elsewhere (Brown & Brooks, 1984; Crites, 1981). Nevertheless, some general comments are in order.

First, no systematic research has been conducted on the role of career development theory in practice—which theory is predominate, how it is used, or even if theory has any influence at all. Moreover, no studies have been conducted that compare the effects of using one theory or the other. Anecdotal evidence supports the impression, however, that career counseling practice is more often than not uninformed by theory.

Second, counselor's need to refamiliarize themselves with all of the various theories available. Each approach deals with different issues (e.g. career development, career choice, career decision-making) and thus no one theory can be expected to offer adequate guidelines for all client situations. Thus the counselor needs theoretical flexibility in order to use the theory that will best fit their client situations.

Third, career development theories have been severely criticized for making assumptions that render them inadequate for ethnic minorities, women, and lower socioeconomic classes (Fitzgerald & Crites, 1980; Fitzgerald & Betz, 1983; Osipow, 1975; Smith, 1982; Warnath, 1975). These criticisms deserve careful attention.

The Status of Career Counseling

This chapter began with the assertion that career counseling is both a misunderstood and underutilized intervention. Admittedly, this position is impressionistic rather than data based. It does seem clear, however, that career counseling occupies second class status among counselors. The publication of articles on ways to make career development more interesting (Bradley, 1983; Miller & Super, 1982; Roark, 1982) suggests that the lack of effective career counseling training is a common and long-standing problem. The findings that counselors view career counseling as dull (Graff & McLean, 1970) and that agencies assign career clients to less experienced counselors (Graff, Raque & Danish, 1974) suggests that career counseling is seen as less captivating and "easier" than personal counseling and psychotherapy. The view of career counseling as a simple endeavor was challenged in a recent recommendation to training programs for counseling psychologists. More specifically, the suggestion was made that "Programs should admit that educational and vocational counseling are indeed more difficult than personal adjustment counseling and order the practicum experiences so that the latter is preparatory to the former" (Myers, 1982, p. 42).

Changing counselor attitudes about career counseling seems necessary but may be a difficult task. Blocher and Biggs (1983) assert that the disparagement of the importance of career counseling is due to a greater fascination with the personal which in turn is caused by "an adolescent voyeuristic view and value system" (p. 264) that rewards counselors when they stimulate clients to discuss taboo areas (e.g., sex behavior).

If a wholesale shift in the values of the counseling profession is needed, as Blocher and Biggs (1983) imply, then increasing the status of career counseling may require a long-term broad-based change effort. Short of such an effort, it is hoped that this chapter successfully portrays career counseling as an engaging and stimulating enterprise. More importantly, however, whether general counselor attitudes become more positive or not, it seems imperative that counselors become skilled in recognizing client situations that call for career counseling. Otherwise, clients are apt to receive either inappropriate or ineffective treatment.

REFERENCES

Abush, R., & Burkhead, E. J. (1984). Job stress in midlife working women: Relationship among personality type, job characteristics, and job tension. *Journal of Counseling Psychology, 31,* 36–44.

Billings, A. G., & Moos, R. H. (1982). Work stress and the buffering roles of work and family resources. *Journal of Occupational Behavior, 3,* 215–237.

Blocher, D. H., & Biggs, D. A. (1983). *Counseling psychology in community settings.* New York: Springer.

Bradley, R. W. (1983). Teaching preservice career counseling classes. *Vocational Guidance Quarterly, 32,* 119–121.

Brammer, L. M., & Shostrom, E. L. (1982). *Therapeutic psychology: Fundamentals of counseling and psychotherapy* (4th ed.). Englewood Cliffs, NJ: Prentice-Hall.

Brown, D. (1984). Issues and trends in career development. In D. Brown & L. Brooks (Eds.), *Career choice and development: Applying contemporary theories to practice.* (pp. 406–416). San Francisco: Jossey-Bass.

Brown, D. (in press). Career counseling: Before, after, or instead of personal counseling. *The Vocational Guidance Quarterly.*

Brown, D., & Brooks, L. (Eds.) (1984). *Career choice and development: Applying contemporary theories to practice.* San Francisco: Jossey-Bass.

Brown, D., & Brooks, L. (in press). Career counseling as a mental health intervention. *Professional Psychology: Research and Practice.*

Caplan, R. D. (1972). *Organizational stress and individual strain: A social psychological study of risk factors in coronary heart disease among administrators, engineers, and scientists.* Doctoral Dissertation, The University of Michigan, 1971, *Dissertation Abstracts International, 32,* 6706B (University Microfilms No 72-14822).

Caplan, R. D., Cobb, S., French, J. R. P., Jr., Harrison, R. V., & Pinneau, S. R., Jr. (1975). *Job demands and workers health.* Washington, D.C.: HEW Publication No. (NIOSH) 75-160.

Carkhuff, R. R. (1969). *Helping and human relations: A primer for lay and professional helpers (vol. 2).* New York: Holt, Rinehart, & Winston.

Crites, J. O. (1974). Career counseling: A review of major approaches. *The Counseling Psychologist, 4*(3), 3–23.

Crites, J. O. (1976). Career counseling: A comprehensive approach. *The Counseling Psychologist, 6*(3), 2–111.

Crites, J. O. (1981). *Career counseling: Models, methods and materials.* New York: McGraw-Hill.

Eaton, W. W. (1978). Life events, social supports, and psychomatic symptoms: A reanalysis of the New Haven data. *Journal of Health and Social Behavior, 19,* 230–234.

Farmer, H. S. (1976). What inhibits achievement and career motivation in women? *The Counseling Psychologist, 6,* 12–14.

Fitzgerald, L. F. (1980). Nontraditional occupations: Not for women only. *Journal of Counseling Psychology, 27,* 252–259.

Fitzgerald, L. F., & Betz, N. E. (1983). Issues in the vocational psychology of women.

In W. B. Walsh, & S. H. Osipow (Eds.), *Handbook of vocational psychology, Vol. I, foundations* (pp. 83–159). Hillsdale, NJ: Lawrence Erlbaum.

Fitzgerald, L. F., & Crites, J. O. (1980). Toward a career psychology of women: What do we know: What do we need to know? *Journal of Counseling Psychology, 27,* 44–62.

Freeman, J. (1975). How to discriminate against women without really trying. In J. Freeman (Ed.), *Women: A feminist perspective* (pp. 217–232). Palo Alto, CA: Mayfield.

Gore, S. (1978). The effect of social support in moderating the health consequences of unemployment. *Journal of Health and Social Behavior, 19,* 157–165.

Graff, R., & McLean, D. (1970). Evaluating educational-vocational counseling: A model for change. *Personnel and Guidance Journal, 48,* 568–574.

Graff, R., Raque, D., & Danish, S. (1974). Vocational-educational counseling practices: A survey of university counseling centers. *Journal of Counseling Psychology, 21,* 579–580.

Haring, M., Beyard-Tyler, K., & Gray, J. (1983). Sex-biased attitudes of counselors: The special case of nontraditional careers. *Counseling and Values, 27,* 242–247.

Holahan, C. J., & Moos, R. H. (1982). Social support and adjustment: Predictive benefits of social climate indices. *American Journal of Community Psychology, 10,* 403–414.

Holland, J. L. (1974). Vocational guidance for everyone. *Educational Researcher, 3,* 9–15.

Holland, J. L. (1977). *The Self-Directed Search.* Palo Alto: Consulting Psychologists Press.

Holland, J. L. (1978). Career counseling: Then, now, and what's next? In J. M. Whiteley & A. Resnikoff (Eds.), *Career counseling* (pp. 57–62). Monterey, CA: Brooks/Cole.

Holland, J. L., Magoon, T. M., & Spokane, A. R. (1981). Counseling psychology: Career interventions, research, and theory. *Annual Review of Psychology, 32,* 279–305.

Holland, J. L., et al. (1980). *The Vocational Exploration and Insight Kit* (VEIK). Palo Alto: Consulting Psychologists Press.

Horan, J. J. (1979). *Counseling for effective decision making.* North Scituate, MA: Duxbury Press.

Ivancevich, J. M., & Donnelly, J. H. (1974). A study of role clarity and need for clarity for three occupational groups. *Academy of Management Journal, 17,* 28–36.

Johnson, J. W., & Stinson, J. E. (1975). Role ambiguity, role conflict, and satisfaction: Moderating effects of individual differences. *Journal of Applied Psychology, 60,* 329–333.

Keenan, A., & McBain, G. D. M. (1979). Effects of Type A behavior, intolerance of ambiguity, and locus of control on the relationship between role stress and work-related outcomes. *Journal of Occupational Psychology, 52,* 277–285.

Kohn, M. L., & Schooler, C. (1973). Occupational experience and psychological functioning: An assessment of reciprocal effects. *American Sociological Review, 38,* 97–118.

Maccoby, M. (1980). Work and human development. *Professional Psychology, 11,* 509–519.

Miller, C. H. (1973). Historical and recent perspectives on work and vocational guidance. In H. Borow (Ed.), *Career guidance for a new age* (pp. 3–39). Boston: Houghton Mifflin.

Miller, M. J., & Super, B. (1982). The art of creating enjoyable career counseling classes. *Vocational Guidance Quarterly, 31,* 144–148.

Mitchell, L. K., & Krumboltz, J. D. (1984). Social learning approach to career decision making: Krumboltz's theory. In D. Brown & L. Brooks (Eds.), *Career choice and development: Applying Contemporary theories to practice* (pp. 253–280). San Francisco: Jossey-Bass.

Moos, R. H. (1981). *Work environment scale manual.* Palo Alto, CA: Counseling Psychologists Press.

Moos, R. H., & Insel, P. (1974). *Work environment scale preliminary manual.* Palo Alto, CA: Consulting Psychologists Press.

Myers, R. A. (1982). Education and training—The next decade. *The Counseling Psychologist, 10*(2), 39–44.

Osipow, S. H. (1975). The relevance of theories of career development to special groups: Problems, needed data, and implications. In J. S. Picou & R. E. Campbell (Eds.), *Career behavior of special groups* (pp. 9–22). Columbus, OH: Merrill, 1975.

Parsons, F. (1909). *Choosing a vocation.* Boston: Houghton Mifflin.

Power, P. G., Holland, J. L., Daiger, D. C., & Takai, R. T. (1979). The relation of student characteristics to the influence of the Self-Directed Search. *Measurement and Evaluation in Education, 12,* 98–107.

Roark, M. L. (1982). More art in the career counseling classroom. *Vocational Guidance Quarterly, 32,* 116–118.

Sheridan, K. (1982). Sex bias in therapy: Are counselors immune? *Personnel and Guidance Journal, 61,* 81–83.

Skovholt, T. M., & Morgan, J. I. (1981). Career development: An outline of issues for men. *Personnel and Guidance Journal, 60,* 231–237.

Smith, E. J. (1982). Counseling psychology in the market place: The status of ethnic minorities. *The Counseling Psychologist, 10,* 61–67.

Spokane, A. R., & Oliver, L. W. (1983). The outcomes of vocational intervention. In W. B. Walsh & S. H. Osipow (Eds.). *Handbook of* vocational psychology: Vol II, application (pp. 99–136). Hillsdale, NJ: Lawrence Erlbaum.

Super, D. E. (1951). Vocational adjustment: Implementing a self-concept. *Occupations, 30,* 88–92.

Tyler, L. E. (1961). The future of vocational guidance. In M. S. Viteles, A. H. Brayfield, & L. E. Tyler (Eds.), *Vocational counseling: A reappraisal in honor of Donald G. Paterson* (pp. 59–70). Minneapolis: University of Minnesota Press.

Van Dijkhuidzen, N., & Reiche, H. (1980). Psychological stress in industry: A heartache for middle management. *Psychotherapy and Psychosomatic Medicine, 34,* 124–134.

Warnath, C. F. (1975). Vocational theories: Direction to nowhere. *Personnel and Guidance Journal, 53,* 422–428.

Chapter 6

GERONTOLOGY:
MENTAL HEALTH AND AGING

JANE E. MYERS

The number of older persons worldwide has increased dramatically in the last 100 years, and particularly since the middle of this century. In the United States in 1900, only 4 percent of the total population was elderly, or over the age of 60. Today, almost 13 percent of the population, some 33,000,000 persons, are in this age bracket (American Association of Retired Persons [AARP], 1993). By the year 2000, it is estimated that half of our population will be over the age of 50 (Brotman, 1982). Roybal (1988) noted that older persons, especially those of ethnic minority background, are especially vulnerable to mental health problems. These include needs for preventive mental health care as well as needs for assistance with significant problem areas. In this chapter, the challenges of later life which combine to make older persons a population at risk are considered, followed by a discussion of the mental health needs and problems of this population. The current status of the mental health treatment system as it relates to older individuals is discussed, including consideration of individual and systemic barriers to effective treatment. The need for mental health counselors to receive specialty training in gerontological issues is addressed.

"Normal" Aging

The challenges faced by older persons are many and varied. Erikson (1963), the first and most prominent life-span developmental theorist, postulated that older persons experience and must resolve the central psychosocial challenge of achieving integrity versus despair. A normative process of life review, commonly observed in the telling of "stories" by persons in later life, is the process by which integrity is reached. Life review occurs with a purpose, that being an integration of life experiences and a sense that the life one lived is the best one could have lived. This is defined as a state of integrity. Older persons who look back on their lives with regret, realizing that they have little time left to make significant changes, may reach a state of depression characterized by despair.

Riker and Myers (1989) suggested that a close study of the decades of life beginning at age 60 could reveal a series of life stages and tasks which had not yet been identified by other researchers. In conducting such a study, they noted two key points: (1) life changes are frequent at all ages and adaptation to change is thus a continuing task, and (2) some tasks are repeated during the various life stages. Some tasks are important for persons of various ages to consider and accomplish, rather than being specific to a particular age. This becomes increasingly true in later life. Successful resolution or achievement of a task is not an end in itself, but a means to continued successful coping with similar or identical tasks in later years.

Riker and Myers suggested three basic assumptions about developmental tasks in later life: (1) life tasks should be positive, (2) participation in activities represents a healthy approach to growing older, and (3) in our lives there tends to be an evolution from a concern about relationships with other persons to a concern about relationships to oneself and to one's God. The developmental tasks for later life posited by these authors all concern reacting to change and building positive life concepts.

The fifties are often a time for questioning work and leisure values and for redefining personal roles in the various life arenas. There is renewed emphasis on relationships with others. In the sixties, persons engage in a careful look at their life habits, replacing busyness for its own sake with personal involvement in helping others, developing one's own capacities, and seeking new life meanings. The seventies are a time when leisure tends to become more important than work, family and friendships grow in significance, and the search for life's meaning intensifies. The eighties provide opportunity for aging persons to strengthen their sense of self and their feelings of personal power. These opportunities may be found through continuing to develop family and friendship circles, expanding creative activities, coping with physical changes, taking more time for reflection, and achieving inner peace. In the nineties, individuals build their sense of spiritual wholeness. This is a time when past problems may become inconsequential, when present relationships and activities are to be enjoyed for themselves, and when the uncertainties of the future can be faced with a sense of composure. People in their 90s and beyond may focus on enjoying their lives through appreciating the events of each day and the people who enter into those days.

Old age clearly is a time of change. While Riker and Myers proposed a positive perspective on roles and relationships and the possibility of continued growth throughout the later years, many authors focus on loss as the central theme of later life. For example, Butler and Lewis (1991) describe loss as the predominant theme characterizing the emotional experiences of older people. Losses may involve either environmental/ extrinsic or intrinsic factors, or some combination of the two. The former include losses such as spouse, friends, and significant others, social and work roles, prestige, and income. The latter may include loss of physical strength and health, personality changes, and changes in sexual abilities.

It has been estimated that 86 percent of all older persons experience physical limitations due to age-related physical changes (Saxon & Etten, 1987). Older adults experience substantial comorbidity, such that the interaction between physical and mental health is an especially common and complicating factor in later life. Physical problems can lead to mental distress, mental distress can exacerbate physical symptoms, and the interaction between the two can lead to an exacerbation of clinical pathology (Cohen, 1990).

Overall, the inevitable losses of aging and death are compounded by individual loss of physical and psychological resilience. Situational crises may arise for older persons as they are faced with a decreasing array of resources to meet an increasing array of needs. Most older persons can cope successfully with these changes. Certainly all have the potential to react to the vicissitudes of aging in psychologically healthful and growthful ways. This is reflected in the fact that most older people are able to remain in community living environments. Only 4–5 percent are in institutional settings at any point in time. Another 10–15 percent are largely homebound due to mental and/or physical disabilities, but are able to continue living independently with some assistance. Unfortunately, the increased stresses of aging create adjustment problems that not all older people meet without some impact on their mental health.

Mental Health and Aging

It has been estimated that almost one-third of older persons have mental health problems that warrant professional intervention (Piacitelli, 1992). This includes older people with clinically significant depression and those diagnosed with major affective disorder or bipolar depression. These estimates are significantly lower than those made even a decade ago, when it was widely believed that the prevalence of serious mental health concerns increased with advancing age. Gatz and Smyer (1992) reviewed epidemiological data, noting the increased availability of such data within the past ten years, and concluded that "older adults have a lower prevalence of mental disorders than do younger adults" (p. 745).

Citing data from several epidemiological studies, Gatz and Smyer (1992) concluded that the prevalence of affective disorder in older adults living in the community is about 4 percent. The prevalence of anxiety disorders averages 7 percent in community studies, with the prevalence of anxiety disorders actually being lower in older adults than younger persons. Anxiety may be more common than depression among older individuals. On the other hand, given the complexities of diagnosis of both depression and anxiety in older people (e.g., the difficulty of differential diagnosis of physical and emotional disorders), it is possible that depression actually is more prevalent than diagnoses indicate, perhaps as high as 15 percent.

Significant cognitive impairment resulting from organic brain disorders ranges between 7 percent and 18 percent in persons aged 85 and older; however mild to severe cognitive impairment in this age group may be as high as 41 percent (Gatz & Smyer, 1992). The incidence of impairment is even higher among residents of long-term care facilities. Forty-three percent of nursing home residents are diagnosed with a psychiatric disorder, according to the 1985 National Nursing Home Survey (National Center for Health Statistics, 1989). In addition, 22 percent of residents in this study were diagnosed with organic impairments. Dementia and/or another diagnosable mental disorder were present in 60 percent of nursing home residents. Gatz and Smyer (1992) estimated that about 22 percent of older adults, living either in the community or in long term care institutions at any point in time, experience some type of mental disorder, including dementia. These estimates are consistent with data presented by Roybal (1988) and others.

Piacitelli (1992) noted that severe cognitive impairment affects 5 percent of the older population, with Alzheimer's Disease being the most common type. He further noted that one-half of older patients with Alzheimer's Disease and one-half of those with multi-infarct dementia are diagnosed concurrently with depression or psychosis.

Suicide rates among older persons are higher than among persons of younger ages (Piacitelli, 1992). Osgood (1992) noted that 95 percent of persons who die of suicide evidence symptoms of major emotional illness within the weeks preceding the suicide. Among older persons, the completion rate for suicide is 4:1, while in the general population it is 20:1. These facts suggest that older persons who are depressed or emotionally distressed do not receive timely intervention. Moreover, outreach and casefinding may be especially important with this population, since the lethality rate for suicide is so high.

The Mental Health System and Older Adults

Unfortunately, existing mental health services for older persons have not met the demand for care. While older persons comprise over 12 percent of the total population, they comprise only 6 percent of the caseload of community mental health centers and 2 percent of the caseload of private practitioners (Flemming, Rickards, Santos & West, 1986). This represents a 2 percent increase over the past decade. Older persons who are homebound have little access to mental health services, and those residing in long-term care settings almost never receive mental health treatment (Roybal, 1988).

Burns and Taube (1990) noted that 44 percent of the mental health care needed by older persons is provided through the general health sector. In other words, physicians are the primary mental health care givers for older individuals, even though they are, as a group, poorly trained to recognize and treat emotional disorders. Further, physicians may be less likely to refer older patients than younger patients for needed mental health care.

While they are underrepresented in outpatient care, older persons are overrepresented in inpatient mental health populations. More than 60 percent of public mental hospital beds are occupied by persons over age 65. More than half of these persons received no psychiatric care prior to their admission, making the mental hospital admission their first contact with the mental health system (Special Committee on Aging, 1983).

Preventive care or early intervention could likely prevent or postpone such hospitalizations.

Gatz and Smyer (1992) note that the deinstitutionalization movement has not resulted in outpatient services replacing inpatient care for older persons. Instead, both outpatient and inpatient care are increasing. Inpatient services are shifting to private psychiatric hospitals and psychiatric units in general hospitals. In addition, nursing homes are replacing public mental hospitals as primary care sites for mentally ill older adults.

The reasons for underservice of mental health care to older persons have been studied and several possible answers proposed. Older persons themselves tend not to seek mental health care for their problems, but rather seek care from their primary physicians. In part, this is due to the lack of a vocabulary for emotional issues in today's older persons. From another perspective, those who are older today hold strong values of independence in resolving personal problems, as evidenced by cliches such as "you don't air your dirty laundry in public." It is also true that today's older persons were raised in a time when mental health services were available only to those with the most severe impairments, and the resultant negative stigma of receiving such services is great.

Additional barriers to service exist among mental health care providers. These barriers include lack of sufficient training to meet the needs of older persons (Gatz & Smyer, 1992; Myers & Blake, 1986; Roybal, 1988), bias against older clients (Butler & Lewis, 1991), and third party payment policies and other systemic factors which prohibit providers from accepting older persons as clients (Knight, 1989; Roybal, 1988). It has been almost 20 years since Cohen (1977) established that therapists may be reluctant to work with older clients due to unrecognized negative countertransference reactions, in that older clients may stimulate the therapist's fears of personal aging or the aging and death of parents. He further suggested that older clients may be perceived as rigid and unwilling or unable to change. The few years they may have remaining can serve as a disincentive to the therapist who feels that his or her time is being "wasted." These issues remain barriers to service delivery today.

Mental health counselors are subject to the same negative perceptions and stereotypes of older persons which are common in our society. Myths such as "old people are all sick, poor, angry, sad, lonely . . ." tend to discourage counselors from working with older clients. Gatz and Pearson (1988) reviewed studies of attitudes toward older people and concluded that global negative attitudes may not be as prevalent as once thought, but that specific biases still interfere with service to older clients. Misperceptions of organic brain syndromes, including prevalence as well as manifestations, tend to discourage mental health providers from active involvement with many older persons.

The net result of the barriers to service delivery is that large numbers of older persons experience significant mental health problems due to lack of suitable preventive and remedial interventions. This is especially true for older individuals experiencing situational adjustment reactions. While the clinical picture of geriatric mental illness is itself depressing, it also is an artifact of our current treatment system. The potential of older persons to respond to mental health interventions is excellent. Recently Knight (1989) determined that psychotherapy is as effective with older persons as with people of any age group. With appropriate, accessible services, major mental illness among older people can be prevented, to a great extent, and treated where preventive efforts are unsuccessful or lacking. The resultant savings in both dollars and human resources is potentially tremendous.

Training Gerontological Mental Health Counselors

As the turn of the century approaches, and the older population increases, their needs for mental health services may be projected to increase as well. If the counseling profession is to respond effectively to the challenges presented by this age group, increasing numbers of gerontological mental health counselors, trained to identify and meet the needs of older people, will be required.

Within the past two decades, counselors have become increasingly aware of the needs of older persons and have begun to direct resources toward meeting those needs. In 1975, only 18 or 6 percent of counselor education programs offered even an elective course in counseling older persons (Salisbury, 1975). By 1988, the number had grown to over 130, or some 36 percent of counselor training programs (Myers, 1989). Some training programs include multicourse sequences and opportunities for supervised practice in settings where older persons may be found. In the early 1980s, Hollis and Wantz (1983) noted that courses in gerontological counseling were the third most frequent new course in counselor education, lagging behind courses.in marriage and family and substance abuse. While a distant third in the 1980s, new courses in this area are declining in the 1990s.

Obviously, the need for increased gerontological training for mental health counselors is both appropriate and timely. As of this writing, the Council for Accreditation of Counseling and Related Educational Programs (CACREP) has approved a specialty in gerontological counseling (CACREP, 1994) and the National Board for Certified Counselors has established a specialty credential (Myers, in press). Still, the job market for geriatric services remains largely within the purview of the medical professions, notably social work. If gerontological mental health counselors are to obtain jobs commensurate with their training, active advocacy by the profession will be required. The job market for gerontological mental health counselors is relatively new, and may be expected to expand through concerted efforts and the documentation of success of mental health interventions with the older population.

REFERENCES

American Association of Retired Persons. (1993). *A profile of older Americans.* Washington, DC: Author.

Brotman, H.I. (1982). *Every ninth American.* (Select Committee on Aging Publication Number 97-332). Washington, DC: U.S. Government Printing Office.

Burns, B.J., & Taube, C.A. (1990). Mental health services in general medical care and in nursing homes. In B.S. Fogel, A. Furino, & G. Gottlieb (Eds.), *Protecting minds at risk.* Washington, DC: American Psychiatric Association.

Butler, R.N., & Lewis, M.I. (1991). *Aging and mental health.* St. Louis: C.V. Mosby.

Cohen, G. (1977). Mental health services and the elderly: Needs and options. In S. Steury & M.L. Black (Eds.), *Readings in psychotherapy with older people.* Rockville, MD: National Institutes of Mental Health.

Cohen, G. (1990). Psychopathology and mental health in the mature and elderly adult. In J.E. Birren & K.W. Schaie (Eds.), *Handbook of the psychology of aging* (3rd edition, pp. 359–371). San Diego, CA: Academic Press.

Council for Accreditation of Counseling and Related Educational Programs. (1994). *CACREP accreditation standards and procedures manual.* Alexandria, VA: Author.

Erikson, E. (1963). *Childhood and society.* New York: Norton.

Flemming, A.S., Rickards, L.D., Santos, J.F., & West, P.R. (1986). *Report of a survey of community mental health centers* (Volume I). Washington, DC: White House Conference on Aging.

Gatz, M., & Pearson, C.G. (1986). Training clinical psychology students in aging. *Gerontology and Geriatrics Education, 6*(2), 15–25.

Gatz, M., & Smyer, M.A. (1992). The mental health system and older adults in the 1990s. *American Psychologist, 47*(6), 741–751.

Hollis, J., & Wantz, R. (Eds.). (1983). *Counselor education directory.* Muncie, IN: Accelerated Development.

Knight, B.G. (1989). *Outreach with the elderly: Community education, assessment, and therapy.* New York: New York University Press.

Myers, J.E. (1989). *Infusing gerontological counseling into counselor preparation: Curriculum Guide.* Alexandria, VA: American Association for Counseling and Development.

Myers, J.E. (in press). From curriculum and competencies to standards and certification: Gerontological counseling comes of age. *Journal of Counseling and Development.*

Myers, J.E., & Blake, R. (1986). Professional preparation of gerontological counselors: Issues and guidelines. *Counselor Education and Supervision, 26*(2), 137–145.

National Center for Health Statistics. (1989). *National Nursing Home Survey* (DHHS Publication No. PHS 89-1758, Series 13, Number 97). Washington, DC: U.S. Government Printing Office.

Osgood, N. (1992). *Suicide in late life: An American Tragedy.* New York: Macmillan.

Piacitelli, J.D. (1992). Beyond therapy: The role of mental health professionals in addressing the needs of the mentally ill elderly. Paper presented at National Press Conference on Aging, Washington, DC.

Riker, H.C., & Myers, J.E. (1989). *Retirement counseling: A handbook for action.* New York: Hemisphere.

Roybal, H. (1988). Mental health and aging: The need for an expanded federal response. *American Psychologist, 43*(3), 189–194.

Salisbury, H. (1975). Counseling the elderly: A neglected area in counselor education and supervision. *Counselor Education and Supervision 14*(3), 237–238.

Saxon, S., & Etten, J. (1987). *Physical change and aging: A guide for the helping professions.* New York: Tiresius Press.

Special Committee on Aging, U.S. Senate. (1983). *Developments in aging.* Washington, DC: U.S. Government Printing Office.

Thompson, L. (1987). Comparative effectiveness of psychotherapy for depressed elders. *Journal of Consulting and Clinical Psychology, 55*(3), 385–390.

Chapter 7

MULTICULTURAL COUNSELING ISSUES

Don C. Locke

The subject of multicultural counseling in mental health settings is broad and encompasses a world of complex detail. On the one hand, we have the various group members who bring with them their own cultural manifestations as well as their unique personal, social, and psychological background. On the other hand, is the multifaceted concept of mental health, a concept which covers a broad psychological spectrum from health to severe psychosis. Obviously, the interaction between these two areas must be considered before a mental health counselor (MHC) can begin to provide services to culturally different clients. If the MHC is to be effective, sources of support available to or denied to particular clients must be understood.

Each MHC must assess both their own personal understanding of self, as well as how much a particular cultural group is understood. Obviously, it is how the MHC perceives the effects of cultural content on a client which determines how the MHC will function in that cross-cultural context. The MHC must have some understanding of the social, political, economic, and cultural contexts in which a particular client functions. The MHC must be expert enough to separate the cultural influences from the influences/behaviors which are preventing the client from becoming fully functioning. The MHC must also be flexible enough to adjust various counseling techniques to the cultural manifestations of a particular client. For example, a counselor must be expert enough to determine if the degree of eye contact or the level of comfort in touching are dependent on cultural reasons or are the result of interpersonal difficulties without regard to cultural group membership.

Finally, the MHC must be capable of adapting counseling models, theories, or techniques to the unique individual needs of a particular client. Such skill requires that the counselor be able to see the client as both an individual as well as a member of a particular cultural group.

Definition of Multicultural Counseling

What is multicultural counseling? The articulation of a clear definition of multicultural counseling is necessary before one can begin to analyze the methods or techniques used in such a relationship. Multicultural counseling is a broad term which encompasses all counseling interactions between persons of different cultural backgrounds. Some writers (Fukuyama, 1990; Pedersen, 1991) have used the term to describe all differences (race, ethnic group membership, age, lifestyle, socioeconomic status, being foreign born, and so forth) which may be apparent in the counseling relationship. For purposes of this discussion multicultural counseling is restricted to a MHC counseling a racial group or ethnic minority group, where the counselor is a member of the majority culture (white, middle-class, English-speaking) and the client is a member of a particular racial group or ethnic minority (African American; Native American Indian; Hispanic, Latino or Chicano; or Asian American) (Locke, 1990). These particular relationships, while in no means inclusive of all multicultural encounters, are representative of the majority of the multicultural contacts between counselors and clients. This specific focus also provides an opportunity to examine similarities and differences between the two populations and study the effects that are manifested in the counseling relationship. Furthermore, this focus affords an opportunity to look at how multicultural counseling differs from counseling in general. Multicultural counseling is a practical area which:

1. **Recognizes the importance of racial group/ethnic minority membership on the socialization of the client.** Such a position requires that the MHC in the multicultural counseling situation consider not only the personal characteristics of the client but the environmental factors as well. Looking only at personal characteristics will probably lead the MHC to assess the personality of the client in terms of a single standard, probably a white, middle-class, English-speaking standard. Much of the early research on "ethnic minority groups" focused on differences between white people and members of these groups. This type of research often led to conclusions that culturally different group members were "deficient" in the area under investigation (Kardiner & Oversy, 1951; Moynihan, 1965; Valentine, 1971). Recent trends in multicultural study suggest that research which compares ethnic majority and ethnic minority groups fails to provide any useful information. Instead, researchers begin with an assumption of "different-

ness" and focus on "within-group" factors. Such a focus provides the opportunity for a look at environmental factors as sources of influence.

2. **Recognizes the importance of and the uniqueness of the individual.** Closely related to the first point is the recognition that racial group/ethnic minority membership is not totally responsible for all the behaviors of a client. Since culturally different persons must interact with the dominant culture, the degree to which the culturally different individual has assimilated parts of the dominant culture varies from individual to individual. This is the principle which necessitates the study of "within-group" differences among culturally different clients. To respond to all members of a particular culturally different population as though they share identical values, beliefs, attitudes, and opinions is to reduce the group members to a mechanistic level. There is considerable evidence that members of specific racial groups have heterogeneous talents, interests, and values (Locke, 1992; Pasteur & Toldson, 1982).

3. **Recognizes that counseling is not value free.** Counselors in multicultural interactions recognize that they bring to the encounter a set of values, beliefs, attitudes, and opinions about the client and that some of these values, beliefs, attitudes, and opinions exist solely because the client is a member of a particular racial group or ethnic population. To argue that counseling is value-free would be to argue in favor of treating all clients alike—probably as if they were from a white, middle-class, English-speaking background. Multicultural counseling requires a MHC to admit higher values explicitly and to use this value recognition as a basis for evaluating everything that takes place in counseling. After all, it is the client's perception of the counselor's value demands and value responses which determines the greatest amount of client behavior.

4. **Recognizes and values the different learning styles, vocational goals, and life purposes of clients, within the context of principles of democratic social justice.** Once the individual and group characteristics are determined, both with the knowledge that the determinations were not made in a value-less context, the counselor and client are ready to begin exploring strategies specific to whatever brought the client to counseling. Whether the culturally different client has very different purposes and goals than those of a client from the dominant culture, or purposes and goals which are quite similar to those of a client from the dominant culture, the MHC must be able to see that neither position is better than the other. Whatever purposes and goals a client chooses are unique to that client and only represent a "difference," not a deficiency.

The counseling techniques then must place a high priority on building a sense of personal worth in the client so that the client feels valued both as an individual and as a member of a particular racial/ethnic group. Once the MHC is aware of and tolerant of behavioral differences, the MHC will understand the processes by which a client learns social behaviors in the content of diverse cultural settings.

Multicultural Awareness Continuum

The Multicultural Awareness Continuum (Figure 7.1) was designed to illustrate the areas of awareness through which a counselor must pass before counseling a culturally different client. The continuum is linear and arranged so that counseling expertise develops only after the counselor has passed through a series of awareness levels. These levels are designed to be developmental since each level builds upon the previous level(s). The process from self-awareness to counseling skills/techniques is flexible since the counselor never achieves absolute mastery of any of the awareness levels. In fact, the continuum is best understood as a lifelong process. As one confronts a culturally different client where some counselor awareness is lacking, the counselor must return to an earlier awareness level, explore the awareness at that level, and then proceed along the continuum to counseling skills/techniques. There is no absolute point to which the counselor must return before proceeding forward. It is important that from the point where one begins to recycle on the continuum subsequent levels must not be skipped.

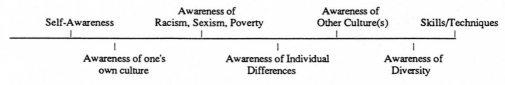

Figure 7.1. Multicultural awareness continuum.

Self-Awareness

The first level through which the counselor must pass is self-awareness. The area of self-understanding is a necessary condition before one begins the process of understanding others. The interpersonal and interpersonal dynamics are very important as they relate to the beliefs, attitudes, opinions, and values which one brings to the counseling process. The process of introspection is important before one explores his/her own culture and adopts a framework from which exploration of the cultural phenomena in subsequent levels can occur (Locke, 1992). This level is critical to the effective development of subsequent levels since the "self does not exist except in relationship" (Ivey, Ivey, & Simek-Morgan, 1993, p. 111).

Awareness of One's Own Culture

Each MHC brings to the counseling process a great deal of "cultural baggage." This baggage may cause the MHC to take certain things for granted and to behave in ways and manners which he/she might not be aware. For example, one might explore the meaning of one's name, looking particularly at the cultural significance of the name. One might note the historical significance related to cultures which are not one's culture of origin. There may be some relationship between one's name and birth order. There may have been a special ceremony when one was named. Thus, the naming process may be a significant part of one's family and cultural history.

The naming process is but one of the many areas where one's cultural influence can be seen. Language, both formal and informal, including body language, is very specific to the cultural group with which one identifies. Language is a primary determiner of the various cultural networks in which one participates. Language, along with many other cultural features, contributes to the values which are cultural specific (Locke, 1992).

Awareness of Racism, Sexism, and Poverty

Racism, sexism, and poverty are aspects of a culture which are understood both from the perspective of how one views these factors as they relate to self as well as how one views others in relation to these factors. These are obviously powerful terms which frequently evoke some defensiveness (Locke & Hardaway, 1980). Even when racism and sexism are not a part of one's personal belief system, one must recognize that these attitudes exist and are a part of the larger culture in which one functions.

The issue of poverty is another area where, even when one does not feel the pangs of poverty personally, a MHC must come to grips with the beliefs held regarding persons who are suffering economic misfortune.

One must wrestle with the question of why some people are poor and how this belief relates to a specific individual or group of individuals. Issues relating to the cause of and the solution to the poverty status of individuals or groups of individuals must be explored by the MHC. A MHC may benefit from exploring the issues of poverty, sexism, and racism from a "systems" approach. Such an exploration can lead the MHC to examine the differences between individual behaviors and organizational behaviors or what might be called the differences between personal prejudice and institutional prejudice. One area where MHCs can see the influence of organizational prejudice is in the attitudes or beliefs of organizations to which the MHC belongs. The awareness that church memberships frequently exist along racial lines and that some social organizations restrict their membership to one sex should help MHCs come to grips with the organizational prejudices they may be supporting solely on the basis of participation in a particular organization (Locke, 1992).

Awareness of Individual Differences

One of the great pitfalls of the novice multicultural learner is to over generalize things learned about a specific culture. A single bit of information is presumed to exist among all members of the group simply because it was observed in one member or a few members of the cultural group. Cultural group membership does not require one to sacrifice individualism or uniqueness. Some counselor education students have been heard to say, "Then we should treat all clients as individuals." We respond to that statement thusly. "We must do both. We must treat the client as an individual *and* as a member of a particular cultural group." The danger lies in the possibility that the MHC may disregard cultural influences and subconsciously believe that he/she understands the client from the point of view of the counselor's own culture. There is a disregard for any culturally specific behaviors which may influence the way a client behaves when the counselor treats the client as an individual only. Such a total belief in individualism disregards the "collective family community" relationship which exists in many cultural groups. The bottom line is that the MHC must be aware of individual differences *and* believe in the uniqueness of the individual before moving to the level of awareness of other cultures.

Awareness of Other Cultures

With the four previous levels of the continuum as background, the MHC is ready to explore the many dynamics of other cultural groups. Most current multicultural emphasis is on African Americans; Native American Indians; Hispanics, Latinos, or Chicanos; and Asian Americans. MHCs must learn the meaning of some of the language of the cultural groups. While this does not require mastery of a foreign language per se, it does require the counselor to be sensitive to words which are unique to a particular culture and to body language which may be characteristic of a particular cultural group. Hofstede (1980), in a research project conducted in 40 countries, concluded that there are four empirically determined criteria by which cultures differ. These four criteria are: (1) power distance; (2) uncertainty avoidance; (3) masculinity/feminity; and (4) individualism/collectivism. These cultural universals have definite implications for the counselor who is studying other cultures. Likewise, Kluckhorn and Strodtbect (1961) identified five areas where cultural groups tend to differ. The five areas are: (1) time, (2) view of human nature, (3) importance of relationship, (4) human activity, and (5) view of the supernatural. Counselors can learn things about a culture by using either the Hofstede or the Kluckhorn and Strodtbect scheme. Such knowledge should help the counselor become effective as he/she understands the values or lifestyles of culturally different clients.

Awareness of Diversity

For years the North American culture has been referred to as the "melting pot." This characterization suggested that persons had come to the United States of America from many different countries and had blended into one new culture. Thus, old world practices had been discarded, altered, or maintained within the new "melting pot." Obviously, some actual "melting" occurred. Yet for the most part, many cultural groups, especially African Americans; Native American Indians; Hispanics, Latinos, or Chicanos; and Asian Americans, did not participate in the melting pot process. Therefore, as time passed, these groups have discovered that the United States American melting pot did not wish to welcome their cultural practices. In fact, these culturally different groups have been encouraged to give up their cultural practices and to adopt the values, beliefs, and attitudes of the "melting pot."

Recently, the term "salad bowl" has come into popular use to describe the United States American culture. The salad bowl concept suggests that aspects from all cultures (the ingredients) are mixed together where each culture maintains its own identity. A well-known African American, Jesse Jackson, used the term "rainbow coalition" to represent the same idea. Such concepts reflect what many have come to refer to as a multicultural society, where certain features of each culture are encouraged and appreciated by other cultural groups. This concept recognizes the strength of diversity and does not require all people to be alike.

Counseling Skills/Techniques

The final level on the continuum is the implementation of what has been learned in other levels in the multicultural process. Before a MHC begins multicultural counseling, he/she must have developed some general competence as a counselor. Passage through the previous levels on the continuum will contribute to this general competence. But it goes much further than simply that. The MHC must have a good knowledge of counseling theories and the accompanying techniques. A MHC must understand how the theory developed, what conditions contributed to its development, and what psychological-cultural factors of the theorist played a role in the development of the theory. The MHC must have developed a sense of worth as a counselor in his/her own cultural group before attempting work with culturally different clients.

Multicultural understanding will not substitute for counseling skills. If the MHC lacks general competence as a counselor, no amount of multicultural awareness will compensate for this inadequacy. In fact, it appears that for effective multicultural counseling to occur, the advantage goes to the MHC who has a great deal of counseling competence and minimum multicultural understanding rather than to the counselor who has little counseling competence and a great deal of multicultural understanding (Nwachuku & Ivey, 1991).

Sources of Conflict in Multicultural Counseling

While the research on the effect of the race of the counselor on the outcome of counseling is inconclusive, there is a trend which suggests that the race of the counselor in a cross-cultural counseling dyad, does influence the process (Williams & Kirkland, 1971; Lorion, 1974; Atkinson, Maruyani, & Matsui, 1978; Sue & Sue, 1990; Parham & Helms, 1981). Race often serves to impede the achievement of therapeutic goals.

Culturally-different counselor/client pairs bring to counseling special factors which result in lowered efficacy in the initial counseling sessions. The major factors contributing to the lowered efficacy are cultural differences, lack of understanding between counselor and client, and prejudice (Vontress, 1971). Many culturally different systems place emphasis on managing personal problems without showing stress. These cultures dictate that one must solve one's own problems, or contain the problem within the confines of the family. As a result, individuals from these cultures are reluctant to self-disclose in the multicultural counseling encounter because they initially perceive counselors from the dominant culture as lacking good will. Culturally-different clients may experience negative or mixed emotions about counseling because they are unsure of what to expect, and what should be verbalized during the counseling sessions. The reluctance to self-disclose is usually an unconscious aspect of the personality which derives primarily from the dominant culture which both socializes and oppresses culturally-different individuals simultaneously.

Different language and communication styles are also important factors which influence the counselor-client relationship. Different patterns of verbal and nonverbal communication create real problems for the counselor and client in a multicultural counseling encounter. Leonard and Locke (1993), in a study of African American and Caucasian communication perceptions, found that black and white college students hold remarkably different views of the communication styles of each other. Black students reported that white students were demanding, manipulative, organized, rude, and critical. White students assigned the traits of being loud, ostentatious, aggressive, active, and boastful to black students. These terms suggest that both groups perceive some degree of threat from the other. Where these beliefs exist, it is unreasonable to expect one group to initiate interactions with the other. Even when communication is initiated, the participants are likely to be hesitant, reserved, and concealing. Such perceptions must be overcome before any kind of effective counseling can occur.

Additionally, counselors often bring to the therapeutic relationship preconceived attitudes and ideas about culturally different clients. These perceptions may be manifested in numerous ways during the counseling process. Block (1981) identified three types of errors made by white counselors when dealing with culturally different clients. The first error is the illusion of color blindness. Here the cultural different client is viewed as just another client without consideration of cultural group membership. The denial of race and/or ethnicity, primarily a factor with African American clients, but becoming important as one hears about the "brown" culture, disregards the central importance of group identification for the cultural different person. It also ignores the undeniable impact of the race of the MHC upon the culturally different client, and it removes the culturally different client from the social environment which can project the client as deviant from the "white middle-class norms," a factor which may lead to the culturally different client being labeled pathological.

The second error is the assumption that all culturally different clients' problems revolve around the conditions of being culturally different in an oppressive society. Being oppressed, or even deprived, may convey to the MHC that the client is permanently limited in personality functioning as a result of environmental factors. Such a view may foster guilt feelings for the counselor who in turn may offer special privileges for the client.

The third error in multicultural counseling is what Vontress (1971) described as the "great white father syndrome." The counselor may communicate to the culturally different client an aura of omnipotence while expressing a desire for doing nothing but good for the client. The counselor will deliver only if the client will put himself/herself in the counselors' hands. If the client does not depend upon the counselor, then the client will be doomed to catastrophe. Such an attitude is often assumed by a counselor who is anxious to prove to the culturally different client that he/she is not prejudiced.

All of these factors can be impediments to effective counseling because they provide a screen through which the culturally different client's actual feelings, desires, and actions are distorted in the therapeutic encounter.

Preparation of Multicultural Counselors

A few years ago, the Association for Counselor Education and Supervision (ACES) (1978) drew up a set of minimum competencies in the area of multicultural counseling. In an attempt to determine how much multicultural knowledge is sufficient, ACES defined several essential elements.

First ACES stipulated that "it is necessary to urge all counselor educators, supervisors, and counselors to establish specific, substantive policies, procedures, and activities designed to improve counseling services for non-white persons" (p. 1).

Whereas the first prescription presented by ACES emphasized the policies necessary to implement counseling services for culturally different clients, the second tended to stress what might be described as "the comparative dimension." It called for a deeper understanding of the other culture, as seen through its history, language, literature, and philosophy. According to ACES, this would bring sensitivity to the other culture(s), increased capacity to analyze issues, enhanced toleration of differences, and more effective counseling. A third point which ACES emphasized referred to a need for research in areas of importance to an understanding of cultural differences. The position paper concluded with some procedures and activities to accomplish the prescribed minimum competencies.

There appear to be five general goals of multicultural counseling: (1) world-view consciousness; (2) awareness of social/economic/political circumstances related to culturally different peoples; (3) multicultural awareness; (4) knowledge of intragroup dynamics; and (5) awareness of human choices.

World-view consciousness (Sue, 1978, Sue & Sue, 1990) involves the recognition of awareness on the part of the individual that he or she has a view of the world that is not universally shared. Four world-view positions were proposed: (1) Internal locus of control—Internal locus of responsibility; (2) External locus of control—Internal locus of responsibility; (3) External locus of control—External locus of responsibility; and (4) Internal locus of control—External locus of responsibility. Sue and Sue postulated that one's world-view is highly correlated with one's life experiences and cultural upbringing. Thus the world-view category into which a client falls can provide a frame of reference for both the client and the counselor.

Awareness of social, economic, and political circumstances involves an awareness of the prevailing conditions which impact upon culturally different persons, individually and collectively. This awareness must be from the perspective that the conditions are different from the conditions which impact upon the dominant culture. This awareness must include acceptance that even identical conditions occurring in the life of a person from the dominant culture and a culturally different person will probably produce different results. Social or economic conditions may produce similar results in clients from different cultural backgrounds but a counselor's awareness must include how society and individuals view the impact of the social-economic factors on culturally different individuals.

Multicultural awareness refers to an awareness of the diversity of ideas and practices found among the culturally different groups in the United States of America. Knowledge of intragroup dynamics means that a counselor has a minimum awareness and comprehension of the key traits of the culturally different system. Finally, awareness of human choices constitutes some awareness of the problems of choice confronting individuals, individually and collectively, in the culturally different group.

The ACES statement is clearly aimed at the reforming faculty, anxious to bring its curriculum more into line with present and future realities. One can readily imagine a committee on the establishment of a core curriculum in graduate counselor education making use of ACES recommendations as the basis for the multicultural element in its program. ACES calls for no radical realignment of the curriculum or revolution in the general approach to counselor education, and its statement stresses the inclusion of certain elements in the curriculum rather than the transformation of the curriculum itself. While there is some attention to outcomes (the need for sensitivity, the need for tolerance), the emphasis falls on programs rather than results. The statement is also based on a set of assumptions about the relationship between a particular experience (location of internship placements) and multicultural understanding. The ACES statement was revolutionary in its emphasis on changing the attitudes of students, persons who would soon become professional counselors. Attitude change is quite difficult to articulate in terms of a particular set of curricular reforms. Such an effort must emphasize programs as well as goals.

This consideration of looking at multicultural counselor education shows that the dimension can be defined in at least two different ways. We can define it as essentially an issue of program content (specific courses and groups of courses), expressed in terms of requirements in the program description. If we look at the matter from this point of view, we are assuming that the courses along with the other program elements, will have the desired outcomes. This relationship between prescription and outcome appears to be ignored in most faculty discussions for curricula changes.

A second view of the multicultural dimension in counselor education takes a rather different approach to the curriculum. There are those who argue that the inclusion of a certain set of multicultural courses in a complete counselor education program may be useful but is not the essence of the issue. These people argue for infusion, or diffusion, of multicultural elements throughout the curriculum. Advocates of this approach suggest that every course can become multicultural to some degree.

Effective multicultural education/training has suffered because a systematic approach to teaching counseling skills relevant to the culturally different has not occurred using the infusion method. While consciousness raising, cognitive understanding, and affective dimensions are important, there is a great need to relate these components to specific skills in working with culturally-different clients. The gap between awareness, understanding, and knowledge, on the one hand, and behavior, on the other, has led to failure in counseling programs and ultimately to ineffective multicultural counseling experiences.

A third approach to multicultural counselor education identifies the problem not so much in terms of changing program content, but in terms of attitude change on the part of those teaching the courses. It may be that what is actually taught is less important than the kind of emphasis that is given to multicultural content. To teach counseling theories and techniques as though all clients are receptive to a given theory or technique clearly does little to provide the student with a multicultural perspective. On the other hand, to teach counseling theory and techniques by drawing all one's examples from culturally different groups may be counterproductive. Perhaps what is more important is for the counselor educator to be constantly aware of the fact that the theory and techniques referred to in the title of the course are not all theory but only certain theory. Counselor education must logically be based on such a relative view. What is needed, in short, among counselor education faculty is "perspective consciousness."

Changes in curriculum are important, but if the curriculum is poorly taught or taught without conviction, it will have little effect on the counseling student. Even with the most enthusiastic faculty member, the key to the whole question is what "rubs off" on the student.

Counselor educators are accustomed to exposing students to certain things and assuming that the things to which they are exposed will be absorbed into their system. Educators talk about people as free agents, yet frequently forget free agency when they want students to learn something. Counselor educators can prescribe curricula as much as they like, but the critical issue is their effect on the students.

If students are to change, faculty members must be predisposed to change. Counselor education is, after all, a process of socialization. Counselor education cannot hope to give their students a multicultural perspective if they do not have such a perspective themselves.

Primary Prevention in Multicultural Counseling

The discussion of multicultural counseling up to this point has taken a rather traditional approach to the issue. The definition of multicultural counseling described the relationship between counselor and client, a rather traditional view which suggested "treatment after the fact." While group counseling was implied, the definition emphasized a one-to-one relationship. The discussion on the awareness continuum emphasized multicultural sensitivity as an element in one's clinical skills, almost as if multicultural awareness is but a counseling technique to be employed under certain conditions with culturally-different clients. The discussion on sources of conflict in multicultural counseling explored the traditional views concerning the influence of race and other variables on the outcomes of counseling. Finally, the section on preparation of multicultural counselors examined how a multicultural emphasis could be included in counselor education programs.

Obviously, each of these ideas is extremely pertinent to a discussion of multicultural counseling. There is an implied belief that if the MHC accomplished all the previous suggestions, the MHC would be an effective multicultural counselor. To some extent, that is an accurate conclusion. Yet, that is not enough. The MHC who works primarily with cultural group clients must demonstrate a contribution to the survival of that culturally different group. Such a position requires the MHC from the dominant culture to understand that injustices perpetrated upon culturally different group members rob them of some of their humanity. Once this understanding is clear, the MHC from the dominant culture must use professional ability and moral sensitivity to insure that justice becomes reality. Kenneth Clark (1974) described the problem thusly:

> Psychology must be a value-laden science, and the fundamental value which must sustain it is a concern with the welfare of man. A social scientist cannot be indifferent to the destiny and the predicament of man and society any more than

medicine could have been indifferent to plagues and diseases. The social scientist must be committed to social change. There is no pure, indifferent, non technologically oriented use of disciplined human intelligence in social science and there is room for none (pp. 138–139).

For community MHCs to accomplish this monumental task means that they must adopt a systems perspective to working with culturally different clients. Such a perspective would be composed of both human and environmental components that would be meshed together in order to understand the interrelations of both. Implied in this systems view, is the notion of a goal-oriented process involving interdependent activities that are coordinated so as to attain certain goals. From this perspective, it would seem that counseling in a multicultural setting would lend itself to a systems-based approach.

The notion of employing a systems-based approach means that MHCs of culturally different clients must attack problems facing their clients on all fronts. First of all, MHCs must see as an appropriate role their involvement in social change. This role requires the MHC to have made a commitment to the idea of social justice. It means responding to the challenge presented by Kenneth Clark. It means that MHCs assume more responsibility than is traditionally recommended by some writers in the field. The MHC must possess effective intervention and consultation skills to effect social change. The MHC must understand change theories and methods and be able to apply and accept appropriate strategies to particular situations.

Second, the MHC must be proactive in dealing with clients and/or potential clients. Once target populations are identified, the MHC must develop and take programs to the culturally different groups. This type of effort means that the MHC can no longer sit and wait for clients to come to the office. Perlmutter (1983) described four areas where the MHC can direct a thrust. The four areas are:

(1) directed at persons or groups **not** defined as patients; (2) directed usually at groups at risk; (3) concerned with contextual rather than individual functioning (e.g., schools, boarding homes, etc., as systems); and (4) designed to maintain health functioning rather than ameliorate pathology (e.g., well baby clinics and vocational counseling) (p. 99).

This idea of productivity has been supported by Sprinthall (1977) when he proposed new primary prevention directions for counseling and by Lewis and Lewis (1984) when they described successful community-based program models of primary prevention. Both of these authors report and emphasize work in the "natural group" to which clients/potential clients belong.

The third component of this approach is that it must be developmental in nature. Adam (1981) identified eight basic human competencies which people in any society need to develop. His list has been modified to include five specific areas applicable to culturally different persons.

1. *Identification with viable role models.* Any developmental program ought to involve persons from the reference group of the identified population. Such an idea has tremendous implications for staffing patterns in mental health centers. Culturally different persons should be employed not only because it is morally right to do so but also because they may serve as role models for culturally different clients.

2. *Responsibility for group processes.* For many culturally different individuals there is a suspicion that the dominant culture decides, independently, what the culturally different group members need. The effective multicultural MHC must involve members of the culturally different group in helping develop programs. Participation in program development will lead to success in the next competency.

3. *Confidence in the ability to solve problems.* Once culturally different group members develop attitudes and skills useful in working through problems, they should also have developed a self-confidence which will be helpful as they tackle future problems.

4. *Intrapersonal and interpersonal skills.* In this area the MHC can develop programs which help culturally different group clients communicate, listen, share, nurture, and empathize with other persons. The client also learns how to communicate with self (self-awareness, self-control, self-discipline). The MHC might provide experiences where clients have an opportunity to express their personal feelings about being a culturally different person and how these feelings might be appropriately communicated to dominant culture persons in an assertive manner. Efforts in the area of peer counseling will benefit culturally different persons in that they begin to develop perspective-taking skills. Peer counseling groups provide strong support networks. Persons who belong to strong support networks can resist much of the stress which often leads to emotional disturbance.

5. *Self-sufficiency skills.* These are skills which allow culturally different persons to function effectively in their environment. Development of these skills emphasize both autonomy and interdependence. Specifically these skills include language, vocational, homemaking, and

leisure-time skills. These areas of skill development must be directly relevant to the life experience of the participants. Too often it appears that skill development efforts have emerged without awareness that they are not what the participants need. Unless the participants perceive some "ownership" of the project by having been involved in the planning, implementation, and evaluation, the effort is sure to fail.

As discussed here, the "change agent counselor" of culturally different clients works on a variety of different levels in the community to eliminate those factors in the environment which limit the full growth and development of clients. The multicultural counselor must select several areas which might make the most impact. An excellent list of possibilities was presented by Kelly (1982). She discussed 12 outstanding programs out of 67 that were nominated for the 1980 Lela Rowland Prevention Award. The 67 programs included 22 for children; 28 for parents, future parents, or families of young children; 7 support groups for the older persons; 7 support groups for adult or family populations at risk because of stress-related disorders; and 3 programs for teachers. Any of these programs can serve as background information for MHCs who wish to develop specific programs for identified racial/cultural groups.

Up to this point, the rationale for primary prevention measures for culturally different populations has focused on a moral or social justice theme. Before leaving the topic, it must be pointed out that because MHCs are not serving all persons in need with the present mental health system, some alternative strategies must be developed. According to the President's Commission on Mental Health (1978), only seven million persons were being seen by mental health professionals each year. Kiesler (1980) cited several surveys which indicated that between 10 and 20 percent (20-45 million) of the population of the United States have serious mental health problems. An even larger group suffers severe life crises resulting from marital disruption, divorce, involuntary unemployment, death of a loved one, and loneliness. Added to this problem is the fact that the President's Commission found that members of culturally different groups, the physically and mentally handicapped, adolescents, and women were being inappropriately served by the mental health system.

These data are enough to produce what Albee (1980) called the fourth mental health revolution. He said that this revolution will

> emphasize social changes aimed at improving the quality of life and reducing avoidable stresses. It will challenge the authority of the mental health establish-

ment and attack the ritualistic devotion to one-to-one intervention. It will expose the fallacies of the illness model (p. 68).

If counseling is to receive acceptance from culturally different groups, it must demonstrate a willingness to engage in primary prevention activities and it must demonstrate the ability to contribute to the quality of life of the culturally different group. This demonstration begins with a recognition of the value-laden nature of the profession. Once this recognition occurs, efforts must begin to influence the various systems which are responsible for the specific societal conditions. MHCs must look at their own self-awareness and their awareness of both their own culture and the culture of the groups with which they work. Counselor education programs must broaden the curriculum to include culturally different group content as well as alternatives to the secondary treatment model.

The primary prevention model seems to offer the greatest promise for counseling culturally different clients. It will not solve all the problems of the culturally different groups or of the profession of counseling, but it does provide a ray of hope for both groups. Primary prevention appears to answer most of the suggestions that counseling and mental health have been inappropriate to the needs of culturally different individuals and groups. MHCs must become part of the revolution. The future of multicultural counseling will be measured by the willingness of all mental health providers to move beyond the rhetoric and become proactive in meeting the needs of all clients.

REFERENCES

Association for Counselor Education and Supervision. (1978). *Position paper: Commission on non-white concerns.* Washington, DC: ACES.

Atkinson, D. R., Maruyani, M., & Matsui, S. (1978). The effects of counselor race and counseling approach on Asian Americans' perceptions of counselor credibility and utility. *Journal of Counseling Psychology, 25,* 76–83.

Adam, C. T. (1981). A description of primary prevention. *The Journal of Primary Prevention, 2,* 67–79.

Albee, G. W. (1980). The fourth mental health revolution. *The Journal of Prevention, 1,* 67–70.

Block, C. B. (1981). Black Americans and the multicultural counseling and psychotherapy experience. In A. L. Marsella, & P. B. Pedersen, P. B. (Eds.), *Cross-Cultural Counseling and Psychotherapy.* New York: Pergamon Press.

Clark, K. B. (1974). *The pathos of power.* New York: Harper & Row.

Fukuyama, M. A. (1990). Taking a universal approach to multicultural counseling. *Counselor Education and Supervision, 30,* 6–17.

Hofstede, G. (1980). Motivation, leadership and organization: Do American theories apply abroad? *Organizational Dynamics, 9,* 42–53.

Ivey, A. E., Ivey, M. B., & Simek-Morgan, L. (1993). *Counseling and psychotherapy: A multicultural perspective.* Boston: Allyn and Bacon.

Kardiner, A., & Oversy, L. (1951). *The mark of oppression: Explorations in the personality of the American Negro.* New York: Norton.

Kelly, L. D. (1982). Between the dream and the reality: A look at programs nominated for the Lela Rowland Prevention Award of the National Mental Health Association. *The Journal of Primary Prevention, 2,* 217–224.

Kiesler, C. A. (1980). Mental health policy as a field of inquiry for psychology. *American Psychologist, 35,* 1066–1080.

Kluckhorn, F., & Strodtbect, F. (1961). *Variations in value orientations.* Evanston, IL: Row, Peterson.

Leonard, R., & Locke, D. C. (1993) Communication stereotypes: Is interracial communication possible? *Journal of Black Studies, 23,* 332–343.

Lewis, J. A., & Lewis, M. D. (1984). Preventive programs in action. *Personnel and Guidance Journal, 62,* 550–553.

Locke, D. C. (1990). A not so provincial view of multicultural counseling. *Counselor Education and Supervision, 30,* 18–25.

Locke, D. C. (1992). *Increasing multicultural understanding: A comprehensive model.* Newbury Park, CA: Sage.

Locke, D. C., & Hardaway, Y. V. (1980). Moral perspectives in interracial settings. In D. B. Cochrane & M. Manley-Casimir (Eds.), *Moral education: Practical approaches* (pp. 269–285). New York: Praeger.

Lorion, R. P. (1974). Patient and therapist variables in the treatment of low-income patients. *Psychological Bulletin, 81,* 344–354.

Moynihan, D. (1965). *The Negro family: The case for national action.* Washington, DC: U. S. Department of Labor.

Nwachuku, U. T., & Ivey, A. E. (1991). Culture-specific counseling: An alternative training model. *Journal of Counseling and Development, 70,* 106–111.

Parham, T. A., & Helms, J. E. (1981). The influence of black students' racial identity attitudes on preferences for counselor's race. *Journal of Counseling Psychology, 28,* 250–257.

Pasteur, A. B., & Toldson, I. L. (1982). *Roots of soul: The psychology of Black expressiveness.* Garden City, NY: Doubleday.

Pedersen, P. B. (1991). Multiculturalism as a generic approach to counseling. *Journal of Counseling and Development, 70,* 6–12.

Perlmutter, F. D. (1983). Partnerships for mental health promotion. *Journal of Primary Prevention, 4,* 96–106.

President's Committee on Mental Health (1978). *Report.* Washington, DC: U.S. Government Printing Office.

Sprinthall, N. A. (1977). New directions for school and counseling psychology. *Counseling Psychologist, 6,* 53–57.

Sue, D. W. (1978). World views and counseling. *Personnel and Guidance Journal, 56,* 458–462.

Sue, D. W., & Sue, S. (1990). *Counseling the culturally different.* New York: Wiley.

Valentine, C. (1971). Deficit, difference, and bicultural models of Afro-American behavior. *Harvard Educational Review, 41,* 131–157.

Vontress, C. E. (1971). Racial differences. *Journal of Counseling Psychology, 18,* 7–13.

Williams, R. R., & Kirkland, J. (1971). The white counselor and black client. *Counseling Psychologist, 2,* 114–117.

HIGHLIGHT SECTION

THANATOLOGY

Steven P. Lindenberg

"Thanatology" is a word that derives its origin from the Greek word **Thanatos,** which translated means "death." "The study of death" has become a field of specialization in health care. Professionals in the field of thanatology include counselors, psychologists, and anthropologists.

The evolution of the field of thanatology has been one that has come about as a result of several forces in modern society. Among those forces is the fact that the life expectancy of populations in Western society has extended considerably. Another factor that has influenced the growth of this field has been the development of medical technology that blurs the formal demarcation between life and death, thus prolonging the dying process. This is particularly notable in cases of trauma and incurable diseases.

A third factor contributing to the development of the field of thanatology are medical advances in the field of organ transplant. Issues involving the transfer of donor organs from one who is dying to one who might live, result in ethical and moral dilemmas that often have psychosocial consequences for individuals and families, both of the donor and the recipient.

A fourth component is the ever increasing burden placed upon society by prolonging life while failing to control populations. Questions concerning intervention to prolong the life of critically ill persons is at one extreme, while issues surrounding abortion cause society to focus more intensely on the rights of individuals concerning not only the "quantity-of-life" but also entitlement to life per se.

Coincidental with these issues are concerns regarding not only the right to life but also the right to death with dignity. For example, does one focus on the "quantity-to-life" regardless of the "quality" of that life?

Closely accompanying the field of Thanatology has been the development of skills, knowledge, and abilities for caring for the bereaved. For instance, in allied health care disciplines, the implications of the stress of sudden versus prolonged death for survivors are quite important. Post-mortem adjustment greatly affects the levels of stress and longevity as well as the physical health of the bereaved person. A classic example is the Anniversary Syndrome. In the Anniversary Syndrome, couples who have had long marriages and experienced interdependency are at risk for increased onset of disease following the death of one of the spouses, particularly during the first year immediately following death.

Also of importance to the emergence of the field of Thanatology and concurrent with its development has been the Hospice movement. (The counselor in the Hospice is described elsewhere in this book.) In Hospice, as well as in other multidisciplinary approaches to health care, issues regarding the quality of life and the meaning of death become paramount to the philosophical and technological care management of the client and the client's family.

The role of the mental health counselor as a Thanatologist is of increasing significance in the overall scope of the delivery of health care services. For instance, concepts that are true in terms of clinical application of techniques for alleviating stress following the death of a family member or beloved friend are also appropos when dealing with other losses. Thus, the techniques developed by the discipline of Thanatology have practical applications in issues dealing with separation, divorce, loss of job, loss of physical abilities, and aging.

Currently, few formal programs leading to degrees for specialization in the field of Thanatology exist. Those that do exist are found primarily in schools of nursing. Historically, nurses have had the most intimate contact with the dying and their families. However, more recently, members of the mental health care disciplines have become involved in the provision of counseling services to the dying, their families, and to the bereaved.

The MHC as Thanatologist counsels the dying, the bereaved, acts as patient advocate, does abortion counseling, and does counseling for posttraumatic stress. The MHC also performs crisis intervention involving sudden death and/or life-threatening trauma and suicide prevention. Counselors may find themselves in situations in which one who is dying must be approached in terms of, for example, organ donation. Hospital-based counselors are also involved in communicating the laws and conditions for autopsy in cases of homicide and accidental death.

Occasionally, the counselor as a member of a Hospice team will be involved in preventive mental health counseling for the family members by helping them through preparatory grief. Such a counselor may also be involved in helping the patient and family plan for the funeral, and act as a coordinator to insure that the family has made appropriate contacts with attorneys and other auxiliary persons regarding preparations for the patient's death.

The MHC is often best at facilitating communications between patients who approach death, their health care team, and their immediate and extended family. The MHC as Thanatologist may also find him or herself involved in life and death decision-making as a facilitator between family members and attending medical personnel regarding the termination of heroic life support measures in the face of incurable disease or hopeless trauma.

Another function of the MHC as Thanatologist is public education concerning customary funeral practices. Counselors may often facilitate decisions regarding interment versus cremation. MHCs are also helpful with regard to minimizing long-term trauma to bereaved parents who have experienced premature neonatal death.

The field of Thanatology is an exciting and challenging field for MHCs. In this field, one has the opportunity to deal with philosophical, theological, moral, and ethical decisions and concepts in a way that is both challenging and rewarding, while at the same time being personally and professionally stimulating.

SECTION III
BROAD–BASED NATURE
OF EMPLOYMENT

Chapter 8

MULTIDISCIPLINARY MENTAL HEALTH TREATMENT TEAMS

LINDA SELIGMAN AND MICHAEL N. CEO

Growth has been rapid in the field of mental health counseling. The American Mental Health Counselors Association, formed in 1976, had over 10,000 members in 1985. This influx of counselors into the mental health delivery system has often been difficult for other mental health professionals as well as for the counselors themselves. As the "new kids on the block," counselors were sometimes viewed with skepticism and disdain, especially since most states had not yet legitimized the counselors' role through licensure legislation. "Counselor" is often thought of as synonymous with "school counselor," and "mental health counselor" can be a confusing and poorly known entity.

Also, the recent changes in some health insurance policies, curtailing benefits for mental health services, has made the mental health field more competitive. This, too, seems to have contributed to negative attitudes toward counselors on the part of some other mental health professionals who resent the competition presented by mental health counselors (MHCs).

Counselors have often had to struggle to establish their credibility and to make a place for themselves in mental health settings. One of the most important ways in which counselors have accomplished these goals is by participating in multidisciplinary mental health care teams. Working along with specialists in other areas of mental health, counselors have the opportunity to demonstrate their capabilities and indicate the special contribution which they can make.

The multidisciplinary treatment team has a number of advantages for both counselors and other mental health professionals. It is a way for counselors to establish their distinct professional reputations, and affords them the opportunity to work with a broad range of client groups. When practicing independently, counselors generally had to refer severely disturbed clients, those with interrelated physical and psychological concerns or those who might require hospitalization or medication, to psychiatrists or other doctoral level mental health professionals. However, as part of a treatment team, counselors can help to facilitate the development and adjustment of even very troubled clients as they collaborate with psychiatrists, psychologists, social workers, and medical professionals.

Participation on a multidisciplinary treatment team may also be beneficial to counselors, because it allows them the luxury of specializing in working with a particular population or aspect of mental health treatment. As independent practitioners, counselors typically work with a broad range of client concerns and develop expertise in individual, group, and/or family counseling. Although counselors on a treatment team must still maintain a high level of competence in the basic counseling skills, they may become the team's specialist in family counseling or career counseling or in working with a particular type of client (e.g., reentry women). Other team members are available to fill in any gaps in the counselor's skills, should the counselor specialize.

Insurance reimbursement for counseling services is also facilitated by the counselors' participation on treatment teams. Some health insurance companies will not provide third-party payments for counselors in independent practice, especially if those counselors are not licensed or certified. However, if counseling services are provided as part of a treatment plan developed and supervised by a psychiatrist or doctoral level psychologist, the counselors' services may well be covered by the health insurance plan, a benefit for both client and counselor.

Counselors' participation on a treatment team can provide balance and add new areas of expertise to the team. Counselors' orientation toward a developmental and preventive model of treatment, emphasizing both person and environment, can offset the pathology-oriented view of the medical model which tends to focus intensely on individual symptomatology (Siegler & Osmond, 1974). Counselors' expertise in career counseling, family counseling, and the use of standardized tests are strengths which are not so prevalent among other helping professionals and represent important skills which counselors can offer the treatment team.

Counselors can also contribute to the team's functioning by their impact on the cost of services. Counseling sessions typically cost less than sessions provided by psychiatrists or doctoral level psychologists; as reflected in the literature (Weikel, Daniel, & Anderson, 1981) and insurance companies' standard payment limits for psychologists and psychiatrists. Treatment which is at least partially provided by counselors will be, therefore, less costly than treatment conducted entirely by psychiatrists or psychologists. This factor will contribute to the increasing trend toward containment of health care costs and will enable some clients to receive treatment which would otherwise have been too costly.

Clients benefit from a team approach not only because of its economic advantages but, more importantly, because it affords them access to a range of mental health professionals with diverse skills and backgrounds. A teamwork approach to diagnoses and treatment should improve the quality of services provided to clients and increase the breadth of services available to meet clients' needs. As Udziela and Whitman state (1982, p. 784), "Through the multidisciplinary team process, the narrow rigidity of each individual discipline gives way to the broader, more colorful strokes provided by a spectrum of viewpoints."

Team Members

The multidisciplinary treatment team is typically composed of three to six people with diverse educational and experiential backgrounds. Working together, they have the expertise necessary to take a holistic approach to their clients; to consider emotional, physical, and intellectual aspects of the clients; and to provide a wide range of treatment modalities. The modalities include: medication; individual, group, and career counseling; and family therapy. The following is a brief description of the professions which often participate in multidisciplinary mental health treatment teams.

Psychiatrists

Psychiatrists have a medical (M.D.) degree and are trained to ameliorate both physical and emotional concerns and to understand the interface between the two. They specialize in the use of psychopharmacological interventions which include medications for disorders such as severe anxiety, depressive symptoms, psychotic patterns, and bipolar disorders. Psychiatrists and other physicians are the only team members who can prescribe medication and electroconvulsive therapy. Psychiatrists can readily gain hospital privileges and, therefore, have easy access to emergency and other hospital services. Some hospitals are reluctant to grant such privileges to nonmedical providers of mental health services. Their attitudes and approaches to psychotherapy vary widely with some advocating medication as the primary form of treatment for mental illness and others being strongly committed to psychotherapy. Most psychiatrists are well grounded in the basic principles of psychoanalysis. However, psychoanalysis is practiced by only a small percentage of psychiatrists with the remainder representing a broad diversity of approaches to the treatment of mental illness.

Nurses

Nurses, especially those with psychiatric training, are sometimes found on treatment teams, especially in hospital or rehabilitation settings. They can play an important role in supervising clients' compliance with medical treatment; observing the impact of medication on clients; and communicating with the physician when the medication is not effective. They can help staff, clients, and their families to understand clients' medical conditions, their prognoses, and the benefits and side effects of the medications which they are taking. Psychiatric nurses are also often trained and skilled in counseling techniques and may provide direct counseling services or serve as cotherapist in a group setting.

Psychologist

Psychologists will typically have a doctorate (Ph.D., Ed.D., or Psy.D.) and training in both psychotherapy and psychological assessment. Masters level psychologists may also be found as members of treatment teams, especially in school settings where the masters degree is the typical credential of the school psychologist. However, the masters level psychologist generally cannot be licensed to practice independently and tends to assume a specialized role in agencies, either serving as psychometrician (administering and interpreting psychological tests) or counselor but rarely demonstrating the expertise in both areas that is manifested by most doctoral level psychologists with degrees in clinical or counseling psychology.

Social Workers

Social workers who are licensed and/or certified (L.S.W. or A.C.S.W.) have met requirements that are similar to those required of licensed or certified counselors qualified for independent practice. The social workers completed two years of full-time coursework (or the equivalent) and have several years of supervised experience. However, social workers tend to be more oriented toward working with a seriously disturbed clientele than are counselors. Many social workers also have more interest in community organization and social policy than do most counselors. The origins of the social work profession were in the settlement house movement and many social workers are still committed to playing an active role in effecting social change. However, social workers do not usually have counselors' expertise in testing and career counseling. The area of overlap of the two professions is substantial, though, with both being skilled in counseling and psychotherapy with individuals, groups, and families.

Mental Health Counselor

Mental health counselors can play a broad and multifaceted role on the treatment team. Specific information on the various roles counselors have occupied on such teams will be discussed in a later section of this chapter. In general, however, counselors as team members tend to be involved in intake interviews; assessment; diagnoses and treatment planning; individual, group, family, and career counseling; and referral.

Activity Therapists

Physical therapists (physiotherapists), occupational therapists, and recreational therapists are all concerned with maintaining both the physical and the emotional health of clients through activity. However, each profession has its own approach to that process and fills a slightly different role on the treatment team. Physiotherapists seek to reduce disease, illness, or bodily weakness in clients through massage, exercise, or other physical activities. They often play an important role in the rehabilitation of physically ill or disabled clients and can contribute not only to clients' physical improvement but also to their emotional adjustment and self-esteem. Occupational and recreational therapists seek to provide diversion to clients; to expose them to new activities, skills, and experiences; and to provide them with opportunities that will be rewarding and productive. Their tasks are often designed to facilitate clients' social interaction with other clients. Both recreational and occupational therapists typically work in in-patient or day hospital facilities. Recreational therapists may specialize in one or more activity areas: dance, music, art, or sports. Occupational therapists are more likely to be involved in teaching crafts or the assembly of a product and often seek to develop work-related skills in clients to enable them to resume employment.

Vocational Rehabilitation Counselors

Vocational rehabilitation counselors are specially trained counselors with expertise in vocational/educational assessment, job development, and job placement. They also have good knowledge of both physical and mental disorders and their impact on clients' levels of functioning. They play an important role in facilitating the adjustment of disabled clients and enabling them to become self-supporting. Vocational rehabilitation counselors work not only with the physically disabled, but also with recovering substance abusers, the mentally retarded, and the emotionally disabled.

Nonprofessional Assistants

Mental health technician, paraprofessional counselor, peer counselor, and counselor assistant are all terms used to designate an individual who is performing some counseling duties but who has not received a graduate degree in a mental health field. Often, paraprofessionals have a history of having dealt with and overcome difficulties similar to those of the clients whom they are assisting. For example, paraprofessional counselors might be former narcotics addicts, now seeking to help clients involved in substance abuse, or they might be Vietnam veterans, counseling veterans with continuing adjustment difficulties. They might also share cultural or ethnic backgrounds with their clients. Because of their commonality with their clients, paraprofessional counselors can offer the treatment team a unique perspective and can sometimes play an important role in reducing client resistance, building trust, and developing rapport between clients and team members.

Teachers

Teachers are sometimes participants in school-based treatment teams. Although not mental health professionals, teachers play an important role in developing individualized educational plans for students with special needs and in promoting the emotional and educational development of those students. Teachers have close on-going student contact that affords them the opportunity to observe and understand students; therefore, teachers can provide the treatment team with important information on the student's needs and changes. Other helping or support professionals may also be included on the team, depending on the nature of the treatment facility and the needs of the clients. These others might be pastoral counselors, dentists, school principals, or lawyers. Expertise in mental health areas is not required for participation on a mental health treatment team; rather, it is the needs of the client which should determine the composition of the team.

Settings for Multidisciplinary Treatment Teams

A review of the literature on multidisciplinary mental health treatment teams yielded articles on over 25 different settings or client populations for whom treatment teams have been used. Although not all of the teams which will be discussed here included MHCs as team members, there seemed to be a place for MHCs on all of these teams. This overview of the literature is provided to give readers a sense of the breadth of the team approach and to provide information on possible settings where MHCs might find employment as part of a mental health treatment team.

Rehabilitation

The greatest number of articles on mental health treatment teams focused on rehabilitation, on taking a team work approach to promoting the physical and emotional health of clients who have been injured or ill or who may have undergone major surgery. Mechanic (1978) and Finch (1975) are only two of a number of authors who recognized the relationship between physical illness and psychological distress. They saw that physical disability could lead to emotional difficulties while mood disorders and other mental illnesses could precipitate or exacerbate physical illness. Carrai and Handford (1983) similarly advocated a biopsychosocial approach and stated, " . . . if professionals treat a handicapped person's physical, emotional, psychological, social, education, and occupational needs, the likelihood of successful rehabilitation is increased considerably" (p. 159).

MHCs participating in multidisciplinary teams in rehabilitation settings need a combination of skills which will enable them to understand and meet clients' needs as well as to function as effective team members. They need to have knowledge of the physiological and psychological implications of disability, of the effects and side effects of medication, and should be able to understand the lifestyle and viewpoints of the physically disabled (Westwood & Nayman, 1981). In addition, they should be skilled in multidisciplinary collaboration, have communication skills and problem-solving techniques, be able to use related resources, and have knowledge of human behavior and development, social variables, and principles of rehabilitation (Steger, 1974).

A broad range of rehabilitation settings using a multidisciplinary team approach have been cited in the literature. Carrai and Handford (1983) wrote of using a team approach with clients with hemophilia. Aitken and Cay (1975) saw a team approach as useful with clients with heart disease, peptic ulcers, or bronchial asthma. Fisch, Conley, Eysenbach, and Chang (1977) saw continuing contact with a treatment team as helpful to phenylketonuric children and their families; the team could provide support, medical treatment, information on dietary recommendations, assessment of intellectual development, and genetic, career, and family counseling. Belcher and Clowers (1978) described a service delivery model in which a treatment team would assist the severely disabled with employment, housing, education, and overall adjustment. Reactions to surgery including fear and anxiety, treatment compliance (appropriate vs. resistant or dependent), defense mechanisms (e.g., delay, avoidance, and denial), and family reactions can all be addressed and the emotional impact of surgery, reduced through a team approach (Furst, 1978). A multidisciplinary team consisting of physician, psychologist, physical therapist, and rehabilitation counselor have also helped patients to reduce chronic pain, increase physical activities, and reduce dependency on medication and medical care (Follick & Ahern, 1982). Children with recurrent physical complaints have also been helped by a team approach. A team approach to the treatment of any potentially life-threatening, disabling, or disfiguring physical disorder seems beneficial in light of the above research studies and the available knowledge on the interaction of physical and emotional aspects of life.

Hospitals

Hospitals provide similar settings for multidisciplinary mental health teams. Articles describe teams operating in both general and psychiatric hospitals. Opirhory and Peters (1982), for example, observed a multidisciplinary team working with the parents of newborns who were "less than perfect." The team facilitated the adjustment of the family and provided them with information on referrals, appropriate parenting skills, and continued support and counseling via home visits, if necessary. Sherr (1975), focusing on a different population, stressed the importance of a comprehensive approach for psychiatric patients including monitoring of the delivery of services, expediting of administrative procedures, responding to patient needs, and effecting behavioral change. Although Sherr saw what she called the rehabilitation psychologist as the key person in managing the treatment process, all of the above tasks could also be performed by a rehabilitation counselor or MHC.

Dentistry

Dentistry is yet another medical arena for the treatment team. Rao (1983) felt that a mental health professional could promote positive interaction between patients and dental clinicians and could encourage dental schools to take a more humanistic approach to patient care. This role of the team member as advocate of change offers counselors the opportunity to have an impact on a wide range of treatment facilities.

Outpatient Medical Facilities

A number of articles are available, describing the operation of multi-disciplinary treatment teams in outpatient medical facilities. Schroeder (1979), for example, described a program in which psychologists worked along with pediatricians, providing telephone and in-person information on child development and behavior management and leading counseling groups for children and their parents. Finch (1975) supported the importance of multidisciplinary team approach in pediatrics, especially in the treatment of children with such disorders as asthma and ulcerative colitis which tend to be aggravated by emotional upset.

Community health centers are also making use of a team approach. In North Carolina, such an approach was used to shift the orientation of a comprehensive neighborhood health center from a place for crisis intervention to a facility where thorough medical and emotional evaluations by multidisciplinary teams helped staff take a preventive approach with its lower socioeconomic clients. This seems like a particularly important shift for working with clients who might avoid the cost and bureaucratic tangles often associated with medical treatment until their medical and emotional difficulties had become severe.

In a similar vein, holistic health care, with its emphasis on wellness, environmental concerns, and responsibility for the self, and its use of such practices as exercise, medication, and natural remedies, has been increasing in availability and acceptance. Such programs afford another opportunity for counselors to work in a multidisciplinary team (Gross, 1980). Recent growth in health maintenance organizations (HMOs) and preferred provider organizations (PPOs) have further established the concept of the treatment team in medical settings.

Human Sexuality

Human sexuality is another focus for collaboration between medical and mental health specialists. The literature describes interdisciplinary health care units, providing counseling, education, and treatment of concerns related to the reproductive system (e.g., genital discomfort, problem pregnancies, infertility, and psychosexual dysfunctions). Such an approach was designed to lead not only to better physical health but to better decision-making, increased self-confidence, and improved marital and sexual interaction (Held, 1977; Maxwell, Hayes, & Martinez, 1976; and Routledge, 1977).

Schools

A great deal of literature on multidisciplinary treatment teams in schools is also available. In a school setting, treatment teams have been used to deal with concerns of the general student body as well as with difficulties presented by young people with special needs.

For many years, a small-scale teamwork approach has been the norm in school settings. Counselors collaborated with teachers, conferred with parents, and referred seriously disturbed children to outside treatment facilities. Now, however, the team approach has expanded and diversified in the schools. A survey of adolescent mental health needs yielded a broad range of concerns: alcohol abuse, employment concerns, and family concerns were among the most important (Nuttall, Nuttall, Polit, & Clark, 1977). A team approach does seem indicated to provide the kinds of services that would be needed. An interesting approach to treatment teams in the schools was described by Contreras (1977) in which a team consisting of an assistant principal, school counselors, teachers, and social workers, team-taught seminars in psychological education to high school students. Team approaches, then, have been used in the schools to accomplish both preventive and treatment goals with the general population of students.

Legislation mandates a team approach in working with special needs children. The first task of such a team is the process of screening and assessment. Cowen, Davidson, and Gesten (1980) described a team approach to the early detection and prevention of school adjustment problems. Multidisciplinary teams are also commonly used in the schools to develop individualized plans to meet the educational and emotional needs of exceptional children. Extensive and long-standing use seems to have been made of treatment teams to help learning disabled children (Alley, Deshler, & Mellard, 1979; Freeman & Thompson, 1975; & Muir, 1975). Activities of counselors on such teams have included psychological, familial, educational, social, and emotional evaluation; family and child counseling; home management counseling; teacher conferences; community, team, teacher, and peer education; serving as an advocate for the child; promoting home-school interaction; treatment planning; and coordination of the team. Counselors have served on treatment teams working with mentally retarded children (Minner & Beane, 1983), assuming a similarly multifaceted role. Counselors in mental health agencies can also participate in school-based treatment teams as consultants, providing needed expertise on diagnosis and treatment of behavioral, intellectual, and emotional disorders of children (Pyle, 1977).

Colleges

A number of articles substantiate use of the treatment team in colleges and universities. In colleges, most often, these are dyads rather than teams and involve collaboration between a psychiatrist or physician and a mental health professional (counselor or psychologist). Team members may be university employees or may be affiliated with area community mental health centers, serving as consultants to the university. An interesting example of a team approach to treating college students involved physicians and a psychologist collaborating in the hypnobehavioral treatment of students with stress-related illnesses such as hypertension, headaches, or asthma (Milne, 1982).

Substance Abuse

Substance abuse, which often has an impact on clients' physical and emotional health as well as on their career development and interpersonal relationships, seems to lend itself very well to treatment via a multidisciplinary team approach. Research suggests that teams working with substance abusers should integrate medical, psychological, and Alcoholics Anonymous perspectives on the causes and treatment of alcohol, with expertise in family counseling being part of the team's repertoire of skills (Coleman & Davis, 1978; Connelly, 1979).

Family Counseling Agencies

Family counseling agencies often need a multifaceted team approach to client treatment. The team, itself, can vary in its composition, depending on the nature of the family's concerns. Fivaz, Fivaz, and Kaufman (1981) described an approach to treating symptomatic families in which a physician, a family therapist, and a developmental psychologist collaborated in helping the family. School counselors and family counselors are another important treatment team for problem families (McDaniel, 1981). Lawyers and counselors can also form a powerful and effective team in doing marital counseling and family mediation and in dealing with issues of child custody (Bernstein, 1976). Genetic counseling is a relatively new aspect of family counseling in which a team approach is common. Typically, a couple meets with a mental health professional and a physician or geneticist to review the family's medical history, perhaps undergo some medical tests, receive information on any genetic risks which have been detected, and, if necessary, receive help from the counselor with any decisions the couple must make about childbearing.

Other Settings

References were found to a number of other settings in which multidisciplinary treatment teams have been used. While teams may be used less extensively in these settings, they are mentioned here to give a sense of the breadth of the team approach.

The corrections field frequently makes use of a team approach in prison, parole, and probation cases. A typical team might include a law enforcement officer, a counselor, and perhaps a teacher, a job placement specialist, a social worker, and/or a psychologist.

Agencies serving the elderly also often use a team approach to be sure that clients' physical and emotional needs are both met. This is particularly important with this population where depression can lead to poor nutrition and illness and where physical disabilities can lead to emotional disorders.

Church settings, too, have begun to use a team approach with pastoral counselors collaborating with psychiatrists in client treatment (Beitman, 1982). A similar collaboration (physician and mental health professional) has been used in the treatment of refugees recently arrived in the United States (Schultz, 1982).

Mental Health Service Delivery Agencies

Of course, agencies providing mental health services often make extensive use of multidisciplinary treatment teams which might include MHC, social workers, psychiatrists, psychologists, and others. Community mental health centers, in particular, developed under a mandate from the federal government to provide a comprehensive range of services, emphasize collaboration and cooperation among the staff.

International Agencies

Multidisciplinary approaches to mental health services are also being developed in many other countries. The literature indicated that such treatment teams, typically consisting of psychiatrists, psychologists, counselors, and social workers, are operating in Israel (Gross, Gross, & Einstein-Naveh, 1983), India (Dwivedi, Dubey, & Kumar, 1983), Canada (Calder, Tyrrell, & Franklin, 1973; Dumont & Torbit, 1976) and Scotland (Ebie, 1971) to cite a sampling.

Clearly, multidisciplinary mental health treatment teams have established themselves in a broad range of settings. Although counselors have not yet found a place for themselves on all of these teams, they certainly have skills which are required by all such teams. Consequently, it is anticipated (and hoped) that MHCs will gain increasing acceptance as integral participants on multidisciplinary mental health treatment teams.

Counselors' Roles on Multidisciplinary Teams

MHCs demonstrate a broad range of skills as participants of multidisciplinary mental health treatment teams. Of course, they are involved in individual and group counseling, intake interviews, and diagnosis and treatment planning. However, they also fill a wide range of more specialized roles. What follows is an overview of some of their real and **potential** roles and activities, as cited in the literature.

Program Evaluation and Development

MHCs have identified personnel needs, evaluated preparation programs, and conducted the planning to fill relevant staffing needs. They have established and coordinated programs that enable the severely disabled to live independently. They have assessed the need for peer support groups and have developed those groups.

Training, Professional Consultation, and Staff Development

Counselors have provided humanistic education and basic counseling skills to dentists and physicians. They have modified the curriculum in professional schools (e.g., medicine, dentistry, law) so that clients' needs are better understood and met. Counselors have provided the treatment team with information on typical human behavior and development and on basic counseling skills. In addition, they have taught team members techniques of stress management for their own use, have trained paraprofessional and peer counselors, have shown teachers and school administrators how to teach human development, have consulted with lawyers in divorce, child custody, criminal, and disability cases.

Community Education and Organization

Counselors have been called on to develop community education and prevention programs for the elderly, to inform clients in remote or rural areas about available services, to help refugees understand and adjust to Western medical care, and to work with pediatricians to provide parents with information on child development and behavior management. Counselors have also taught principles of human development to adolescents, provided adolescents with information on sexuality and birth control, offered consultation to community organizations, and taught communication skills to couples.

Identification, Assessment, and Placement of Special Clients

Other tasks asked of counselors have included developing individualized educational plans for special clients (e.g., mentally retarded, learning disabled, physically handicapped) and organizing and implementing programs for the early detection of school adjustment problems. They also have administered and interpreted inventories of ability, interest, and personality and made occupational and educational placement recommendations for a variety of clients.

Specialized Counseling Techniques

MHCs have used hypnotherapy to help individuals with stress-related illnesses. They have facilitated patients' management of chronic pain, provided career counseling to disabled individuals, used biofeedback to promote stress management, and provided crisis counseling to substance abusers and rape victims.

Adjunctive Mental Health Services

Counselors have provided information and facilitated stress management, adjustment, and planning for families of disabled individuals, and for parents of children with birth defects. They have facilitated the decision-making of individuals who seek information at genetic counseling centers, provided counseling and stress-management to pre- and postoperative patients, provided information and counseling to families of clients engaged in substance abuse, worked with families and employers to plan and implement environmental changes for hospitalized or institutionalized clients who were returning to their homes and jobs, monitored and encouraged patient compliance with medical treatment, and referred clients to appropriate agencies.

Administrative and Management Tasks

Counselors have performed a broad range of administrative and management tasks. They have been known to coordinate services (e.g., meditation, fitness, nutrition, counseling) for clients at a holistic health center, sought funding for programs via grant writing and interaction with governmental agencies, coordinated functioning of multidisciplinary treatment teams, coordinated implementation of children's individualized educational plans, and served as case managers, overseeing clients' treatment.

Issues in Multidisciplinary Treatment Teams

The preceding review of the literature has made it clear that MHCs play a significant and multifaceted role in mental health treatment teams. It also seems clear that such teams are beneficial for both team members and their clients.

However, there are also some challenges and concerns raised by the operation of such teams. This section will explore these, in an effort to help MHCs to anticipate and minimize any difficulties which they might encounter as participants of multidisciplinary treatment teams.

Common Orientation

It is important for team members to have a shared conception of the approach they will take to treatment and an understanding of their client population, the service delivery model they will use, and the team's goals. A frequent conflict, on such teams, is between the psychiatrist who espouses a medical model, oriented toward treatment of illness and pathology, and the nonmedical mental health professional who is more likely to advocate a preventive or developmental approach to treatment.

Such a possible conflict was highlighted by the research of Pihl and Spiers (1977) who administered three inventories including the Rokeach Dogmatism scale to professionals and students from four helping professions. Pihl and Spiers found significant differences among the groups. These findings and other less well documented articles indicate that conflicting orientations among treatment team members is a common source of tension and diminished effectiveness.

In light of this, it seems advisable for teams to devote time, both early in their development and at subsequent points, to developing a shared perspective on their philosophy and functioning, to become in all senses, a true team. It also seems important that the team present a clear and cohesive image to the public; this would be very difficult to accomplish if the group were not, in fact, working together in a consistent and cooperative way.

Mutual Understanding

It is also important for team members to understand each others' roles and competencies, and both their differences and similarities. This should maximize their effectiveness as a team by enabling them to know what the team can and cannot do and which team members have expertise in which activities. Role overlap is inevitable in such teams and members need to realize that " . . . no particular discipline possesses sole ownership of wisdom and procedure in explaining and dealing with behavioral problems" (Pihl & Spiers, 1977, p. 269).

It has been suggested that programs training prospective members of a multidisciplinary treatment team should acquaint students with the variety of human service providers (Myers, 1982). This seems like a worthwhile suggestion. However, until it is universally implemented, team members will need to find other ways to become acquainted with each others' professions. Vassil and Balgopal (1982) have suggested role exchange as a way for helping new health professions to become acquainted with each others' attitudes and activities. Staff development workshops and in-service training programs provide other vehicles for expanding team members' understanding of their colleagues' roles. Finally, an environment which encourages open interaction between team members and provides time for interaction to take place is probably most important in helping team members to understand each other as both individuals and professionals.

Distribution of Power

The distribution of power is often a source of stress for team members, especially if it is unclear or seems inequitable to some members. Typically, teams will have a manager or leader. This is often the psychiatrist but may be one of the nonmedical human service workers. Some teams have consultants who serve as team managers. The manager's style of handling power and authority as well as the team's satisfaction with that person as leader will have a considerable impact on the team's satisfaction with the balance of power. Treatment teams, of course, also have unofficial leaders as do all groups; this may be the most capable member, the most verbal member, or perhaps the most aggressive member. The team's clients also have power; some groups are largely directed by the expressed needs of their clients while other groups seems to impose their own needs and direction onto their clients.

That imbalance will exist in a team seems inevitable and to strive for equity in power seems unreasonable. However, it does seem possible to establish a team in which all members see themselves and are seen as powerful and important contributors to the team and where the power balance is sufficiently flexible to accommodate a range of client and professional needs. Communication and problem-solving skills can help team members to develop an attitude of sharing and interdependence as well as a clear sense of their own place on the team.

One approach to establishing an effective team is the development and team acceptance of a process for assessing the functioning of the team. Approaches to such evaluations have been described in the literature (Fleming & Fleming, 1983). The use of an on-going process of team self-evaluation can promote feedback and communication within the team and prevent entrenchment of members' roles and hierarchies. The team's power structure also seems likely to receive more acceptance if bureaucratic constraints are minimized for both team members and clients, if members have developed a sense of respect and appreciation for each other, and if open dialogue on the team's strengths and weaknesses is possible.

Cooperation

Lowe and Herranen (1981) found that teamwork in health care delivery was an evolutionary process with distinct developmental stages. It takes time, then, for a team to develop itself into a cooperative and smoothly running entity. Competition certainly exists between mental health professionals and if team members feel lacking in power and importance on the team, they can become absorbed with their individual roles and gains and can lose sight of the power and importance of the team. However, given a positive community and institutional environment, a team that is willing to collaborate and communicate, and the time for assessment and development, a multidisciplinary treatment team can evolve that is synergistic and of benefit to both clients and team members.

REFERENCES

Aitken, C., & Cay, E. (1975). Clinical psychomatic research. *International Journal of Psychiatry in Medicine, 6,* 29–41.

Alley, G. R., Deshler, D. D., & Mellard, D. (1979). Identification decisions: Who is the most consistent? *Learning Disability Quarterly, 2,* 99–103.

Beitman, B. D. (1982). Pastoral counseling centers: A challenge to community mental health centers. *Hospital & Community Psychiatry, 33,* 486–487.

Belcher, S. A., & Clowers, M. R. (1978). Service delivery model for the severely disabled individual: Follow-up. *Journal of Applied Rehabilitation Counseling, 9,* 174–177.

Bernstein, B. E. (1976). Lawyer and counselor as an interdisciplinary team: The timely referral. *Journal of Marriage and Family Counseling, 2,* 347–354.

Calder, B., Tyrrell, M., & Franklin, G. (1973). The case for counsellor technicians and counsellor assistants. *Canadian Counsellor, 7,* 133–138.

Carrai, E. B., & Handford, H. A. (1983). Problems of hemophilia and the role of the rehabilitative counselor. *Rehabilitation Counseling Bulletin, 26,* 155–163.

Coleman, S. B., & Davis, D. I. (1978). Family therapy and drug abuse: A national survey. *Family Process, 17,* 21–29.

Connelly, J. C. (1979). Current issues in the hospital treatment of alcoholism: The role of the alcoholism counselor. *Journal of the National Association of Private Psychiatric Hospitals, 10,* 32–34.

Contreras, P. (1977). Staff and organizational development in psychological education: An example. *Counseling Psychologist, 6,* 64–67.

Cowen, E. L., Davidson, E. R., & Gesten, E. L. (1980). Program dissemination and the modification of delivery practices in school mental health. *Professional Psychology, 11,* 36–47.

Dumont, F., & Tarbit, G. (1976). The expanding role of the counsellor: Fitting means to ends. *Canadian Counsellor, 11,* 24–27.

Dwivedi, P., Dubey, B. L., & Kumar, V. (1983). Role of social scientists in extending health services to the community. *Indian Journal of Clinical Psychology, 10,* 85–91.

Ebie, J. (1971). Features of psychiatric relevance at an experimental multi-disciplinary social casework centre in Edinburgh. *Social Psychiatry, 6,* 122–128.

Finch, S. M. (1975). Psychophysiologic disorders in children and adolescents. *International Journal of Psychiatry in Medicine, 6,* 213–225.

Fisch, R. O., Conley, J. A., Eysenbach, S., & Chang, P. N. (1977). Contact with phenylketonurics and their families beyond pediatric age: Conclusion from a survey and conference. *Mental Retardation, 15,* 10–12.

Fivaz, E., Fivaz, R., & Kaufman, L. (1981). Dysfunctional transactions and therapeutic functions: An evolutive model. *Journal of Marital and Family Therapy, 7,* 309–320.

Fleming, D. C., & Fleming, E. (1983). Consultation with multidisciplinary teams: A program of development and improvement of team functioning. *Journal of School Psychology, 21,* 367–376.

Follick, M. J., & Ahern, D. K. (1982). Outpatient behavioral management of chronic pain. *Behavioral Medicine Update, 3,* 7–10.

Freeman, S. W., & Thompson, C. R. (1975). The counselor's role with learning disabled students. *School Counselor, 23,* 28–36.

Furst, J. B. (1978). Emotional stress reactions to surgery: Review of some therapeutic implications. *New York State Journal of Medicine, 78,* 1083–1085.

Gross, A. M., Gross, J., & Einstein-Naveh, A. R. (1983). Defining the role of the social worker in primary health care. *Health and Social Work, 8,* 174–181.

Gross, S. J. (1980). The holistic health movement. *Personnel & Guidance Journal, 59,* 96–100.

Held, J. P. (1977). The evaluation of sexual health services in a medical setting. *Journal of Sex & Marital Therapy, 3,* 256–264.

Lincoln Community Health Center. (1977). Delivering mental health services to an ambulatory, low-income population. *Hospital & Community Psychiatry, 28,* 846–848.

Lowe, J. I., & Herranen, M. (1981). Understanding teamwork: Another look at the concepts. *Social Work in Health Care, 7,* 1–11.

Maxwell, S. L., Hayes, G., & Martinez, A. (1976). Reaching rural adolescents with programs in sexuality. *Personnel & Guidance Journal, 54,* 387–388.

McDaniel, S. H. (1981). Treating school problems in family therapy. *Elementary School Guidance & Counseling, 15,* 214–222.

Mechanic, D. (1978). Effects of psychological distress on perceptions of physical health and use of medical and psychiatric facilities. *Journal of Human Stress, 4,* 26–32.

Milne, G. (1982). Hypnobehavioral medicine in a university counseling center. *Australian Journal of Clinical & Experimental Hypnosis, 10,* 13–26.

Minner, S., & Beane, A. (1983). Professional dilemmas for teachers of mentally retarded children. *Education and Training of the Mentally Retarded, 18,* 131–133.

Muir, M. (1975). The consideration of emotional factors in the diagnosis and treatment of learning-disabled children. *Journal of Pediatric Psychology, 3,* 6–9.

Myers, R. A. (1982). Education and training: The next decade. *Counseling Psychologist, 10,* 39–44.

Nuttall, E. V., Nuttall, R. L., Polit, D., & Clark, K. (1977). Assessing adolescent mental health needs: The views of consumers, providers, and others. *Adolescence, 12,* 277–285.

Opirhory, G., & Peters, G. A. (1982). Counseling intervention strategies for families with less than perfect newborn. *Personnel & Guidance Journal, 60,* 451–455.

Pihl, R. O., & Spiers, P. (1977). Some personality differences among the multidisciplinary team. *Journal of Clinical Psychology, 33,* 269–272.

Pyle, R. R. (1977). Mental health consultation: Helping teachers help themselves. *Professional Psychology, 8,* 192–198.

Rao, A. P. (1983). Social work in dentistry. *Health and Social Work, 8,* 219–229.

Routledge, D. (1977). Program development and human sexuality. *Journal of Leisurability, 4,* 9–12.

Schroeder, C. S. (1979). Psychologists in a private pediatric practice. *Journal of Pediatric Psychology, 4,* 5–18.

Schultz, S. L. (1982). How Southeast-Asian refugees in California adapt to unfamiliar health care practices. *Health and Social Work, 7,* 148–156.

Sherr, R. L. (1975). Developing direct psychological services that incorporate the insider's position. *Rehabilitation Psychology, 22,* 124–128.

Siegler, M., & Osmond, H. (1974). *Models of madness, models of medicine.* NY: Macmillan.

Steger, J. M. (1974). Multidisciplinary model for undergraduate education in rehabilitation. *Rehabilitation Counseling Bulletin, 18,* 12–20.

Udziela, A. D., & Whitman, B. Y. (1982). The psychologist on the multidisciplinary developmental disabilities team. *Professional Psychology, 13,* 782–788.

Vassil, T. V., & Balgopal, P. A. (1982). Role exchange: An innovative strategy for teaching and learning in the health field. *Indian Journal of Social Work, 43,* 139–146.

Weikel, W. J., Daniel, R. W., & Anderson, J. (1981). A survey of counselors in private practice. *AMHCA Journal, 3,* 88–94.

Westwood, M. J., & Nayman, J. (1981). Counseling persons with a disability: A professional challenge. *Canadian Counselor, 15,* 158–161.

Chapter 9

WORK SETTINGS OF THE MENTAL HEALTH COUNSELOR

KATHLEEN H. JONES AND ARTIS J. PALMO

Mental health counselors (MHCs) are engaged in waging a continuing and increasingly effective battle for recognition as primary providers of mental health services in the United States. The identification of counselors primarily with educational settings is gradually being displaced. For example, Weikel and Taylor (1979) surveyed 332 American Mental Health Counselors Association (AMHCA) members and found that MHCs were employed in community mental health centers, private practice, college counseling centers, private agencies, and state agencies. The myth that counselors work only in schools is being slowly replaced by the reality of professional counselors finding employment in most areas of mental health care.

The leadership of AMHCA has sought to sensitize their membership to their right to professional recognition (Wilmarth & Beck, 1984), yet many issues of professional rivalry and legally sanctioned exclusionary obstacles still remain (Asher, 1979; DeRidder, Stephens, English, & Watkins, 1983; Randolph, 1978). The primary professional rival for MHCs employed in community and private agencies is the profession of psychology. Although there is disagreement among professional psychologists regarding the employment of master's level psychologists versus doctoral level psychologists in agency settings (Albee, 1977), Dimond, Havens, Rathnow, and Colliver (1977) report that the large majority of agencies employ the master's level psychologist. In addition, Dimond et al. state that the demand for employment will continue. This increase in the utilization of master's level professionals in mental health agencies has provided increased employment opportunities for MHCs, but not without difficulties.

Leaders from AMHCA, the Association for Counselor Education and Supervision (ACES), and the Council for the Accreditation of Counseling and Related Educational Programs (CACREP) have stressed the need for the development of comprehensive, mental health counseling programs that are separately identified from school counseling programs (Weikel, Seiler, Wittmer, Sheeley, Stone, & Brooks, 1985). As a result of this encouragement from various professional groups, more and more graduate programs are defining clear standards for the training of the MHC that will enable the MHC to find employment in the professionally competitive settings of community and private mental health centers.

Needs of Community Mental Health Centers

Anderson, Parenté, and Gordon (1981) state that "Mental health practitioners from various disciplines provide remarkably similar services" (p. 848). The "disciplines" discussed by Anderson et al. include the traditional core providers, psychiatrists, psychologists, social workers, and psychiatric nurses as well as counselors. Anderson et al. reported in their survey of all of the five mental health care providers listed, that the need for master's level mental health providers will continue into the 1990s. Even though the disagreements among the five professional groups will more than likely continue, it is apparent that there is agreement regarding the continued need for master's level mental health care providers.

Bloom and Parad (1977) examined the professional activities of community mental health center staff members as well as their perceived training needs. Although the primary emphasis of the survey was on the activities and training needs of psychologists, the survey provides important information regarding the activities of counselors in mental health care centers. Bloom and Parad surveyed 55 of 87 federally assisted centers located in 13 Western states. Those surveyed included psychiatrists, psychologists, social workers, nurses, and "other mental health professionals" (counselors, physicians, rehabilitation specialists, and social scientists).

The results reported by Bloom and Parad showed that psychiatrists, psychologists, social workers, and nurses spent more time in the overall category of clinical activities than "other mental health professionals." However, a breakdown of the categories within clinical activities demonstrates that the professionals in the counselor category (other mental health profession) spent as much time or more in individual, family, and group treatment compared to the other four groups. The four primary groups spent on the average, more time in patient and ward management, diagnosis, and crisis/emergency care than did other mental health professionals.

Bloom and Parad also report that the "other mental health professionals" spent greater amounts of their time in consultation, after care, interagency collaboration, training, supervision, and staff conferences. It is apparent from Bloom and Parad's report that the MHC has a place in the mental health center as a provider of important therapeutic services not totally provided by the other core providers. In addition, the report demonstrates that the primary skill of the MHC, counseling, is highly utilized within the mental health care center setting. Finally, Bloom and Parad note that the significant differences found among the core providers in the way their time was allocated were, in reality, often unimpressive in actual time units. It seems that the various services offered by mental health care centers are often performed by various mental health care workers in a shared fashion.

Feldman (1978), citing the lack of relationship between mental health center services and the training of those who provide the services, has called for the training of mental health professionals not tied to one discipline. The needs of the clients of mental health centers, according to Feldman, include "brief psychotherapy, crisis intervention, group and family therapy, and treatment approaches for patients from diverse ethnic groups" (p. 87). It appears evident that the training of the MHC fits the needs of today's mental health center.

Although it is apparent that the well-trained MHC has a place in community and private mental health centers, several barriers still exist. Randolph (1978) surveyed community mental health directors in the southeastern United States to determine their preference for the titles, training, and skills of prospective doctoral level employees. A strong bias in favor of mental health professionals calling themselves psychologists was evident. The title counselor was ranked very low. In fact, Randolph reported several instances of doctoral level counselors not being considered for positions for which they were qualified due to their degree title. Part of this difficulty centered on the inaccessibility of counselors to psychology licensure in many states. Licensure is necessary to receive third party payments which are used to reimburse community mental health centers for services provided. Other findings reported by Randolph (1978) were that coursework with a strong psychology emphasis was preferred. Preferred skill areas included individual, family, and group therapy, crisis intervention, consultation, intake, assessment, and diagnosis.

Good communication skills and personal warmth were highly rated personal attributes. In another article, Randolph (1979) analyzed the data for master's level practitioners and found the same standards to apply. The major point being made is that although the MHC may possess the training and skills necessary for agency employment, other factors (i.e., psychology licensure) may prohibit the MHC from employment in certain positions. Although it may be too early to make a definitive statement, counselor licensure in several states may be a significant help to the employment status of MHCs.

One other aspect of the changing role of the mental health professional needs to be mentioned. The Community Mental Health Amendment of 1975 (Feldman, 1978) placed the burden of proof of effectiveness of services squarely in the hands of the agencies. This meant that community mental health centers had to prove that their services were effective in order to maintain funding. As a result, the mental health care provider was placed in the position of not only being an effective therapeutic agent, but also, a skilled researcher. As Anderson (1981) notes, counselors often find that the basic research techniques learned in graduate programs may be insufficient for the tasks required in the center. The highly skilled MHC also needs sound training in program evaluation and assessment, a skill sometimes neglected in counselor training programs.

It can be seen that community mental health counselors require skills in individual counseling, group counseling, family counseling, consultation, crisis intervention, brief psychotherapy, assessment, diagnosis, and research skills. While these qualifications are not specific to only community mental health counselors, they form the base by which the MHC can meet the professional role expectations of community mental health centers.

Other Mental Health Agency Needs

The settings in which MHCs work are many and varied. Previous discussion has centered on the role of the MHC in community mental health centers. Other settings demand differing skills and define counselors' roles according to a wide array of applications and expectations.

Gellman and Murov (1973) discussed the psychodevelopmental and sociocultural focus being fostered by private community agencies. These authors reported that the primary services provided by counselors are "tri-dimensional . . . —familial, individual, and social" (p. 158). Other skills needed by the MHC included needs assessment of clients and skills in milieu therapy. Leung (1975) contrasted the role of clinical counselors with community agency counselors. According to Leung, clinical counselors work in hospital emergency rooms and detoxification units. In working with these clients, the clinical counselor's role is to support clients as they arrive, clarify what has happened, assist in determining therapeutic goals, and help them to determine future behavior. Clinical counselors also serve as the referral source back to the community.

Evans (1983) described the role of the counselor as treatment specialist within the criminal court system. The treatment specialist provides defendants and courts with a neutral third party who can identify needs, match appropriate resources, and make referrals. Evans listed requisite skills as interviewing techniques, assessment, and knowledge of, evaluation of, and liaison with referral sources. Oral and written skills are needed for presentation and testimony.

Gerontological counseling is a growing area of mental health counseling requiring specialized skills. (See Highlight Section—Gerontology.) Myers and Blake (1984), in a follow-up of counseling graduates specializing in gerontological counseling, found these counselors were employed in area agencies on aging, community mental health centers, state/community social service agencies, senior citizen centers, and other diverse settings. Myers and Blake presented three important conclusions from their follow-up study: (1) counselors are employed in settings where "a substantial portion of their time is spent working with older persons" (p. 335); (2) many different agencies employ "gerocounselors;" and (3) counselors are employed in agencies that provide services for all ages of clientele as well as agencies whose primary function is serving the older person. MHCs trained in gerontological counseling have a wide variety of employment opportunities available to them.

Leung and Eargle (1980) delineated some of the skills needed by the MHC for working with the elderly in public housing. Beyond establishing a trusting relationship, the counselor must be able to help the client to solve practical problems through such skills as assertiveness. Also, techniques unique to the elderly such as life review therapy, as well as skills dealing with anxiety and death, are needed.

One of the more recently developed employment settings for the MHC, as reported by Harvey and Schramski (1983), is working with special populations diagnosed as mentally retarded and mentally ill. The authors saw this as an opportunity for MHCs to develop specified programs for this group. Counseling for improved interpersonal functioning as well as job training allows clients to grow toward deinstitutionalized independence.

The chronically mentally ill represent a client population who do not typically respond to traditional therapies. Marlowe, Marlowe, and Willets (1983) reported that case management is the primary intervention utilized with the chronically mentally ill. Case management, as defined by Marlowe et al., included assessment, planning, linking, monitoring, and advocacy. "Assessment is the process of identifying a client's strengths, deficits, needs, level of functioning, and extent of impairment" (p. 187). The MHC as a case manager synthesizes all the data gathered from all important sources, and then begins the second step in case management, planning. "The objective of planning is to construct an individualized service plan (ISP) for the chronically mentally ill (CMI) client" (p. 187). An important aspect of the case manager's role in planning is the utilization of as many community resources as possible. Therefore, the MHC must be fully aware of all the resources available within the community milieu.

The third aspect of case management, linking, assures that the CMI client receives the services outlined in the ISP. Monitoring, the fourth aspect of case management, requires the MHC to be continuously assessing the plan throughout the client's development to assure necessary and appropriate services are being provided. Finally, the MHC as an advocate in case management means assuring that the client's rights are not violated. Whether the client is in an institution or not, the client has certain rights that allow for expression of complaints and resolution of grievances. Advocacy can also mean rights for legal representation or rights for public benefits.

Marlowe et al. feel that MHCs can fill an important void in the mental health system with the CMI client by being effective case managers. Utilizing the skills outlined above, MHCs can provide a service that permits the CMI client to live a more satisfactory life in the community.

As mentioned by Marlowe et al., consultation is a major aspect of the MHC's role in the services provided to clients. Werner (1978) described a successful consultation program using six levels of consultation, each of which require making an assessment of the consultee's request and an exploration of appropriate interventions. Another view of consultation moves beyond the agency itself and into the community. Lewis and

Lewis (1977) advocated the role of the counselor as a social change agent working with community groups to seek change in the community. This leads to an increased sense of power for their clients. Special contributions counselors can make are based on their skills in assessment, coordinating efforts, training others in social effectiveness, and open advocacy for change perceived as necessary for the health of their communities.

Employees in agency settings require and expect varied expertise from the counselors they employ. While there are many skills common to any counselor function, specialized skills in specialized settings seems to be the key to successful functioning for the MHC in an agency setting.

Counselor Education and the Roles of the Mental Health Counselor in the Community

Bradley (1978), in a review of the counseling literature for the ten years between 1968 and 1978, questioned whether counselor education programs were responding to the needs of the clients and institutions which counselors serve. Programs which stress therapy over prevention, individual rather than group or consultation skills, isolation from rather than involvement in the social milieu of the client, do not serve the needs of many institutions and agencies where counselors are presently employed. Bradley feels that the role identity problems that counselors experience may be a partial function of the divergence in expectations emanating from training and the reality of the actual work role.

Aware of such criticisms, and as a response to the trend toward community counseling, counselor education programs are reviewing the academic and experiential components of their programs to produce the competencies which are perceived to be required by community mental health centers. As recently as 1983, Caulfield and Perosa endorsed a training program for counselors which emphasized common competencies and a broadened curriculum leading to employment in either a school or community setting. However, most counselor education programs have felt impelled to design separate programs for community mental health counselors. While certain core competencies are common to the profession of counseling, counselor educators have appropriately perceived the need to respond to the role requirements of mental health counseling in the community by initiating diverse and separate programs, much as they have done for rehabilitation counseling.

Stadler and Stahl (1979) surveyed master's level counselor education programs to determine trends in community/agency counselor training. They reported that this training emphasis is rather new (67% reported their programs in existence for 6 years or less). They also found that curricular choices did not necessarily reflect probable agency needs. Coyne (1980) surveyed community counselor master's programs to determine how they would be evaluated against a community counseling model stressing prevention and a systematic community focus. His findings supported this model as an ideal and as a current trend in master's level community counseling programs. Another study of counselor education programs was done by Wantz, Scherman, and Hollis (1982). This analysis of trends over the past ten years found that counseling specialization is increasing. Courses most frequently added were marriage and family counseling, consultation, gerontological counseling, and career and life planning courses.

To determine the specific master's level competencies required by community agencies, DeRidder, Stephens, English, and Watkins (1983) surveyed administrators and directors of eleven different types of agencies in the state of Tennessee. The purpose of the survey was to form the basis for a community counseling program responsive to the needs of the future employers of its graduates. The agencies represented a variety of settings including employment, family, mental health, aged, court, and family planning agencies. The results of the survey delineated four competencies as core to all settings: (1) understanding human development and the barriers to learning and adjustment; (2) competency in global counseling skills; (3) knowledge of ethics; and (4) clear communication skills. The individual agencies rated various other competencies as specifically desirable, including competencies in areas such as abuse, assessment, consulting, career development, and supervision.

A program, described by Randolph, Sturgis, and Alcorn (1979) at the University of Southern Mississippi to train community counselors, has been designed to account for the major role requirements desired by mental health centers as determined by Randolph (1979). This program emphasizes training in the delivery of both direct and indirect professional services in agencies. The state requirement for a two year degree for professional employment in some agencies led to an expansion of the program with an increased psychological emphasis. The title of the degree was changed to counseling psychology as a response to employment requirements.

The competencies required by the roles of the MHC in the community are of necessary concern to counselor educators. While program revisions are occurring in the present, the future trends predicted to influence MHCs must also be considered.

Future Trends

Delphi polls have been used by several authors to predict future trends that will influence counselor roles. In projecting trends in the mental health professions for the next twenty years, Anderson, Parenté, and Gordon (1981) and Anderson and Parenté (1980) found that mental health professionals (MHCs, psychologists, psychiatrists, administrators, nurses, and social workers) predicted that master's level training will become more specialized. Certification will become mandatory at the master's level. Master's level practitioners will also find themselves working in supervised positions. Other than psychologists, mental health professionals predicted that master's level counselors will receive third-party reimbursement. Psychologists reported that it is unlikely that the master's level mental health professional will receive third party reimbursement on a routine basis. Graduate program accreditation will also become mandatory.

Counselor educators, in a 1983 Delphi poll (Daniel & Weikel, 1983), predicted that masters' training will become longer and more specialized. It was also predicted that increasing numbers of counselors will be employed in private counseling agencies and business/industry settings. Prevention, one of the main foci of community psychology (Goodyear, 1976), is predicted to become a major role for MHCs.

Summary

Beyond the basic counseling skills common to all counselor training, community mental health counselors need to be sensitive to the specialized skills their specific work setting may require. While undoubtedly some of these skills are developed on the job (Randolph, 1978), others can be attained through coursework and graduate training. This will lead to increased employability of the MHC. The complex roles that MHCs serve are professionally demanding. The recognition of the profession of mental health counseling hinges on the past record of excellence and the willingness of the profession to remain responsive to the growing demands of the mental health community.

At this point in the development of the profession, MHCs are employed throughout the community in a broad array of settings. Two points seem particularly important to make at this time. First, the MHC has an unlimited number of available work settings—from hospitals to private agencies. The creativity shown by MHCs in their employment settings has produced a continuing demand for broadly trained professionals, which appears to be growing each successive year.

Second, if the MHC is to continue to be an important part of the community mental health movement, the MHC must maintain an attitude of continuous professional development. The traditional core providers have a very firm grip on certain aspects of community mental health programs. If MHCs are to achieve parity with the other core providers, they must continue to demonstrate the effective skills suggested in the previous sections.

REFERENCES

Albee, G. W. (1977). The uncertain future of the MA clinical psychologist. *Professional Psychology, 8,* 122–124.

Anderson, W. (1981). How to do research in community mental health agencies. *Personnel and Guidance Journal, 59,* 517–523.

Anderson, J. A., & Parenté, F. J. (1980). AMHCA members forecast the future of the mental health profession. *American Mental Health Counselors Association Journal, 2,* 4–12.

Anderson, J. K., Parenté, F. J., & Gordon, C. (1981). A forecast of the future for the mental health profession. *American Psychologist, 36,* 848–855.

Asher, J. K. (1979). The coming exclusion of counselors from the mental health care system. *American Mental Health Counselors Association Journal, 1,* 53–60.

Bloom, B. L., & Parad, H. J. (1977). Professional activities and training needs of community mental health center staff. In I. Iscoe, B. L. Bloom, & C. D. Spielberger (Eds.), *Community psychology in transition* (pp. 229–240). Washington, DC: Hemisphere Publishing.

Bradley, M. K. (1978). Counseling past and present: Is there a future? *Personnel and Guidance Journal, 57,* 42–45.

Caulfield, T. J., & Perosa, L. M. (1983). Counselor education-quo vadis? *Counselor Education and Supervision, 22,* 178–184.

Coyne, R. K. (1980). The "community" in community counseling: Results of a national survey. *Counselor Education and Supervision, 20,* 22–28.

Daniel, R. W., & Weikel, W. J. (1983). Trends in counseling: A Delphi study. *Personnel and Guidance Journal, 61,* 327–331.

DeRidder, L. M., Stephens, T. A., English, J. T., & Watkins, C. E., Jr. (1983). The development of graduate programs in community counseling: One approach. *American Mental Health Counselors Association Journal, 5,* 61–68.

Dimond, R. E., Havens, R. A., Rathnow, S. J., & Colliver, J. A. (1977). Employment characteristics of subdoctoral clinical psychologists. *Professional Psychology, 8,* 116–121.

Evans, J. (1983). The treatment specialist: An emerging role for counselors within the criminal court system. *Personnel and Guidance Journal, 61,* 349–351.

Feldman, S. (1978). Promises, promises or community mental health services and training: Ships that pass in the night. *Community Mental Health Journal, 14,* 83–91.

Gellman, W., & Murov, H. (1973). The broad role of the community agency counselor. *Personnel and Guidance Journal, 52,* 157–159.

Goodyear, R. K. (1976). Counselors as community psychologists. *Personnel and Guidance Journal, 54,* 513–516.

Harvey, D. R., & Schramski, T. G. (1983). ADAPT: A day program for the dually diagnosed clients. *American Mental Health Counselors Association Journal, 5,* 44–48.

Leung, P. (1975). Clinical counselors. *Personnel and Guidance Journal, 54,* 113–114.

Leung, P., & Eargle, D. (1980). Counseling with the elderly living in public housing. *Personnel and Guidance Journal, 58,* 442–445.

Lewis, M. D., & Lewis, J. A. (1977). The counselor's impact on community environments. *Personnel and Guidance Journal, 55,* 356–358.

Marlowe, H. A., Marlowe, J. L., & Willetts, R. (1983). The mental health counselor as case manager: Implications for working with the chronically mentally ill. *American Mental Health Counselors Association Journal, 5,* 184–190.

Myers, J. E., & Blake, R. H. (1984). Employment of gerontological counseling graduates: A follow-up study. *Personnel and Guidance Journal, 62,* 333–335.

Randolph, D. L. (1978). The counseling-community psychologist in the CMHC: Employer perceptions. *Counselor Education and Supervision, 17,* 244–253.

Randolph, D. L. (1979). CMHC requisites for employment of master's level psychologists/counselors. *American Mental Health Counselors Association Journal, 1,* 64–68.

Randolph, D. L., Sturgis, D. K., & Alcorn, J. D. (1979). A counseling-community psychology master's program. *American Mental Health Counselors Association Journal, 1,* 69–72.

Stadler, H. A., & Stahl, E. (1979). Trends in community counselor training. *Counselor Education and Supervision, 19,* 42–48.

Wantz, R. A., Scherman, A., & Hollis, J. W. (1982). Trends in counselor preparation: Courses, program emphases, philosophical orientation, and experimental components. *Counselor Education and Supervision, 21,* 258–268.

Weikel, W., Seiler, G., Wittmer, J., Sheeley, V., Stone, L., & Brooks, D. (1983, April). American Mental Health Counselors Association and Association for Counselor Education and Supervision panel: Common concerns for credentialing. Symposium presented at the Annual American Association for Counseling and Development Convention, New York City.

Weikel, W. J., & Taylor, S. S. (1979). AMHCA: Membership profile and journal preferences. *American Mental Health Counselors Association Journal, 1,* 89–94.

Werner, J. L. (1978). Community mental health consultation with agencies. *Personnel and Guidance Journal, 56,* 364–368.

Wilmarth, R. R., & Beck, E. S. (1984). The professional counselor: A new activist identity or following our own advice. *American Mental Health Counselors Association Journal, 6,* 104–105.

HIGHLIGHT SECTION

MENTAL HEALTH COUNSELING IN EDUCATIONAL SETTINGS

EDWARD S. BECK

The origins and history of the counseling movement are well-chronicled. Depending upon the training one receives, the associations to which a chronicler belongs, and the philosophical assumptions about the nature of counseling that are made, there is a plethora of literature dealing with the evolution of counseling and counselor roles in educational settings. The literature is replete with references to the historical evolution of school psychological, mental hygiene, and social work services as functions of the student personnel department. Chroniclers of the guidance and counseling movement are quick to agree that the structure of counseling services for students in educational settings varies from district to district and institution to institution. In addition, the counseling services are sensitive to economics, demographics, and ethnographics, as well as the local acceptance of an understood functional definition for the counseling professional (Barry & Wolf, 1957; Dinkmeyer & Caldwell, 1970; Faust, 1968; Ferguson, 1968; Hilton, 1979; McDaniel, 1966; Miller & Prince, 1976; Patterson, 1971; Shertzer & Stone, 1974; Van Hoose & Pietrofesa, 1970; Wrenn, 1962).

Hoyt (1970), a pioneer in counseling, summarized the historical and etiological development of counseling by suggesting that:

1. Counseling has deep roots in the study of psychology of individual differences, learning, vocational development, and personality development.
2. Counseling has deep roots in education; the nature and structure of education in America, educational philosophy, educational goals, and principles of curriculum development.
3. Counseling has deep roots in the domain of statistics, measurement, and research.

Although Hoyt discounts the roles of sociology, economics, and anthropology as contributors to the field of guidance, it is clear, that within the last several decades these fields have made significant contributions to our understanding of the mental health counseling needs of students within the educational system.

Educational institutions' preoccupation with the mental hygiene of students is well-documented. In narrating the evolution of the elementary school counseling, Faust (1968) points to the works of Burnham (1924) and the influence of the White House Conference on Child Health and Protection in 1930. The concern of educators for the mental well-being, for the psychological adjustment of students in schools, and for preparing them to take their places in society, were beginning to emerge in a flurry of pragmatic responses within the school system. With the societal shift of families from an agrarian orientation to an industrial society and with the massive influxes of immigrants from all over the world, the schools found themselves in a process of not only educating students to curriculum, but of "Americanizing" students from diverse cultural and ethnic backgrounds. Schools became the focal point for societal change and cultural assimilation. The role of the student-support professional began to emerge.

As the need for support professionals became recognized throughout the entire educational structure and with the quickly emerging industrial manpower needs of the pre- and post-World War I and II periods, guidance support was evolving in all arenas of education. Post World War II, the adjustment to a rapidly-changing world with an exponentially increasing technological and communications base became part of the educative lessons in school. Psychological education for life became as important as reading, writing, and arithmetic. New roles dealing with mental health and hygiene were beginning to emerge for school counseling and other community mental health professionals in educational settings.

Population expansion, industrialization, prosperity, war, and peace brought important societal changes to which traditional mental health providers had difficulties in responding. The public's increasing demand for equal educational opportunity for all of its citizens raised complicated issues of evaluation, tracking, and specialized curricula. The recognition of the importance of human relations, values clarification, socioethnic differences, and vocational training quickly brought psychoanalytically and psychometrically-oriented mental health professionals into a new awareness. Psychological life skills of an individual became an important educational goal, although not as important as high achievement scores and graduation with a diploma. Traditional delineated forms of psychosocial school guidance intervention and psychoanalytic skills became quickly recognized as ineffective for the school counseling professional and the concentration in graduate training institutions became focused on short-term and group counseling, prevention, coping skills, and program development.

From this complex, uniquely American phenomena emerged the student personnel and guidance professional. Typically recruited from the classroom, after years of teaching or coaching, the role of dean of students or guidance counselor emerged. Early traditional roles included tracking of student attendance and discipline. As society became increasingly mobile following World War II, guidance counselors became additionally concerned with the development of vocational awareness in students. Vocational guidance became the primary emphasis. With the growing social awareness raising from civil rights concerns, the feminist movement, environmental movements, and the Vietnam conflict, school guidance personnel became increasingly aware of the importance of helping students develop social and psychological awareness skills to cope with the demands of the era. With increasing questioning of existential values and attitudes, the increased rate of teenaged pregnancies, child abuse, widespread substance abuse and suicide, counselors found themselves having to respond to students whose academic problems were symptoms of far more complex psychosocial problems.

From the rigorous demands made on school and university student personnel professionals during the 1960s and early 1970s, when schools became society's battleground, concepts of prevention, holism, psychological education, developmentalism, and the attainment of coping skills as important cocurricular activities to be offered by school counseling professionals, began to emerge. Communities looked to school counseling professionals to develop both preventive programs and effective community links to mental health agencies. Counselors were called upon as consultants to treat increasingly complex mental health and developmental problems of students in educational settings. Their work took on functional dimensions of teacher, psychotherapist, consultant, psychologist, and social worker, in addition to the routine guidance function.

This transition and process, in turn, led to the creation of counselors within educational settings who identified more strongly with mental health counseling than the traditional school guidance personnel. Counselor education programs were incorporating much more mental health counseling and psychological content in the training.

The role of the counseling professional in educational settings quickly expanded, yet the economic realities of the 1970s and 1980s obstructed the maximizing of the full potential of this new awareness. With soaring oil prices, rapid inflation, heavy tax burdens, decreased dollar purchasing power, and other economic and political realities of the time, little money was appropriated to schools. What money that remained was committed to a "return to basics" approach whereby basic education was reemphasized instead of affective education. School guidance personnel at all levels found themselves being asked to augment their roles and services, while at the same time they were being cut in funding and staff lines. With counselors being "riffed" from both educational and agency settings, a new independent, more entrepreneurial service provider arose—the mental health counselor. The professional counselor would, working through private practice and consultation models, come to provide many direct and indirect services to school districts and higher education institutions.

Elementary and Secondary Counseling

Several patterns of response have evolved. In many school districts, school counseling professionals were severely cut and the remaining staff have been forced to try to absorb larger loads. Realizing that there comes a point of diminishing returns and, yet trying to remain responsive to student needs, many school counseling professionals have sought to provide more effective links to services through community agencies, private practitioners, clergy, and community groups. While these outside providers have also been beset by the same economic realities as the schools, there has evolved a close working relationship between the schools and the professional counseling providers in a number of communities. Referrals and the development of professional relationships with outside providers has, in many ways enhanced the availability of comprehensive guidance and psychological services available to students in educational systems. Consultation, referral, and support by counseling professionals in the community to school and university systems is becoming more integrated. This has arisen as a result of economic realities, as well as from a genuine embracing of interdisciplinary approaches to the mental health hygiene needs of students at all levels of education.

Where school systems can no longer afford student personnel services with health care, psychological, social work, and counseling professionals to the same extent as in the 1960s, more and more make use of service providers outside of the school. The referral with a consultative link to the institution is becoming more widely adopted. These developments have prompted the U.S. Bureau of Labor Statistics to note that though the employment outlook for counselors will be slow in educational settings, there will be increased opportunities for mental health counselors in private practice (*Occupational Outlook Handbook, 1984–1985*).

These developments force the remaining school counseling staff to assume a more general role, serving as a direct service provider in some instances (usually within the counselor's area of expertise and functional responsibility) and as a coordinator or monitor of a referral link in other cases. What is becoming clearer, however, is that the traditional training and definitions of counselors by work settings have become inadequate to respond to the trends of the future with respect to service delivery to school populations. Lindenberg (1984) suggests that the response should be to define the profession of counseling in terms of being mental health care providers first and to develop the appropriate standards for training and practice and finally to develop the appropriate subspecialities. He criticizes the current professional tact of developing uneven professional standards based upon counselors functioning within isolated work settings rather than starting out with a professional body of knowledge and then picking up subspecialties as appropriate. He argues that the current student personnel service professional will be obsolete as the role of the professional counselor moves from the traditional role through the "generalist" role and eventually to the health care provider role.

Those "guidance" personnel in the school systems will evolve into mental health care specialists incorporating developmental, preventive, and life skills education with an educational orientation. By the same token, they will be relying far more heavily on their clinical mental health counseling colleagues in agencies, health maintenance organizations, private practice, and community agencies to provide the bulk of the therapeutic and specialized services which will become increasingly financed by private group and individual insurance plans, prepaid health care plans or offered through programs for business and industry for the families of employees.

The consequences of this change will necessitate new alliances, patterns of referral, and professional identity among school and college counseling personnel, as well as counseling professionals in private practice, employees' assistance programs, health maintenance organizations, and community agencies. For example, a teenaged adolescent alcoholic of the future may not necessarily be treated by the school counselor, within the school psychological services, but referred back through his/her parent's employee assistance program, as part of business response to the complex needs of the employee's family. Yet, at the same time, the school counselor may be running substance abuse prevention programs within the institution and seeking to educate and, hopefully, to help those who step forward to receive these desperately needed services.

In 1962, C. Gilbert Wrenn, and his associates from the Commission on Guidance in American Schools, were charged by the American Personnel and Guidance Association (now the American Counseling Association) to "look into the future of society, of education, and of the role and preparation of the professional counselor." The commission asked secondary and elementary school counselors about what "counselors will be expected to do in the future" focusing in on the 1980's. While 57 percent of all the respondents from the American School Counselors Association indicated they saw themselves as direct providers of counseling services, about 10 percent suggested that counseling would rely on accessibility to many resources. A majority of elementary school counselors saw the counselor as "serving as a coordinator of many counseling facilities in the school and in the community." They tended to see themselves as resources for parents and teachers and not necessarily as direct providers of service. Counselor educators tended to view the importance of counselors being increasingly aware of: (a) student developmental needs; (b) self-understanding within the context of the culture; (c) the mental hygiene implications of making educational and vocational plans; (d) the importance of mental health and psychological appraisal as it is effected by the use of tests; (e) cultural and vocational changes within our society as it effects the development of students; (f) the role of consultation with teaching staff, administrators, and parents; (g) the mental health implications of the curriculum; and (h) community resources (i.e., community agencies) (Wrenn, 1962).

Nearly a quarter of a century later these prophetic results have become a reality for many counselors. Economics, perhaps as much as professional insight has caused the realization of some of these prophesies. Nevertheless, it is clear that the role of the counselor in educational settings has evolved more as a coordinator and facilitator of services, than as a direct service provider.

Higher Education

In higher education, the trends and patterns are less distinguishable. The existence of college counseling centers at most institutions of higher education was virtually unknown until after World War II. In response to the returning veterans, supported by the G.I. Bill educational benefits, counseling centers were formed to provide academic and career advisement in a civilian world. Dependent upon the mission of the college, the socioeconomic level of the student body, and the regional values where the institution was located, college counseling services were: (a) career planning and placement services; (b) mental health services; (c) academic advising center and/or (d) (more recently), student development centers. Larger institutions tend to have each of these functions in separate quarters, staffed by distinct personnel. Large institutions with departments of psychiatry, counselor education, clinical and counseling psychology typically staff the mental health centers with interns under the supervision of the full-time staff. Smaller institutions and schools without counseling training programs are, with ever increasing regularity either cutting back on or blending their mental health services into other health care services or relying more heavily on community referral by other support personnel. Though undergraduate and professional school populations have high suicide and suicide attempt rates, pure mental health services within the college environment have not only been cut back, but are frequently argued against by misguided interpreters of student development theory who suggest that prevention must prevail over treatment. Administrators feel forced to choose between treatment or prevention, rather than seeking a balance between the two.

Considering the economic climate of the 1980s, it is clear that prevention may survive, but at a decreased level. With this in mind, counseling center directors look more and more to the medical model and have embraced the clinical/counseling doctoral level, license-eligible psychologists who label students with psychiatric diagnoses from the fourth edition of the **Diagnostic and Statistical Manual** (American Psychiatric Association, 1980) in order to make the counseling self-sufficient. Rather than incorporate the developmental and preventive philosophies of the mental health counseling movement in dealing with student concerns, students are subject to a medically-oriented counseling program. Consequently, treatment rather than prevention or adjustment is where the fiscal resources are shifting.

This unfortunate development negates many of the advances of the student development movement and is forcing mental health counselors to adopt the "psychologist" identity rather than retain the counselor or student development specialist model. It is forcing solid training programs in counselor education to abandon counseling identities and respond to the market by seeking psychological accreditation. In any event, while mental health services should be provided by traditional providers on campus, not every client needs a DSM–IV diagnosis, no matter how benign. In fact, in my experience of over fifteen years as a mental health counselor in a college counseling center, I would say that only 5–10 percent of my clients have needed traditional psychiatric out-patient or in-patient services. Most have needed accurate information, help with decision-making, clarification and structure, reassurance and an objective but friendly listener. It is easy to label all cases with insurance-reimbursable diagnoses which would justify the professional counselor's need to see him/herself as one who "cures the sick." Diagnosing all counselees, however, negates the role of the clinical mental health counselor who is both a prevention and clinical provider, not one or the other.

Changes and the Future

A real problem exists with respect to recording the history of and prophesizing the future of mental health counseling in educational settings. Considering the metamorphosis that is transpiring in the helping professions (i.e., the establishment of professional identity by function and not by work setting), it is difficult to calculate how many counselors actually recognize they are functioning as mental health counselors in educational settings and declare themselves as such. Until such time as professional counselors are willing to define themselves categorically and not assimilate into other professions, there will continue to be confusion as to a role and identity for mental health counselors in education.

Yet, it is clear that there continues to be a need for: (1) mental health services to be delivered directly by educational systems; (2) counselors, regardless of professional identification to either focus entirely or partially on mental health counseling as a professional function within educational settings; (3) educative, preventive, and consultative mental health services available either from within or linked with educational systems; and (4) perpetual justification of the need for mental health services within educational systems.

What is sad is that those professional counselors identifying with the extremely important guidance and counseling movement may find themselves providing fewer and fewer services in the future until they realize and adapt to the economic and educational realities of modern life. Accreditation, certification, licensure, and even third-party reimbursement, which heretofore had negative connotations to many counseling professionals now have deliberate professional meaning. The public and allied professions are demanding accountability and excellence in education, yet at the same time allocating less and less resources. A buyers' market currently exists. Why hire a 37-hour master's-level counselor from an ill-defined "counseling" program, when you can get a Ph.D. from an accredited program for not much more. The challenge goes out then to the profession to upgrade its training standards for the limited number of positions envisioned in educational institutions to compete and regain the hold on professional counseling.

REFERENCES

American Psychiatric Association. (1980). *Diagnostic and statistical manual of mental disorders*. Washington, D.C.: APA.

Barry, R., & Wolf, B. (1957). *Modern issues in guidance—Personnel work*. New York: Teachers College, Columbia University.

Burnham, W. (1924). *The normal mind*. New York: D. Appleton & Co.

Dinkmeyer, D., & Caldwell, E. (1970). *Developmental counseling and guidance: A comprehensive school approach*. New York: McGraw-Hill.

Faust, V. (1968). *History of elementary school counseling: Overview and critique*. Boston: Houghton Mifflin.

Ferguson, D. G. (1968). *Pupil personnel services*. New York: The Center for Applied Research in Education, Inc.

Hilton, T. L. (1979). *Confronting the future: A conceptual framework for secondary school career guidance*. New York: College Entrance Examination Board.

Hoyt, K. B. (1970). This I believe. In W. H. Van Hoose & J. J. Pietrofesa (Eds.),

Counseling and guidance in the twentieth century: Reflections and reformulation (pp. 102–117). Boston: Houghton Mifflin.

Lindenberg, S. P. (1984). Mental health counseling: Approaching the 21st century. *Counseling and Human Development, 16*(7), 1–12.

McDaniel, H. B., & Shaftel, G. A. (1966). *Guidance in the modern school.* New York: Holt, Rinehart & Winston.

Miller, T. K., & Prince, J. S. (1976). *The future of student affairs.* San Francisco: Jossey-Bass.

Patterson, C. H. (1971). *An introduction to counseling in the schools.* New York: Harper & Row.

School relationships with the home in the interests of mental hygiene. Unpublished section of 1930 report, Washington, D.C.: White House conference on child health and protection, 1930.

Shertzer, B., & Stone, S. C. (1974). *Fundamentals of counseling: Second edition.* Boston: Houghton Mifflin.

U.S. Bureau of Labor Statistics. (1984). *Occupational Outlook Handbook: 1984–1985 edition.* Washington, D.C.

Van Hoose, W. H., & Pietrofesa, J. J. (1970). *Counseling and guidance in the twentieth century: Reflections and reformulations.* Boston: Houghton Mifflin.

Wrenn, C. G. (1962). *The counselor in a changing world.* Washington, D.C.: American Personnel and Guidance Association.

HIGHLIGHT SECTION

MENTAL HEALTH COUNSELORS IN HOSPITAL AND CLINIC SETTINGS

E. DUANE RIEDESEL

The task of identifying the role of mental health counselors (MHCs) in hospital and clinic settings from a historical perspective is virtually impossible due to the paucity of information about MHCs in the related literature. MHCs have, however, found limited employment opportunities in hospital and clinic settings throughout the United States. In as much as there is a limited amount of historical material, this presentation will be developed largely from personal experience and information developed through association with others who are employed in these types of settings.

There are several reasons for the limited number of MHCs employed by hospital and clinic settings. Perhaps the most important is that MHCs per se are relatively new members of the health-care team and because of this, personnel office staffs at hospitals and clinics are unfamiliar with the services that MHCs can provide. Since MHCs have only been professionally recognized since 1976 (Weikel, 1985), the actual number of active MHCs is not known. Consequently, it is difficult to assess the number who are employed in clinic and hospital settings. It is known that membership in American Mental Health Counselors Association topped the 10,000 mark in 1985 and that this number represents approximately 10 to 25 percent of all MHCs. Of the current AMHCA members, only a small percentage are currently employed in hospital and clinic settings on a full-time basis.

It has long been clear that MHCs are providing professional services of high quality, but as is pointed out in an American Mental Health Counselors Association Journal article (Wilmarth & Beck, 1984), MHCs had never identified themselves as a distinct profession that could or should coexist with social workers, psychologists, psychiatrists, and psychiatric nurses. Wilmarth and Beck further indicate that MHCs have been treated as second-class citizens by their professional colleagues and by federal, state, local, and private agencies in which they were employed.

Another key, and important factor to explain the low numbers of MHCs employed in hospital and clinic settings, is the historical and traditional alignment of the social work profession with the medical staff in hospital and clinic settings. Hospitals for many years have employed social workers to do nursing home placement, public assistance applications, funeral arrangements, patient advocacy, discharge planning, and more recently, counseling services on a one-to-one, family, or group basis. It is the good fortune of social worker professionals to systematically be sought for employment in these work places. The reason for this is not so much that social workers are offering better care, but it is more often the case that MHCs have not taken the initiative to proclaim their expertise in these areas to the persons responsible for hiring.

Traditional work settings for MHCs were identified in the past (Weikel & Taylor, 1979), and at that time, few MHCs reported employment in a hospital setting. Of those persons surveyed, 39.16 percent identified themselves as being employed in a community mental health clinic. The next largest segment reported private practice as their primary work setting. Others reported, in descending order of percentage, were college counseling centers (9.04%), college professor/teacher (6.93%), private agency (7.83%), state agency (6.93%), student (1.50%), and other (9.64%). Those who were not employed in a counseling setting, but identified themselves as a MHC, were less than one percent. In addition, Seligman (1983) reports in her survey that in recent years counselors have increasingly been employed in such nonschool settings as community mental health, health centers, hospitals, and substance abuse centers. If hospital and clinic personnel managers or human resource personnel do not ever see resumes from MHCs, they will more than likely never know the profession exists. Since little is known about MHCs as health-care providers, MHCs have had to make a sales pitch for the profession of mental health counseling as well as for their own competencies within the field of mental health. While this is a cumbersome approach for gaining employment, it is essential to the growth and recognition of the profession. The National Institute of Mental Health (chief federal funding agency for community mental health centers) and the National Register of Health Service Providers recognize only four professional disciplines (psychology, psychiatry, social work, and psychiatric nursing), of which counseling is not included. Until mental health counseling becomes recognized as a fifth core profession, the other core providers will probably continue to enjoy some job market advantages over counseling (Randolph, Sturgis, & Alcorn, 1979).

It is no longer an accepted universal truth in the hospital and clinic settings that only social workers are hired. It is no longer an accepted univeral truth that only Ph.D. clinical psychologists or psychiatrists are capable of understanding and treating human pain and suffering in a therapeutic relationship. MHCs can and do make significant therapeutic contributions in the treatment of the chronically, as well as the acutely, mentally ill in our communities. MHCs are making a much larger impact on the community by providing health care alternatives to the general population in need of counseling intervention but not hospitalization. MHCs are becoming a group of health-care professionals with which to be reckoned. Although there is still resistance and we continue to hear the phrase, "We are looking for a social worker or psychologist to fill this position," employment opportunities for MHCs are increasing. They are increasing because MHCs are challenging the status quo in the health-care industry and, when given the opportunity, are making significant contributions in health-care facilities.

A major step forward is the recent inclusion of mental health counselors in the 1985 edition of the *Occupational Outlook Handbook.* The prospects for employment in hospital and clinic settings will undoubtedly increase as the recognition increases. But, the hard work of breaking down the traditional barriers at the local level will continue to be the sole province of the professionals living and working in the towns and cities across the country.

MHCs will find themselves more employable in hospitals and clinics if they have a specialty interest and developed skills that relate to hospital or clinic settings. For instance, MHCs can take their counseling skills into chemical dependence facilities if they have also received additional training in this area. Rape and domestic assault facilities can use the counseling expertise of MHCs with crisis intervention training. The same holds for MHCs interested in working in trauma centers or hospital emergency departments. Crisis intervention and short-term treatment skills and interventions are essential to clientele seen in these kinds of settings. MHCs are uniquely trained to provide essential proactive interventions, and when coupled with additional, more specialized training, the MHC becomes even more employable.

Familiarization with the hospital or clinic's protocols for dealing with rape, incest, domestic violence, child abuse, substance abuse, violent behavior, and involuntary psychiatric detention are essential. More than simply counseling someone, the MHC needs to be aware of the chain of command procedures for seeing patients, legal ramifications of charting, and legal ramifications of proper sequence of staff intervention. These procedures will vary from setting to setting. The nature of hospital work is basically crisis intervention and short-term treatment.

One of the main considerations for MHCs working in medical settings is learning the language of medicine. A large part of that language for MHCs is contained in the *Diagnostic and Statistical Manual-IV (DSM–IV)*. For some counselors, the process of attaching a diagnostic label to a client is uncomfortable; it is antithetical to their view of the counselor as an individual who promotes positive growth and who does not emphasize past emotional difficulties (Seligman, 1983). Clinic and hospital settings will require the use of diagnosis from the DSM–IV. Familiarization with it and how it is used is a must in order to be able to effectively communicate with the professional colleagues with whom the MHC will be working. That is not to say that you have to agree with the procedure, but MHCs will need to know it and understand it.

In order for MHCs to have any impact among professionals and consumers, they must continue to prepare themselves thoroughly and competently, with expectations of excellence. Professional identity is an important consideration for the development of employment opportunities in hospitals and clinics. This can most effectively be accomplished through knowing what is happening professionally with other MHCs at the local, regional, and national levels. The fledgling MHC should locate a MHC professional organization nationally and in their state in order to build their professional identity. Counselors must encourage their professional organization to lobby the Joint Commission on the Accreditation of Hospitals (JCAH) for inclusion of MHCs as core providers of health-care services. Someday recognition of MHCs by government and private institutions will be commonplace. It will then no longer be the collective struggle of a profession seeking to gain an identity, but a personal struggle for individuals to compete openly and fairly with competent professional colleagues for all employment opportunities in hospitals and clinics.

REFERENCES

Randolph, D. L., Sturgis, D. K., & Alcorn, J. D. (1979). A counseling community psychology master's program. *American Mental Health Counselors Association Journal, 1*(2), 69–72.

Seligman, L. (1983). An introduction to the new DSM-III. *The Personnel and Guidance Journal, 61*(10), 601–605.

Weikel, W. J., & Taylor, S. S. (1979). AMHCA: Membership profile and journal preferences. *American Mental Health Counselors Association Journal, 1*(2), 89–94.

Weikel, W. J. (1985). The American Mental Health Counselors Association. *Journal of Counseling and Development, 63*(7), 457–460.

Wilmarth, R. R., & Beck, E. S. (1984). The professional counselor: A new activist identity or following our own advice. *American Mental Health Counselors Association Journal, 6*(3), 104–105.

Chapter 10

MENTAL HEALTH COUNSELORS IN PRIVATE PRACTICE

ARTIS J. PALMO AND LINDA A. PALMO

As the mental health field continues to grow and change, private practice has become more and more the occupational choice for many mental health counselors (MHC). Recent survey articles (Bubenzer, Zimpfer, & Mahrle, 1990; Zimpfer & DeTrude, 1990) show that large groups of counselors have chosen private practice. The generic definition of private practice is seen as providing direct mental health services to the general public. There are problems with this simplistic definition. First, "What are the direct mental health services provided to the public?", and second, "How can the mental health services be rendered to the public?" The purpose of this chapter is to discuss: (1) the broad array of services that actually comprise private practice, (2) pragmatic issues in delivering services to the public, (3) the advantages and disadvantages of private practice, and (4) professional issues related to the operation of a successful and ethical private practice.

Important Characteristics of the Private Practitioner

As in all career choices, the first step in determining the appropriateness of private practice for an MHC is to take time to reflect on the personal characteristics desired for a successful practice and then compare those characteristics with the personal characteristics of the MHC. An accurate understanding of the demands of the private practice work setting is essential for the potential success of a MHC in this career area.

A strong commitment to the choice of private practice is the most important aspect of operating a successful mental health counseling practice. Regardless of whether the MHC decides to enter full-time or part-time practice, he/she must be willing to devote significant time and energy to the initiation and development of the practice. When trying to determine the amount of time you need to devote to a private practice, the "rule of thumb" is for every hour you spend with a client, you will spend another additional hour working on that case. Therefore, if you desire to carry a weekly caseload of 10 clients, you will most likely spend 20 hours per week in private practice. If you desire to carry a weekly caseload of 25 clients per week, you will most likely spend 50 hours per week! Before entering private practice, the MHC must be realistic about the time and energy commitment that accompanies the establishment of a private practice.

One of the most important characteristics for the private practitioner is the ability to develop a structure and boundaries for their practice. The MHC must discard myths such as "you can make your own hours," "you don't have to answer to anyone," and "you can be your own boss." Certainly these myths have some semblance of reality. However, in truth, the private practitioner must develop an organized system of delivery of client services including set hours, answering to client demands and ethical limitations, and struggling to maintain an appropriate balance between work time and personal time. Although there may be no administrative superior to dictate hours, vacations, or meetings, the successful MHC may work harder with longer hours than those required by an agency or institutional setting.

Finally, the MHC desiring to enter private practice needs both patience and self-confidence. Unlike other positions in mental health agencies, the financial stability of the private practitioner is directly related to the number of clients seen each week. If your practice is budgeted on the basis of serving 25 clients per week, and you are faced with winter storms in January and February that reduce your caseload to 12 clients per week, what do you do to overcome the devastating losses? With this example, the importance of patience and self-confidence becomes obvious.

Potential private practitioners must be confident in their own abilities to effectively serve the public through their counseling and consultation skills while having the patience to develop an effective referral base in the community. The MHC must also have the confidence and patience to believe he/she will recover from the snags and setbacks they may encounter in private practice. Although private practice can eliminate administrative superiors, it increases the MHC's dependency on the general public as consumers of services. Beginning a private practice is a professionally challenging task as well as a financially scary proposition. In order to overcome the challenges involved, the MHC has to have patience and self-confidence to withstand the pressures and demands of a practice.

Components of Private Practice

The mental health services provided by private practitioners can be as individually unique as the private practitioner themselves. As MHCs develop practice goals, they need to consider four general components of private practice: **(1) Counseling Services, (2) Consultation Services, (3) Supervision, and (4) Community Involvement.** Each MHC needs to integrate these components and define the general and specific areas of practice that most interest him/her and meet his/her level of ability.

Counseling Services

The basic component to any private practice is counseling services. Regardless of the services provided in a varied practice, counseling usually is the primary focus of the activities and skill that generates the most consistent revenue in the practice. The MHC can offer individual, group, family, and/or marriage counseling depending on his/her training and experience. It is possible to specialize in unique services such as career counseling, adolescent or child counseling, rehabilitation counseling, or drug and alcohol counseling. But as mentioned above, a broad array of counseling skills is needed to keep the practice functioning in addition to a specialty area focus.

The key to providing counseling services is to know one's own counseling specialties/skills and to recognize the potential needs of the population to be served. First, a MHC may gain expertise in a counseling specialty by academic or experiential training. In either case, it is the responsibility of the MHC to recognize and develop the counseling services he/she can offer as a private practitioner as well as market these specialties to potential consumers. Second, surveying the community needs prior to establishing a practice is always a good idea. Talk about your plans with ministers, social agencies, school counselors, private practitioners, medical doctors, and employers before beginning the practice in order to gain some insight into the needs of community.

Third, the MHC will need to be realistic about whether or not there is a sufficient client base to support a practice in their areas of interest/expertise or whether the interest/expertise areas will need to be expanded.

For example, one MHC wanted to have a practice that specialized in eating disorders of women, a specialty the MHC had developed while working in an in-patient hospital setting for eating disorders. However, the MHC quickly learned that maintaining these clients in an out-patient setting was much more difficult than in the hospital setting. For this MHC, a rethinking about practice goals and professional skills was in order. Professional development of various treatment modalities and counseling specialties is a key to success.

Consultation Services

A second major component of private practice services is consultation. There are typically two types of consultation services that can be incorporated into a private practice: (1) unpaid consultation with MHCs and professionals from other types of mental health settings, and (2) paid consultation with other groups, agencies, businesses, or institutions. In the first type of consultation, the MHC is seeking further information by a free exchange of data and impressions with others involved with the client. Of course, this exchange is always done with the appropriate releases of information. The consultation process is a very important aspect of a successful practice, since the process links the MHC with a broad range of other professionals who may be able to offer services for your clientele and vice versa. The sustenance of a growing private practice depends partially on the ability of the MHC to benefit from interaction with others in the mental health community.

The second type of consultation, establishing paid consultative relationships with other organizations who desire and need your expertise, can offer some exciting and fulfilling alternatives for the MHC in private practice. Specific consulting relationships can be developed with schools, agencies, industries, hospitals, or other professionals needing your services. For example, one MHC was hired as a counseling consultant to offer individual and group counseling for students at a small private school. The school could not afford to hire a full-time counselor, so the MHC was hired to do 12 hours of counseling per week. Another MHC was hired to offer parenting classes at a community center for parents desiring assistance with handling prekindergarten children. One MHC, with a specialty in the elderly, was hired to offer group counseling at a nursing home. These examples are but a few of the multitude of consulting opportunities available to the ambitious and creative MHC in private practice.

Supervision

A third component to private practice is supervision. Being able to give and receive supervision can enhance the viability of a practice. Supervision is a means for the MHC to gain areas of expertise and additional credentials for providing specific services in the mental health field. In addition, no matter what level of training has been reached, every professional MHC needs a system of checks and balances. Therefore, seeking the advice and direction of another professional regarding certain cases being carried in the practice is a necessity on an ethical, professional, and personal level.

Supervision can play a major role in the practice for an MHC in a number of ways. One, the demands that have been placed upon private practitioners by professional boards, insurance carriers, and managed care organizations dictate the need for supervision between and among professionals. In our offices, a group of 10 mental health professionals from various fields, meet once a month in peer supervision groups of 5 to discuss cases and review treatment plans. In this way, we are meeting our own professional needs and the requirements of our certificates and/or licenses. Another form of peer group supervision that has been done by solo practitioners has been to form a group among solo practitioners from one geographical area. This has worked for many of our own professional acquaintances.

A second important form of supervision involves the reimbursement of MHCs by certain insurance groups or managed care companies. Some companies will only recognize certain professional degrees or titles, such as psychologist or psychiatrist. In these instances, the MHC is not accepted as preferred provider of services and cannot receive reimbursement. However, the MHC is accepted with some insurance arrangements if he/she is supervised by a psychologist or psychiatrist. Some MHCs may not accept this arrangement for supervision because they feel their independence is compromised, but that is a decision that needs to be made carefully since finances are a big part of the decision. Depending upon the licensure and insurance regulations in a state, the supervision requirements may vary for MHCs; therefore, each MHC will need to carefully examine his/her state's regulations before entering into private practice.

The third form of supervision within a private practice can be the supervision by an MHC of another counselor's work for financial remuneration. Many new MHCs desire some professional advice and supervision of their caseload, especially when they are beginning to practice. Also, if an MHC has a specialized area of expertise, he/she may be able to market this expertise to others in supervision groups or individual supervision. The sharing of professional techniques and insights is rewarding and expands the domain of private practice to a broader definition of mental health services. Supervision can be professionally stimulating, an opportunity to meet with others, and a way to avoid professional isolation within the practice.

Community Involvement

The final component of the private practice services is community involvement and public relations. Since the general public is the consumer of mental health services, the private practitioner will benefit from developing a visible and definitive image within the community. Community involvement can sometimes mean delivering free services for local groups and organizations, such as the PTA, Diabetes Support Group, Singles Group at the local church, and so on. There is a great benefit gained through taking the opportunity to present and educate the public to the necessity and importance of mental health services. In short, the community service and public relations work done by MHCs on a voluntary basis will promote respect for each individual counselor and the mental health field in general, as well as, develop a broad-based referral network.

Community service is an important professional component and obligation for all MHCs, whether in private practice or another setting. In order to meet the requirements of the MHC's code of ethics and the definition of a profession as outlined in Chapter 3, MHCs should devote some part of their professional life to giving something back to the community. Although this is at times a difficult task for the private practitioner, community service is a necessity for all MHCs.

In summary, the four general components to private practice services can be individually organized and translated by each MHC. It is obvious that part of the autonomy of private practice is the individual's choice of services to be offered. A private practitioner can simply offer counseling services or broaden his/her scope to incorporate a variety of mental health services. The definition of private practice need only be limited by the skills and confidence of the MHC. But one of the fears that may inhibit an MHC from developing a private practice is the "fear of being in business." The pragmatics of a private practice can be dealt with as effectively as any other life problem. Simply pinpoint the issues to be faced in a privately owned business and begin to make choices. Viewing the pragmatics of private practice as business choices diffuses anxiety and enhances the freedom to change directions as one's career develops.

Private Practice Work Settings

There are three different private practice work styles for MHCs: incorporated groups, expense sharing groups, and sole proprietors. Each private practice style has unique characteristics that can meet the particular needs of any MHC. The choice of a particular type of work setting can depend on personal goals, professional goals, and/or simply taking advantage of an opportunity.

In contrasting the incorporated groups, expense sharing groups, and sole proprietors, the differences focus on the structure of the private practice. Incorporated groups may include a diverse group of mental health providers such as psychologists, psychiatrists, social workers, and MHCs or simply a group of MHCs. More than likely in today's mental health market, the incorporated group is a broadly defined group of mental health professionals rather than a singular professional group. The group is bound by a legal document which makes each group member a legal partner in the business. The nature of the legal document creates a dependency between partners for the success or failure of the business. All moneys earned are given to the corporation. Each partner earns a weekly or monthly "draw" (salary) depending on their contribution of time, status, or initial investment. The legal document also clearly defines the procedures for leaving the business.

In expense sharing groups, there may also be a diverse group of mental health professionals or simply a group of MHCs, but there is no legal document that binds the group together as a corporation. Each individual makes his/her own salary and functions as a sole proprietor, but the group shares office expenses or consulting fees for other professionals. Within this structure, the group may eventually become incorporated or an individual may leave and develop his/her own private practice as a sole proprietor. The expense sharing groups usually have contracts defining the specific financial and business responsibilities each professional shares as a part of the group. In this way, there are no misunderstandings of each professional's responsibilities to the group.

Finally, sole proprietors usually work alone in their private practice and develop consulting relationships with other mental health providers. Even though the colleagues of a sole proprietorship are not physically present in the office, the sole proprietor is dependent on a network of mental health providers within the community. Sole proprietors earn their own salary and pay their own expenses. One of the interesting transitions that has taken place over the past few years has been the development of mental health groups comprised of sole proprietors who have chosen to function as a group for generating and maintaining clients, but not losing their autonomy or having to leave their individual offices. These groups are sometimes referred to as "groups without walls" (*Psychotherapy Finances*, published by Ridgewood Financial Institute, Inc., 1016 Clemons St., Ste. 407, Jupiter, FL 33477). Changes in managed care and preferred provider networks have forced private practitioners to examine new and creative professional arrangements to survive in the field of mental health.

As the MHC considers the possibility of establishing a private practice, a complete knowledge of various business and professional relationships is a necessity. Therefore, the authors suggest that the reader attend various workshops sponsored by the American Counseling Association, American Mental Health Counselors Association, or any of the affiliate associations. In addition, there have been books published by both organizations that speak to the establishment of a private practice. In addition, one of the most valuable resources for the private practitioner was mentioned above, *Psychotherapy Finances*. Read as much as you can, talk to other professionals in private practice; and seek the advice of professional financial advisors.

Remember, the initiation of a private practice can be a frightening undertaking; therefore, seek as much advice as possible. In addition, private practice for the MHC is a relatively new career for the majority of MHCs. A review of the past 20 years of the *ACA Journal* will show that there are only a few articles related directly to private practice. For MHCs, they will need to have much patience and self-confidence as they approach the building of a private practice, and not lose focus on the importance of personal integrity for themselves or their clients.

Networking Within Mental Health

The "aloneness" factor can be a major surprise for the MHC in private practice. If one's previous work setting was an agency or educational setting, the lack of continuous daily contact with other professional colleagues can change solitude to loneliness. While there are no distractions, there is also no immediate outlet for the intense demands of continuous counseling cases. If a MHC chooses to work as a sole proprietor in private practice, it is important to recognize the need for professional associations and outlets through local, state, and national counseling organizations. The purpose in establishing a professional network of mental health colleagues is to continue personal growth as well as limit professional burnout.

The concept of working in a group setting of MHCs has several distinct advantages. First, several MHCs working in a group can offer support and encouragement to each other. The group can also provide opportunities for professional growth through discussion of cases and assisting with difficult cases, i.e., cotherapy or psychological evaluation. The ability to conceptualize professional cases and improve counseling skills can only come with continued discussion of cases with other professionals.

Second, MHCs can join in a group with other mental health providers who have complementary skills. For example, within a group of three MHCs, one may have a specialty in child counseling, one in marriage counseling, and the third in vocational assessments. By joining together in private practice, they can offer a broader range of services to the public as well as learn from each other's area of expertise.

Third, the MHC in private practice is dependent upon other mental health providers for consultation and referral. It is advantageous to be able to offer a range of mental health services within one private practice setting. For example, a private practice may consist of a psychiatrist, MHC, and psychologist. If the MHC has a client in need of a psychiatric or psychological evaluation, this can be completed within the group practice. Without the resources of these colleagues within the practice, the MHC would have to refer the client to other agencies or individuals to attain these specialized services. In addition to the consulting role of the psychiatrist and psychologist, they can also serve as a referral source for the MHC and vice versa.

Although there are several advantages to working in a group setting, there is also a risk involved. The association with colleagues within a group practice can have legal and financial ramifications. Being business partners or simply business associates calls for a high level of trust. Before entering or initiating a group practice, an attorney and an accountant should clarify the legal and financial responsibilities of each group member. In this way, later misunderstandings can be avoided. Having a well-written document outlining the association among practitioners is a must.

One final note about networking needs to be made. Whether you become involved in a formal group practice or group without walls, it is very important for the individuals to set specific times and days for meetings, consultations, and/or supervision. Frequently, colleagues in the same office only have contact between counseling sessions or on a haphazard basis, leaving many decisions to hurried moments in-between appointments. Professionals dedicated to networking have to commit to setting aside time for meetings, supervisions, and general conversation.

Pragmatic Needs of the Private Practitioner

Beginning a Private Practice

Relatively few essential items are needed in initiating a private practice office. Unlike other professions, such as dentistry, the MHC may need to make a relatively small financial investment in acquiring the supplies and services necessary to initiate a practice. The essentials for the MHC in practice are office space, office equipment, phone service, answering service/machine, FAX, office supplies, and liability insurance.

The MHC has two choices in selecting appropriate office space: renting or purchasing a professional setting. Most neophyte private practitioners choose to begin practice on a part-time basis and consequently rent office space. In a part-time practice, it is most efficient to rent office space for the time it will be used. If the part-time practitioner chooses to rent office space from an established mental health provider, the benefits can be numerous. The MHC can gain not only office space, but also the use of office equipment, established phone service, and the professional "mentoring" of the more established mental health provider. Renting office space from an established practitioner is also applicable for a MHC entering private practice on a full-time basis. Some practitioners we know have actually rented space in physician's offices or with a group of attorneys.

The other approach for selecting office space in private practice is to purchase an office building or office space. This can be accomplished by an individual or group of professionals. There are several important considerations in determining whether to rent or purchase office space that need to be discussed. First, what are the financial resources available to the MHC? Private practice is a business and success will be dependent on income being greater than expenses. A MHC needs to determine how much he/she is willing to spend for office space, and then decide whether to buy or not. Second, what are the short-term and long-term professional goals of the MHC? Some MHCs have no desire for a full-time private practice while others begin part-time with expressed desire to become full-time. Professional goals are imperative in determining the financial investment in acquiring office space. Third, what professional mental health support systems can be facilitated in this office space? Some MHCs may desire to work with the mentoring of an established practitioner, while others desire more autonomy. The location of office space makes a statement about the MHC's professional identity in the mental health community and with individual clients. By identifying the MHC's individual needs, the choices regarding office location and the option to rent or purchase office space can become quite clear.

Finally, many neophyte practitioners are tempted to establish a private practice within their homes to reduce financial expenses. It takes great self-control to maintain the home as a personal part of the MHC's life when the private practice demands professional time in the home. The ramifications of practice in the home impact on every member of the MHC's family. The MHC must consider the many types of clients he/she will serve and question, "Would I want these individuals to know where I live and have access to my personal home?" The disadvantages of establishing office space in a home are the increase in the feelings of being "trapped" by the practice, the additional feelings of "loneliness" from the mental health community, and the decreased ability to set professional "boundaries" with clients. These disadvantages need careful consideration before selecting this approach to private practice.

Depending on the approach to securing office space, an MHC may need to make decisions about acquiring office equipment and phone/communication systems. In the beginning, a less sophisticated office may be necessary, but as the practice grows, the needs can change drastically. The usual needs for a private practitioner include a desk, several chairs and/or sofa, pictures, tables, lamps, and framed diplomas/certificates. This equipment can also be rented or purchased depending on financial resources and professional goals. Office supply stores or furniture outlets can assist the neophyte in cutting costs. In acquiring office equipment the MHC should strive for professionalism and comfort. The ambience of the office will set the tone for the client-counselor relationship. The office equipment reflects the MHC's identity as a professional. It is important for the MHC to be comfortable within the setting he/she creates, as well as creating a comfortable environment for the clients.

The most important piece of equipment a MHC will purchase is the phone and the type of answering services to accompany the phone. The authors suggest the practitioner secure a professional answering service for the practice versus an answering machine. The answering service seems more personal, is more professional, and provides a means of being contacted in case of emergencies. If the MHC does not have the financial resources to obtain an answering service, then a sophisticated answering machine can be substituted. Be aware that the initial investment in a phone and answering system is high, but a real necessity for a smoothly functioning office.

When using an answering machine, the practitioner has to be sure that the clients reach a professional in times of emergencies. Some of our professional colleagues leave a message for clients indicating one or all of the following: "If this is an emergency and I cannot be reached, (1) call my associate Mr. Frank B. at 555-5555; (2) leave your number with my pager at 555-5555; and/or (3) call Crisis Intervention at 555-5555 for immediate assistance." It is very important that the client have an avenue for receiving assistance in case of a crisis; therefore, the answering machine needs to provide as much information and help as possible.

Office supplies are the necessary materials to be utilized on a day-to-day basis in the office. This material includes: professional cards and stationery, files for record-keeping, intake forms for clients, receipts for services rendered, and any other materials needed in a professional office. These types of materials are a necessity for public relations, billings, and keeping information in appropriate forms at the office. As a beginning, the practitioner should have business cards, stationery, and envelopes, intake forms, file folders, and billing forms. Office supplies are an absolute necessity for the business and professional demands of a private practice.

As a part of today's legalistic society, the MHC must secure professional liability insurance for his/her professional security and employment. Liability insurance not only protects against the possibility of errors of commission or omission, but also is a requirement of many preferred provider and managed care groups who will seek your business. Information regarding various types of liability insurance can be obtained from either ACA or APA. In addition, depending upon whether or not the office is in the MHC's home or another building, the MHC should be sure he/she is covered for any accidental injuries that could occur on the premises, such as someone falling and hurting himself/herself. Since the office eventually becomes a large investment, insurance coverage is necessary to protect against loss of furniture, equipment, and other office materials.

Finally, the amount of money needed to initiate a private practice can vary greatly depending on the needs and desires of the individual MHC. Some professionals begin with a significant amount of financial backing, for example $10,000, while others begin with only several hundred dollars. The MHC must decide how much of a financial risk he/she is willing to take in investing in the pragmatics of initiating a private practice. Financial expenses range from renting office space and equipment to purchasing an office building and equipment. Determining the amount of money to be spent can only be done after a clear set of professional goals has been written. Success is dictated by the professionalism of the MHC, not the financial resources available to the MHC. Private practitioners are in business to provide services to the general public. The office atmosphere is the "icing on the cake."

Attorney and Accountant

Over the tenure of a private practice, the most important professional advisors for the practitioner (in addition to colleagues) are an effective attorney and accountant. As early as possible, the practitioner needs to secure the services of both. Being in private practice means being in business, and it is the MHC's responsibility to protect his/her professional interests, both legally and financially. Private practice is not only doing cases, but also the operation of a business, hopefully, a successful business.

An attorney can serve important roles for the MHC. As professionals,

MHCs are susceptible to the demands of consumers; therefore, to be an effective professional, the MHC must be able to determine what is best for consumers within the ethical guidelines of mental health counseling. Frequently, the process of determining what is best for the client/consumer involves the interpretation of legal as well as ethical guidelines. Having an effective attorney will provide the MHC with the security to provide services that meet the highest ethical standards as well as meeting legal necessities.

In addition, the attorney can provide the necessary advice, determine guidelines, and produce legal documents for the business aspects of the practice. It is necessary to have written agreements before entering any cooperative arrangements with other professionals. In order to do this most efficaciously, the MHC should enroll the services of an attorney.

Finally, with the tremendous growth in family law caused by the increase in divorce and disintegration of the family, attorneys have sought the counseling services of MHCs to handle the resulting personal problems faced by their clients. More and more, a strong relationship between attorneys and counselors is developing because of the needs of children and divorcing adults. Maintaining an effective consultative relationship with an attorney(s) is very important aspect of private practice for counseling professionals. From providing child custody evaluations to handling divorce mediation/counseling to counseling abused spouses, the MHC will find that a full involvement with the legal community is an important aspect of the practice.

Regarding the financial protection of the business, the MHC will need to purchase the services of an accountant. The accountant/business advisor can assist the practitioner in business arrangements with other professionals or agencies; develop an effective accounting/billing system for the practice; take care of the Internal Revenue Service; provide advisement for financial investments; determine retirement plans; and on and on. Since most MHCs do not have a business and finance background, securing the services of a financial advisor is a necessity.

In addition to financial advisement, the accountant can assist the MHC in determining realistic business goals for each upcoming year. For example, the accountant can assist the MHC in determining an appropriate goal for amount of income to be earned in the coming year. Projecting income on a yearly basis assists in the planning of future activities of the practice. The projections can help determine the amount of time to spend with direct counseling services to clients versus consultation versus other professional activities.

If a MHC does not have ready access to an accountant or the financial resources to secure such services, the local banking institutions employ advisors that can be of tremendous assistance. The bank can provide similar types of advisement's regarding investments and future financial planning. The new private practitioner must quickly realize that the practice is a business and take the necessary steps to protect and enhance the business components. As the IRS states, if a business does not make money in three years, it becomes a hobby. An accountant or financial advisor assists the MHC to develop a business rather than a hobby.

Complications. Finally, in order to understand more completely the necessity for maintaining professional contacts (networking) with other mental health professionals, an attorney, and a business advisor, a brief case study will be presented to demonstrate the types of problems that can arise in a practice that necessitates the securing of advice from allied professionals.

> An MHC in private practice was faced with a clear-cut case of child abuse. As a result, the parents of the child were reported to the county office of child abuse. The problems that arose for the MHC as a result of this case were numerous. First, shortly after reporting the abuse, the parents withdrew from the counseling, but the child wanted to remain in counseling with the MHC. Second, the parents had their attorney file papers against the MHC for reporting the abuse. Third, the county children's services demanded significant amounts of time from the practitioner in order to appropriately pursue the abuse charges and provide services for the family. Fourth, the family was referred to another counselor suggested by the agency, but the child refused to attend.

There is obviously much more to this case than is presented in one paragraph, but the brief description of the difficulties provides the necessary information to demonstrate the need for assistance from other professionals. In cases such as the one above, the private practitioner needed advice regarding the best possible ethical, legal, and financial avenues to follow. The MHC utilized two other counseling professionals for advice in addition to consults with the children's agency. Because the case involved abuse, the MHC consulted an attorney to determine her rights legally as well as to obtain advice regarding the necessary services to be provided under the ethical guidelines of the profession.

For the private practitioner involved in a case such as this, another factor soon enters into the picture—finances. First, much of the time spent on the case was not based on receiving fees. Second, the child chose to remain in counseling with this practitioner without the emotional or financial support of the parents. Because of the nature of the case, the child could not ethically be referred to another counselor for fear of further psychological damage. Third, the agency began demanding more time from the practitioner by requesting written reports and attendance at legal hearings. As you can see, the case also began to infringe upon the financial aspects of the practice. If the practitioner were to have several cases such as this at one time, the drain of the financial resources of the practitioner would be outstanding.

The moral to the case that is presented is simple. In order to operate an effective private practice, MHCs must do adequate planning and surround themselves with a set of advisors who will assist them in determining ethical practices, in understanding legal requirements, and in establishing a well-functioning "business" practice. If an MHC is considering a part-time practice as an adjunct to a full-time job, they should remember this case. We have been associated with several part-time practitioners who have faced such circumstances and found them to have a major dilemma on their hands. The demands of abuse cases did not fit with the demands of their full-time jobs, which made them very vulnerable, legally and ethically. Anyone considering part-time practice needs to keep in mind that some cases can be very difficult and quite time consuming.

Referral Sources

The most common error made by the MHC initiating a practice is to neglect the building of an effective referral base. Although the financial investment in the practice is important, it is not the most important aspect of establishing a private practice. If the practice is to grow, the MHC must allocate the time and resources for the development of a strong referral system.

Sources of referral in the community are numerous. They include schools, private and public agencies, churches, businesses, industries, other mental health professionals, hospitals, doctors, rehabilitation centers, and on and on. Gaining access to these agencies and individuals is not always easy; therefore, the planning of methods to gain entry into their offices is a must.

Entry can be accomplished by various means. MHCs can send publications about their practice to the directors of the organizations or to established professionals like doctors, lawyers, school counselors, and judges. In addition, the MHC can direct letters to the heads of various organizations (churches, agencies, hospitals, etc.) requesting to meet with them. Obviously, it is important to attend these meetings as well prepared as possible regarding those services you can provide the individual or organization. It has been the authors' experience that the best access to many of these organizations is through volunteering your services for special programs that you can present. Churches, community agencies, and schools are often very willing to invite a counseling professional to present on topics such as stress, family issues, drugs, parenting, wellness, and other contemporary topics.

Throughout the initiation of a practice, the MHC must always remember that the investment in referral building is an investment in the practice. Doing the work with referral sources sets the stage for the beginning of a successful practice in the community. Although it has not been true 100 percent of the time, most free or nominal fee presentations we have done have created new referrals in the practice. If at all possible, we attempt to make ourselves available for presentations that will add to the referral base for the practice.

Goal Setting

Probably one of the most important activities that a private practitioner can do for himself/herself is to plan, on a yearly basis, the goals for the practice. The planning of goals should be in certain specific areas, including: (1) professional goals; (2) financial goals; (3) skill development; and (4) personal/family goals.

Professional goals include establishing guidelines for the types of activities you will attempt to accomplish over the period of a year. This can include: (1) the number of cases you would like to carry during an average week or month; (2) the types of cases (individual, couples, families, and groups) you want to be carrying; (3) the extent and type of consulting or training you would like to provide; and (4) the amount of supervision you want to do with other professionals. Each of these aspects of a practice needs to be defined within the MHC's skills, desires, and professional aspirations.

In conjunction with the establishment of professional goals, the MHC will also need to set certain parameters for the financial growth of the practice. The number of cases carried, the types of consulting opportunities available, and any other activities to be attempted must be put within the context of the financial aspects of the practice. For example, in order to meet the professional goal of increasing consulting for the year, the MHC may have to do more voluntary types of activities (such as a parenting program for a local agency) while at the same time increasing the number of counseling sessions per week in order to meet established financial goals. The point to be made is that the setting of one professional goal may mean the alteration of other previously established goals.

Third, the MHC in private practice needs to establish a direction for his/her own skill development. In order to continue to grow professionally, the year's activities for training will need to be carefully planned in terms of time away from the practice and the financial investment. The greatest difficulty for the practitioner is the professional loneliness factor. To combat the loneliness, the MHC needs to plan both training and professional organizational involvement to remain a truly effective professional.

Finally, the MHC must establish separate personal goals for himself/herself to remain a well-rounded individual and professional. As counselors continually recommend to their clients, "Take care of yourself!", the practitioner must insist upon establishing a personal life plan for the year. This means setting guidelines and boundaries for the amount of time to spend on the practice each week, the planning of vacations, involvement with the family, and other personal needs. The effective MHC in private practice is the individual who not only attends to the "business" but also attends to his/her own personal life. Modeling "wellness" is an important goal for the practitioner, since the clients watch very closely the activities of the counselor.

Keeping It Together

The mental health of an MHC in practice is central to the ability to deliver effective mental health services to clients. It is impossible to help clients "get it together" if the MHC cannot "keep it together." The MHC in private practice needs to establish limits between personal and professional time to provide for his/her own needs. This is far easier said than done in a full-time practice. The amount of bonding and nurturing inherent in a positive client-counselor relationship can threaten personal development. So much time can be given to others, that there is little time remaining for oneself. The inability to limit professional time can cause both personal and professional failures.

In order to have the level of energy necessary to work with many people on intense and demanding life problems, a MHC must have moments out of the limelight. The "pleasure factor" in adult life is particularly important to the MHC in private practice. It is extremely difficult for the neophyte private practitioner to see how much personal "playtime" can be lost when initiating a practice. A MHC must be a master at identifying his/her own needs for time, space, and nurturing. Because of this, these authors believe that each MHC, at some point in his/her life, should consider therapy for himself/herself. Sitting in the client's seat can deter burnout, foster appropriate limit setting, and enhance personal growth and awareness.

The topics in this chapter cover many issues important for the MHC considering a private practice. Creativity will generate referral sources, while skill and fortitude will sustain the practice. Financial resources can be an advantage but are certainly not a necessity. Self-awareness is a necessity. When the MHC becomes stressed, clients and colleagues sense the hesitancy and the practice falls off. The number of MHCs entering the world of private practice is growing. Within the arena of private practice, the rewards can be numerous, the stimulation evident, and the satisfaction immeasurable. With knowledge, motivation, dedication, and confidence, the MHC can take his/her rightful place among the ranks of mental health providers in private practice.

REFERENCES

Bubenzer, D. L., Zimpfer, D. G., & Mahrle, C. L. (1990). Standardized individual appraisal in agency and private practice: A survey. *Journal of Mental Health Counseling, 12*, 51–66.

Zimpfer, D. G., & DeTrude, J. C. (1990). Follow-up of doctoral graduates in counseling. *Journal of Counseling and Development, 69*, 51–56.

Suggested Reading

Psychotherapy Finances, Ed. Gayle Tuttle, Ridgewood Financial Institute, Inc., 1016 Clemons Street, Suite 407, Jupiter, FL 33477.

HIGHLIGHT SECTION

THE MENTAL HEALTH COUNSELOR
AND HOSPICE

STEVEN P. LINDENBERG

The term *Hospice* derives its origin from the medieval practice of providing shelter to the wounded, infirmed, and weary by monks. It was a place where one who was seriously ill or lost could seek safe haven. In modern times, hospice is synonymous with the concept of caring for the terminally ill. Hospice is a multidisciplinary approach to the palliative care of the dying patient and his/her family. Hospice care treats the patient and the patient's family with pain control as a paramount concern. The phrase "death with dignity" could be called the hospice motto. In the hospice philosophy, the patient manages his/her dying process with the assistance of others. The emphasis is on the "quality" as opposed to "quantity" of life. Hospice is **not** euthanasia (humanely and actively terminating a patient's life in the face of hopeless physical circumstances), since hospice care does nothing to assist the patient in hastening death.

In order for a patient and family to be eligible for treatment, the patient must have a trajectory which projects death to occur in approximately six months. The patient must be aware that his/her disease is incurable and that death is imminent. He/she agrees that interventions will be palliative and not curative. The patient is free to withdraw from treatment at any time. Also, hospice will not abandon the patient or family should the patient live longer than six months. At the time of death, no resuscitation is performed. Orders to this effect appear in the patient's chart. Consent is obtained from the patient documenting his/her understanding and willingness to participate in the hospice program.

Volunteer involvement in the care of the patient is the primary service delivery system. Recruiting, training, and supervising volunteers is the major focus of the professional staff and takes considerably more time than evaluating, admitting, staffing, and managing the actual cases.

Professional intervention is minimal. Medication is generally administered by a hospice nurse under orders from either an attending physician or the hospice medical director. The family participates in caring for the patient to the highest degree possible and is encouraged to be present at the patient's death. Bereavement counseling for surviving family members by specially trained volunteers lasts as long as 14 months on a schedule of decreasing frequency monitored by the staff.

Counseling is a key component of hospice care. In the United States, the Tax Equity and Fiscal Responsibility Act of 1982 (TEFRA) identified the mental health counselor as one of the mental health professionals qualified to provide the counseling/psychosocial services in a Medicare eligible hospice program.

The mental health counselor functions at many levels and is a key member of the multidisciplinary team within the hospice. Administration is one of the counselor's responsibilities and the counselor often has the responsibility for being the patient-care coordinator.

The counselor is often directly involved in hands-on care, especially when the counseling skills needed to communicate or to alleviate emotional pain exceed those skills possessed by the volunteers assigned to the case. More often than not, the skilled professional counselor intervenes to augment and support the volunteers. It is usually in those cases where there are more serious conflicts and sequellae that direct intervention by the mental health counselor is mandated.

Individual, family, and bereavement counseling are the most important components of health care delivery for the hospice. Additionally, the mental health counselor working in the hospice setting, acts as patient advocate and "gatekeeper." For instance, the counselor may consult with a social worker concerning facilitating hospital or nursing home placement for short stays as warranted on a case-by-case basis. Also, the hospice counselor may see the need for psychiatric consult in the event of complications such as organic brain involvement or intractable anxiety and/or depression. Counselors often use their skills to facilitate referral and negotiate palliative medical interventions through team meetings with the attending physician, hospice nurse, and/or medical director.

The hospice counselor participates in the recruiting, training, and supervision of volunteers. Debriefing and monitoring the emotional and psychological well being of the volunteers as well as other staff members is also a component of the counselor's role in the hospice.

The professional mental health counselor is an important fulcrum around which ethical issues are balanced concerning the dying patient. He/she has an integral role in monitoring standards and reviewing cases. The counselor gives the hospice program professional credibility. He/she is the team member best qualified to counsel the dying. As such, the mental health counselor is often the key person in the hospice team.

Chapter 11

COUNSELING IN BUSINESS AND INDUSTRY

MICHAEL SHOSH

P rivate practice, human service agencies and educational institutions have traditionally been the setting for professional mental health counseling; however, since the mid-1940s, mental health counselors have found increasing opportunities to work in business and industry. Two pioneering counseling programs were at the Hawthorne Plant of Western Electric in Chicago and at the Prudential Insurance Company in Newark. The Hawthorne program followed the classic study of Roethlisberger and Dickson (1940) and was available to employees on the plant floor. The Prudential counseling unit was a formal counseling service established by Dr. John Bromer (both programs were terminated by the mid-1950s).

Another key impact on the growth of mental health counseling in business and industry came with the development of Employee Alcoholism Programs, also occurring in the mid-1940s. Originally following the concept of Alcoholics Anonymous' Twelfth Step of "reaching out in recovery," the EAP movement has grown and changed significantly. The focus on alcoholism and drug abuse has broadened to include a wide range of behavioral health issues. In 1972, 25 percent of Fortune 500 companies had some kind of EAP; in 1981, over 50 percent had some sort of counseling program; and by 1990, over 85 percent provided this service to employees.

Professional mental health counselors have played a primary role in the growth of EAPs, as well as in the growth of the field of Industrial/Organizational Psychology. This section will focus primarily on describing the nature of employee assistance counseling and will discuss more broadly on the roles for mental health counselors in other functions in business and industry.

History of EAP

The first recognized Employee Alcoholism Programs were established in the mid-1940s at E.I. DuPont de Nemours, Eastman Kodak, and at Kemper Insurance. These programs were initiated because it was recognized that, through participation in Alcoholics Anonymous, a poorly functioning alcoholic employee could be returned to formerly productive behavior. These programs were generally staffed by volunteers or alcoholism counselors who were themselves recovering alcoholics. These programs required few company resources to operate and were generally successful. Through the next two decades, these programs were modified to include other drug dependencies, and supervisors were often trained to identify symptoms of addiction in their employees and to make referrals to the programs. The passage of the Hughes Act in the mid-1970s provided grant money for the development of employee alcoholism programs and encouraged employers to refrain from discharging employees diagnosed with alcoholism. This opened the door for growth in the field of EAP development and operation. A number of problems were identified with the approach of focusing EAP on chemically-dependent employees: (1) employees using the EAP were stigmatized as addicts; (2) employees did not access the EAP until the late stages of addiction; (3) supervisors were generally poor diagnosticians and were both uncomfortable and resistant to playing the role; (4) the programs focused on identifying an illness instead of a job performance; (5) personal problems unrelated to addiction, but negatively impacting work performance, were often ignored. To address these problems, EAPs began to change their focus. Job performance problems were identified as the focus in making referrals to the program; a "broadbrush" approach (working with a broad range of personal problems) was adopted and EAP came to mean Employee Assistance Program instead of Employee Alcoholism Program. The "broadbrush" approach required EAP staff to have broader training in the areas of mental health assessment and counseling, and the staffing of EAPs became more professionally trained. There was also a recognition that effective EAP professionals needed knowledge outside the clinical arena. In the mid-1980s, the Employee Assistance Professionals Association (EAPA, formerly known as the Association of Labor-Management Administrators and Consultants on Alcoholism) developed a professional certification process to assure that employee assistance professionals could demonstrate knowledge in business and labor management, policy and procedural development, and the identification and treatment of addictions in addition to typical mental health counseling skills. The 1990s have witnessed the continued expansion and modification of EAP staff responsibilities. Issues like workplace wellness, drug testing, and the advent of the HMOs and managed health care have had a significant impact on the role played by EAPs in their organizations.

Types and Models of EAPs

Two types of EAP have evolved over the years: internal and external. Internal EAP is generally located in work organizations with over 2000 employees. Staff of an internal EAP are employed by the work organization and are generally attached to the Human Resources function of a company. They are often housed in the Corporate Medical Department, or they may function independently, answering to top management of the Human Resources function. External EAP provides services to smaller organizations on a contract basis. Staff of an external EAP may be employed by the provider organization or may be employed as independent contractors or consultants. EAP provider organizations vary significantly in size, nature, and sophistication and therefore present various opportunities to mental health professionals.

Most EAPs operate in an assessment/referral model. A client meets with an EAP professional to discuss his/her problem, evaluate the severity and significance of its impact, and to develop a plan of action to address the problem. If some sort of treatment is required as part of the problem-solving process, a referral is made to appropriate professionals outside the EAP. In this model, most clients will receive one to three sessions, although clients requiring educational interventions (stress management) or supportive counseling (grief work) may continue within the EAP. Many clients in this model find that they receive enough perspective, clarity, and/or new information in the assessment/referral process to enable them to manage their problems without additional therapy. A second EAP model is a short-term counseling model which provides clients with up to eight to twelve sessions of brief therapy. This model encourages the EAP professional to establish a therapeutic relationship with a client and strive for problem resolution defined by and using models of brief therapy.

Why Organizations Have EAPs

Companies will generally adopt an EAP for some combination of the following reasons:

Business or Financial Impact: It has been documented in numerous studies that an EAP can have a positive impact on problems like attendance, on and off-the-job accidents, and overall productivity. There is also some evidence suggesting that EAP can significantly reduce the negative impact of chemical dependency on the job by providing early intervention and diagnosis with referral to appropriate levels of treatment. Unfortunately, research in the EAP field is fraught with all of the design problems plaguing most behavioral health research, and data supporting EAP effectiveness is often vulnerable to challenge.

Human Interest: It is not unusual to have a company's management team become interested in having an EAP after their sensitivity to human interest concerns is stimulated. The suicide of a highly visible employee; diagnosis and treatment of alcoholism in a top executive; divorce and the ensuing decline in job performance of a highly valued employee; these situations and others motivate managers to identify effective ways to "help." EAPs may be viewed as the most effective way to systematically provide help for many employees.

Social Pressure: In the business community, most leading companies provide some sort of EAP services to their employees. In addition, the AFL–CIO and their affiliated unions have all spoken out in support of EAP services for their members. These two factors combine to create motivation for company managers to integrate EAPs into their own organizations.

The EAP Counseling Process

Most EAP services are made available to employees and their immediate dependents. Clients may have contacted the EAP on their own, or at the recommendation of a family member, coworker, or friend. These contacts are generally made without anyone else in the work environment being aware. Some clients will be referred to the EAP by a supervisor or manager. These referrals are often made as the result of failing job performance related to a personal problem. In these cases, the referring supervisor and/or human resources manager may be aware that a referral has been made and will expect confirmation of follow through.

Although use of the EAP cannot generally be made a condition of continued employment (outside the exception of drug testing programs), it is not unusual for work organizations to use some form of constructive motivation in difficult cases.

The assessment will be conducted with the client and a plan of action will be developed. The assessment must consider the interaction of drug or alcohol abuse with the presenting problem. It must also consider the relationship between the client's work and the problem, determining the impact of one on the other. The development of a plan to address the problem must involve the client in a significant way to ensure the maximum chance of a positive outcome. Follow-up with the client and any referral resources utilized will help to determine the appropriateness and effectiveness of any plan. In any case where a client is removed from the work environment for a period of time, follow-up may involve reintegrating the individual to the work environment. In the case of supervisor or manager referred clients, follow-up with the referring supervisor is a key to maintaining the integrity of the EAP.

EAP and Confidentiality

Client confidentiality is a major issue in all EAPs. Unless clients feel their contacts with the EAP are confidential and the information they share is carefully protected, utilization of the EAP will be very low and its overall effectiveness seriously thwarted. At the same time, companies purchasing EAP services for their employees may not understand or be sensitive to the need for confidentiality. Isolation of the EAP from the rest of the organization, resulting from too strictly keeping the canon of confidentiality, can also lead to a program's demise as it did in the Hawthorne Plant Program of Western Electric (Levinson, 1983). Counselors working in EAPs are obligated to abide by all the federal and state laws and guidelines regulating the management of information shared by clients diagnosed with behavioral health problems or chemical dependencies. The ethical dilemma presented by clients who present a danger to themselves or the public is one faced by all clinical practitioners. The best ways to avoid problems with confidentiality are to develop policies and procedures which support the maintenance of client confidentiality and to educate all EAP professionals regarding the procedures and importance of maintaining client confidentiality.

EAP Services

Providing direct clinical services in the form of assessment/referral and short-term counseling are the core of any EAP. Many EAPs will also provide additional clinical services in the form of 24-hour crisis intervention and organizational trauma debriefing. Trauma debriefing is perhaps the newest process and was developed in recognition of the emotional impact a traumatic event can have on participants and bystanders alike. Accidents on-the-job resulting in serious injury or death; suicide or the unexpected death of a valued, visible employee; these are examples of situations where trauma debriefings may be useful. In other times of significant organizational stress such as down-sizing or mergers, the EAP may be called on to provide advice and direction to management and/or support for work groups or individuals.

Training and education programs may also be offered through the EAP. Health and wellness programs, smoking cessation, weight loss, and stress management courses may be offered. Prevention and education programs related to drug or alcohol abuse are often associated with the EAP. Almost any topic related to behavioral health is fair game for the EAP professional.

Training in the areas of communications skills, leadership skills, and managerial development, as well as team building, conflict management, and group problem solving are areas where the EAP begins to cross the bridge into Organization Development (OD). Consulting with supervisors and managers on the handling of troubled or problem employees may also cross the EAP/OD bridge.

The EAP may also provide services in the area of career counseling. Career counseling is often viewed as a service unto itself, but the EAP professional may frequently deal with issues related to job design and functions, career development, outplacement counseling, relocation counseling, preretirement counseling, etc.

Industrial/Organizational Psychology and Organization Development

This section on Industrial/Organizational Psychology (I/O Psych.) and Organization Development (OD) is presented here because they provide a significant area for growth and development to individuals trained as mental health counselors.

Although the first graduate degrees in Industrial Psychology were awarded in the early 1920s, the field failed to gain significant recognition until the 1940s, and it was not until 1973 that the American Psychological Association developed a Division of Industrial/Organizational Psychology. The broadly stated goal of this Division was to understand the relationships between people and work (Landy and Trumbo, 1976). I/O Psychology combined three separate movements which all arose independently in the industrial arena. The testing movement gained visibility through the use of intelligence testing in the placement of recruits during World War I. Its roots were based in differential psychology which studied individual differences in personality traits, abilities, aptitudes, interests, etc. The experimental/industrial engineering movement used methods of experimental psychology and industrial engineering to conduct time-and-motion studies and evaluate the impact of the design of machines and work, as well as work environments on the productivity of employees. The final movement to contribute to I/O Psychology was the human relations movement. This movement focused on the feelings, motivations, and interpersonal relationships of workers, and it was out of this movement that the famous Hawthorne study originated. Each movement reached a significant degree of recognition on its own before the interdependence and overlapping impact on productivity caused them to unite under one goal.

Organization Development is an evolving field with its roots in the human relations movement in I/O Psychology. It represents one of today's leading edges of applied behavioral science and is attracting more talented practitioners every day. One definition of OD is that it attempts to improve organizations through planned, systematic, long-range efforts focused on the organization's culture and its human and social process (French and Bell, 1984). It uses techniques and methods associated with group therapy, action research, survey research and feedback, and laboratory training. Individuals trained as mental health counselors and working with business and industry may find the move into OD work as an easy transition filled with challenge and satisfaction. In fact, the work of the EAP professional and the OD professional often overlaps. Consider the following situation:

The EAP counselor for a medium-sized manufacturing company witnessed a sharp rise in the number of clients he was seeing. The increase was made up of employees involved in work on the plant floor and, although each employee presented his/her own personal problem, each talked about changes at work as adding significant stress. The counselor discussed his observations with the Human Resources manager, who explained that the plant was beginning to change its manufacturing process. It was moving away from in-line manufacturing, where a product essentially moved down an assembly line, to a team concept where products would be assembled in total by small groups of employees. This move was seen as necessary to keeping the company competitive by making its manufacturing process more flexible and responsive to customer demands. What was not considered was the impact this change would have on workers who were comfortable with the old process and did not understand the value of teams, or who were not interested in sharing responsibility with a team. The EAP counselor joined the company's training department and additional OD consultants in developing a process to enable the people most affected by this change to make the transition with less fear and resistance and more understanding and positive energy. Ultimately, this process directly reduced the amount of work stress experienced by plant employees, thus completing the loop.

In order for this situation to have occurred, the EAP counselor needed to be sensitive to the relationship between a client's presenting problem and his/her work environment. The EAP counselor needed to feel comfortable with operating managers in the organization and they needed to regard the counselor's input as credible. This means that the counselor needed to use language and concepts which could be understood by management and to present ideas which were related to the company's values. This requires a level of training and experience which often goes beyond pure clinical skills.

Summary

The aggressive business environment of today has put significant pressure on organizations to get the greatest level of productivity out of each employee. This increased concern in worker productivity makes each employee a more highly valued resource and has increased the demand for professionals who understand human motivation, interpersonal behavior and group dynamics. Counseling professionals specialize in this kind of understanding. Counselors contribute to business and industry by working with troubled employees and returning them to full productivity. More proactively, they provide training, education, and management consultation aimed at creating and maintaining healthier work environments and emotionally healthier employees. Graduate programs conscious of this market for counselors in business and industry are providing degrees of various aspects of I/O Psychology, Organization Development, Human Resource Management, and even workplace counseling. Business and industry represent a fertile environment for mental health counselors interested in broadening their vision and their influence.

REFERENCES

Cairo, P.C. (1983). Counseling in industry: Selected review of the literature. *Personnel Psychology, 36* (1), 1–18.

French, W.L., & Bell, C.H., Jr. (1984). *Organization development: Behavioral science interventions for organization improvement.* Englewood Cliffs, NJ: Prentice-Hall.

Kets, deVries, M.F.R. (1991). *Organizations on the couch.* San Francisco: Jossey-Bass.

Landy, F.J., & Trumbo, D.A. (1976). *Psychology of work behavior.* Homewood, IL: Dorsey Press.

Levinson, H. (1983). Clinical psychology in organizational practice, *occupational clinical psychology.* New York: Praeger.

Manuso, J. (1983). *Occupational clinical psychology.* New York: Praeger.

Masi, D.A. (1984). *Designing Employee Assistance Programs.* New York: Amacom.

Parsons, R.D., & Meyers, J. (1984). *Developing Consultation skills.* San Francisco: Jossey-Bass.

RESOURCES

Professional Organizations:

1. Employee Assistance Professionals Association (EAPA)
   2101 Wilson Blvd., Suite 500
   Arlington, VA 22201
2. Employee Assistance Society of North America (EASNA)
   2145 Crooks Rd., Suite 103
   Troy, MI 48084
3. American Society of Training and Development (ASTD)
   600 Maryland Ave., Suite 305
   Washington, DC 20024
4. NTL Institute
   1501 Wilson Blvd., Suite 1000
   Arlington, VA 22209

5. OD Network
   52 Treaty Elms Lane
   Haddonfield, NJ 08033

HIGHLIGHT SECTION

THE MENTAL HEALTH COUNSELOR
AS CONSULTANT

JAMES A. BOYTIM

During the 1979 American Personnel and Guidance Association Convention (now the American Counseling Association), Dickel, Huston, and Boytim presented the program, "Consulting: New Roles, New Clients, New Trends." The presenters observed that when they were enrolled in their doctoral programs in the late 1960s and early 1970s, there were no elective courses in the consultation process, "how to" books on the topic were not readily available, and key journals had not yet used the theme of consultation for special issues. Since then, much has been written on the subject (see sample resources listed at the end of this section) and training opportunities for counselors to learn about the consultation process have increased. These changes suggest the reasonableness of a paragraph written by the author to a colleague shortly after the convention program:

> Fee for service, part-time consultation is likely to increase in the future roles assumed by counselors. Prevention and growth are stressed in mental health agencies, the holistic approach to medicine is increasing, and trained professionals will seek new avenues of service under the general label "consultant." Qualified, ethical, responsible consultants will open new opportunities for employment for human service workers. (Boytim, personal communication, May 18, 1979)

What is consulting? Lippitt and Lippitt (1978) have described consultation as a two-way interaction, as "a process of seeking, giving, and receiving help. Consulting is aimed at aiding a person, group, organization, or larger system in mobilizing internal and external resources to deal with problem confrontations and change efforts" (p. 1). Miner (1992) suggests that most consulting is very much a "feast-or-famine matter," partly because business conditions may dictate a client's willingness to pay for it. He believes that success requires "giving clients what they want so that they will come back for more, and doing a certain amount of marketing of one's services" (p. 12).

Organizations hire consultants for a variety of reasons. In his book, *The Consultant's Kit,* Lant (1981) offers several examples: to augment staff, provide expertise, provide objectivity, identify problems, act as a catalyst, to instruct, and to influence others (pp. 4–5). Gelso and Fretz (1992) believe that consulting is very cost-effective as a strategy for providing preventive, remedial, and developmental services and is congruent with using individuals' assets and strengths within all types of organizations. Kurpius (1985), in concluding an article on consultation interventions, suggests these approaches will be central to mental health services in work settings:

> It is quite possible that in the future a large portion of mental health services will be provided at the work place in the form of prevention and development rather than remediation. . . . If we believe completely what we espouse, that people do make the difference, maybe consultation with the many existing interventions could intervene in a positive way and make the difference that is desired by so many (p. 386).

The services a mental health counselor (MHC) offers in consultation will depend on that individual's special interests, talents, knowledge, reputation, and experience. Additionally, the opportunities that exist within the community and the openness of organizations to the use of outsiders will vary. Sample organizations that may use MHCs as consultants include:

Educational units —universities, colleges, schools (public or private at any grade level), preschool programs, adult education programs, in-service programs, special populations or departments, state departments of education, alternative education units, literacy programs, professional unions or associations, parent groups, or student service personnel departments;

Professional office groups —medical corporations, dental partnerships, hospitals, hospices, nursing homes, legal firms, and service providers such as realtors, financial institutions, insurance firms, retailers, recruiting and outplacement firms, preretirement planners, and professional associations;

Industrial and business organizations —major corporations with multiple production, research, or service locations, single operation plants or offices, small business firms, the hospitality industry, and home-based entrepreneurships;

Branches of government —federal (including military installations), state, county, local, special programs funded by tax revenues (such as those provided by area agencies on aging);

Volunteer or community service units —United Way affiliates that provide youth services, recreation, support for the homeless or abused, or other community programs and volunteer efforts designed to address local concerns;

Religious system outreach programs —sponsored counseling clinics, retirement homes, nursing facilities, day care services, or foster care programs;

Support groups —self-help groups of all types, informational groups, awareness groups, and community improvement organizations.

Perhaps Lant (1981) captured the opportunities that may exist for counselors when he said, "The only limitation in consulting is a person's imagination. No matter how obvious the solution to problems might seem, people can use help in solving them, and they are willing to pay for that help" (p. 4).

MHCs seeking consultation opportunities may wish to consider these suggestions as they get started:

1. Determine those skills, talents, interests, experiences, and unique qualities in your possession that provide the base for offering services to specific organizations.

2. Consider how much time you have to devote to this aspect of your career and set aside time to develop the necessary skills.

3. Decide, within current ethical guidelines, how you will market your skills. You need to let others know of your availability, your interests, your successes, and your abilities.

4. Broaden your reading to include new areas that will enable you to communicate with the groups you serve.

5. Establish new contacts among potential client organizations. Also, develop a network of consultants upon whom you may call if you need specialized help.

Sample Cases

Dental Office Consulting. This author served as a consultant for a dental office group for a period of twelve years (Boytim, 1983). In general, this concerned six issues within the office: (1) prevention or reduction of personal stress; (2) protection or improvement of mental health within the office staff; (3) development of coping strategies that are humanistic in orientation; (4) improvement of the employee selection process; (5) development of greater group cohesion among all staff members; and (6) enhancement of the practice of participatory management. While the time devoted to this consultation differed from month to month and the topics changed as new issues were considered, the writer's services were used on a regular basis during an extended period.

A partial list of projects undertaken included:

Staff Training — provided new insights and procedures to reduce stress generated by anxious patients, time pressures, cancellations, economic pressures, esteem issues, family problems, and isolation; taught basic counseling skills to staff so that employees viewed patients in a more holistic manner; provided models to help understand personality and to improve listening skills (Glasser, Maslow, Berne, Gordon, others); used a variety of self-assessment instruments to have staff members recognize personal strengths and appreciate differences among the employees.

Office Management — developed new hiring procedures that involved all employees in the interviewing and selection process; introduced participatory management opportunities (agenda building, special project leadership assignments, and revision of the office procedure manual and job descriptions); revised information letters for new patients; established yearly schedules for employee evaluation, fee revision, and budget review.

Direct Consultation — helped the dentist to write a professional practice philosophy; assisted in developing long-range plans; discussed implications for dental practice of insurance policy changes, marketing trends in dentistry, and local demographic changes.

Industrial Consulting. For fourteen years, the writer was a consultant for a manufacturer of industrial crystals and oscillators. This was an informal, on-call arrangement with the president of the firm to "help me, help the company," as he expressed the tasks at the outset. Among the areas of service provided were: (1) direct consultation with the president, personnel director, senior engineers, sales director, and others holding key management positions; (2) training and consultation with supervisors; (3) counseling services for employees; and (4) activities designed to reduce or prevent work-related problems or stress among employees.

Among the services provided were:

Direct Consultation — met with the president and his senior staff members twice yearly in preparation for employee plant meetings; reviewed employee suggestions for possible implementation; provided recommendations for resolving occasional employee-supervisor or supervisor-supervisor conflicts; suggested modifications in the employee handbook to clarify work conditions and benefits.

Supervisor Training — discussed management styles; lectured on topics requested by the president (for example, "Stress in the Work Place," presented to all salaried personnel); used self-assessment inventories to improve staff interactions.

Counseling Services — provided short term counseling sessions for employees upon request of the president, personnel director, or plant manager (held either in plant or at the author's private office).

Family Business Consultant. The third example will be briefer than the first two, in part because it took less time and in part because the number of people involved was very limited. For several months, I worked with a husband-wife team, owners of a retail/service business with fewer than twenty employees, who were planning for their retirement and were selling the business to a son who had worked for the firm for several years. The major issues were the transfer of power and decision-making responsibilities and finding common ground between two philosophies of business and two management styles. Several meetings were used to establish goals and timelines, practice conflict resolution and problem solving skills, resolve values clashes, and review progress. The outcome was an orderly transfer of company leadership, the eventual retirement of the new owner's parents, and continued success of the business.

In closing, the number of MHCs engaging in consultation will continue to grow as the next century approaches. Preparation will improve and competition for contracts will increase. The reader who wishes to expand activity in this area of service should heed this comment from the preface of Lippitt and Lippitt:

> The process of consultation is challenging, awesome, rewarding, and humbling. It is not a science, but as a performing art, it requires the constant growth of those who practice it.

At the same time, one needs to be aware of the new emphasis being placed on consultation in counselor training and a recent challenge given by Brown (1993) to those who would be professional practitioners of this art:

It is . . . abundantly clear that we as a professional group need to take a stand on the training of counselors and insist that counselors of the future be fully trained as consultants or that they refrain from engaging in the process (p. 142).

REFERENCES

Boytim, J (1983). The counselor as dental office consultant. *Arizona Counseling Journal, 8* (1), 28–34.

Brown, D. (1993). Training consultants: A call to action. *Journal of Counseling and Development, 72* (2), 139–143.

Dickel, C., Huston, R., & Boytim, J. (1979, April). Consulting: New roles, new clients, new trends. Presentation given at the American Personnel and Guidance Association Convention, Las Vegas, NV.

Gelso, C. J., & Fretz, B. R. (1992). *Counseling psychology.* Forth Worth: Holt, Rinehart and Winston.

Kurpius, D. J. (1985). Consultation interventions: Successes, failures, and proposals. *The Counseling Psychologist, 13* (3), 368–389.

Lant, J. L. (1981). *The consultant's kit.* Cambridge, MA: JLA Publications.

Lippitt, G., & Lippitt, R. (1978). *The consulting process in action.* La Jolla, CA: University Associates.

Miner, J. B. (1992). *Industrial-Organizational Psychology.* New York: McGraw-Hill.

RESOURCES

Boytim, J. A., & Dickel, C. T. (1990). Helping the helpers: Teacher support groups. *Resources in Education,* 25 (12). (ERIC: ED 321-199). As Employee Assistant Programs become commonplace in business and industry, counselors in school settings are encouraged to use some professional time to help teachers and other school personnel through the development of in-school support groups. Ideas can be used in other work situations by EAP counselors.

Dorn, F. J. (1986). The road to workshop consultation: Some directions for the new traveler. *American Mental Health Counselors Association Journal, 8* (2), 53–59. This article provides mental health counselors with an overview of how to become involved in delivering staff development workshops to specific audiences.

Dougherty, A. M., Dougherty, L. P., & Purcell, D. (1991). The sources and management of resistance to consultation. *The School Counselor, 38* (3), 178–186. Issues related to resistance in school settings are reviewed. Understanding the sources of resistance may lead to increased opportunities for consultation with a greater proportion of school personnel.

Kormanski, C. (1988). Using group development theory in business and industry. *Journal for Specialists in Group Work, 13* (1), 30–43. The author examines and compares theories of group development and identifies trends in business and industry that characterize the group process.

Kurpius, D. J. (1982). Conceptualizing group process consultation as an OD intervention.

Journal for Specialists in Group Work, 7 (1), 12–20. Many of the common stages of group development that occur in counseling groups can be seen during group consultation. This article provides a discussion of group consultation as an important intervention for organizational development specialists.

Woody, R. H., Hansen, J. C., & Rossberg, R. H. (1989). *Counseling Psychology: Strategies and Services.* Pacific Grove, CA: Brooks/Cole. See Chapter 9—Consultation, pp. 171–185.

JOURNAL SPECIAL ISSUES ON CONSULTATION

The Counseling Psychologist (July 1985), 13 (2). Contains four major articles followed by related reactions/extensions with Duane Brown and DeWayne J. Kurpius as guest editors.

Elementary School Guidance and Counseling (February 1992), 26 (2). Consists of two editorials and eight articles assembled under the direction of Edwin R. Gerler, Jr., editor.

Journal of Counseling and Development (July/August 1993), 71 (6). DeWayne J. Kurpius and Dale R. Fuqua serve as guest editors for a special issue on the conceptual, structural, and operational dimensions of consultation. Sections include: (1) conceptual and operational foundations of individual, group, and organizational consultation (seven articles); (2) assessment and organizational diagnosis (two papers); (3) the impact of organizational culture on change (two selections); (4) how contextual differences influence consultation programs (three offerings); and (5) quantitative and qualitative dimensions in consultation research (three contributions).

Journal of Counseling and Development (November/December 1993), 72 (2). DeWayne J. Kurpius and Dale R. Fuqua edit the second special issue, this time with the focus on prevention, preparation, and key issues. This continuation of the above sections and the number of articles in each include: (6) primary prevention consultation: conceptual orientation and special programming (two); (7) professional preparation of consultants: supervision and standards (two); and (8) trends and topical issues in consultation (eight).

The Personnel and Guidance Journal (February 1978), 56 (6). Includes an introduction and overview of consultation, six articles on consultation models and operational procedures, and five examples of field-tested consultation programs in schools, colleges, and mental health clinic programs with DeWayne J. Kurpius as guest editor.

The Personnel and Guidance Journal (March 1978), 56 (7). Nine articles on topical issues and features in consultation and four on training consultants with guest editor DeWayne J. Kurpius.

HIGHLIGHT SECTION

MENTAL HEALTH COUNSELING AND ALCOHOL AND OTHER DRUG ABUSE

DAVID VAN DOREN

M ental health counselors (MHCs) can provide important services in the area of alcohol/drug abuse and dependency. The role of the MHC varies depending on the setting, the stages of abuse or dependency, and the expertise of the MHC. Because of the many frustrations of dealing with manipulative and highly defensive clientele, counselors may attempt to avoid working with clients with alcohol and other drug problems. However, since these problems pervade all counseling settings and all types of clientele, this escape is impossible. The counselors who fail to recognize chemical abuse issues do a great disservice to their clients and to the profession. MHCs need to be a significant part of prevention, intervention, rehabilitation, relapse prevention, and recovery for the chemical abuser and his/her family.

INCIDENCE AND PREVALENCE

Schuckit (1989) estimates that between 5 and 10 percent of drinkers in the United States develop some type of drinking problem. Alcohol abuse was found to be the most common of 15 major psychiatric disorders with a prevalence rate of 11.9 percent for men and 2.16 percent for women and lifetime prevalence rates of 23.83 percent for men and 4.75 percent for women (Helzer, Burnham, & McEvoy, 1991). Kaplan and Sadock (1988) estimate there are 400,000 to 600,000 heroin addicts. Peluso and Peluso (1988) report an estimate of two million cocaine addicts. The U.S. Department of Health and Human Services (1990) estimates that 3.3 million use marijuana daily. Each of these individuals has a direct impact on the lives of significant others, which leads to many more millions of people in the United States directly affected by alcohol abuse, alcoholism, and other drug abuse and dependency.

The MHC cannot escape dealing with chemical abuse and its aftermath. Family therapists, employee assistance personnel, school counselors, counselors in community counseling centers, and private practitioners all must be aware of the signs and symptoms of chemical abuse and dependency and take an active role in addressing this societal concern.

ASSESSMENT AND INTERVENTION

Denial is a major defense mechanism used by chemically-dependent clients and their families. MHCs have a role in the assessment and intervention of chemical dependency, requiring the examination of clients' chemical use patterns and related damage. Affective disorders, anxiety disorders, conduct disorders, antisocial personality, and other mental health problems are diagnoses often given to the chemically dependent client who is seeking help for behavior problems while protecting the chemical use. It is vital to confront the substance abuse or dependency disorder prior to or concurrent with treatment of other disorders. In some cases, the symptoms of these other disorders will dissipate with a healthy chemical dependency recovery process.

The three most common psychiatric disorders associated with alcoholism are affective disorders, anxiety disorders, and conduct disorders (antisocial personality). Forty-seven percent of alcoholics have a diagnosis of a second psychiatric disorder. The lifetime prevalence of major affective disorders among alcoholics is between 18 and 25 percent, while prevalence of depressed mood, sleep or appetite disturbance, and cognitive disturbance in the alcoholic population ranges from 20 to 90 percent (Helzer et al., 1991). Alcoholics are 21 times more likely to be diagnosed as having antisocial personality than nonalcoholics (Helzer & Przybeck, 1988).

Estimates of substance abuse among chronically mentally ill young adults range from 15 to 60 percent. Drug users also have high rates of alcoholism. Thirty-six percent of cannabis users, 64 percent of stimulant users, and 84 percent of cocaine users met diagnostic criteria for alcoholism. Antisocial personality, mania, and schizophrenia are highly associated with alcoholism and other drug dependence (Helzer et al., 1991).

The therapeutic effectiveness of the MHC demands the recognition of the widespread abuse of chemicals and the high percentage of mental health clients who are affected by abuse and dependence. Differential diagnosis and dual diagnosis require an understanding of the chemical dependency process as well as an understanding of mental health disorders.

When other disorders are addressed without acknowledging and confronting alcoholism and/or other chemical dependency, the MHC enables the abuse to continue. Attempts to address chemical dependency without treating an appropriate dual diagnosis greatly increases the possibility of relapse. Effective mental health counseling includes (1) the recognition of chemical dependency and confrontation of this dependency process, (2) the assessment of other diagnoses, and (3) the implementation of a treatment plan which addresses all relevant diagnoses.

AODA TREATMENT

Within chemical dependency treatment programs, various roles exist for the MHC. The treatment of chemical dependency necessitates the confrontation of the client's abusive behavior pattern. Exploration of the damage connected with the use/abuse of chemicals and the recognition of the loss of control over the chemical facilitates growth and development of the chemically-dependent client. Intensive treatment programs are usually provided in outpatient facilities. However, when related health problems, detox, or other significant factors threaten recovery, inpatient treatment may be necessary.

Within the context of intensive treatment, MHCs may facilitate the client's recognition that specific personal issues are related to the abuse of chemicals. Acknowledging these other personal concerns (e.g., sexual abuse, depression, anxiety, poor self-concept, poor interpersonal skills) and exploring their connection to the client's chemical use facilitates relapse prevention. Although these other concerns may need to be addressed, chemical dependency must be the primary focus of treatment. After the recovery process has begun, the MHC can further explore these other issues. A primary focus upon other problems may allow the client to delay or avoid an acceptance of chemical dependency. Effective mental health counseling requires differentiating primary and secondary chemical dependency and providing a treatment plan which incorporates dual diagnoses and/or other related symptoms.

Following an intensive treatment program, MHCs can play a significant role in effective aftercare which will enhance ongoing recovery. Ten percent of the recovery from chemical dependency takes place in the initial intensive treatment, while 90 percent occurs afterwards (Royce,

1989). Lifestyle changes are needed and emotional and behavioral concerns must be addressed in order to cope without the chemical. Many alcoholics and other chemically-dependent individuals seek help to develop sober/straight lifestyles through Alcoholics Anonymous, Narcotics Anonymous, or other self-help groups. MHCs need to learn about these programs and integrate the use of support systems into the overall counseling experience.

Personality issues which led to chemical dependency or issues developed during the dependency process need to be addressed during ongoing recovery. Sexual abuse, affective disorders, violent behavior, anxiety disorders, marital problems, or other issues may be associated with chemical abuse and dependency. Some of these concerns may be resolved through the elimination of chemical use, but often further counseling to deal with these concerns is needed to facilitate continued sobriety. If not successfully addressed, the behavior problems may lead to a relapse.

All human beings struggle at times to cope with problems. The MHC must recognize that the prime coping mechanism for chemically-dependent clients has been to escape through the use of chemicals. Personal problems need to be approached directly and new means of coping developed. It is necessary to acknowledge that early sobriety may be threatened by the personal struggles in the client's life unless new forms of coping are developed.

RELAPSE PREVENTION

Relapse rates ranging from 50 to 90 percent of individuals recovering from chemical dependency have been reported in the literature (Gorski, 1986, 1989; Marlatt & Gordon, 1985). Gorski (1986) suggested that only 10 to 20 percent of recovering alcoholics have experienced a successful recovery without any relapses.

Relapse is a process, a progressive pattern of affect, behavior, and cognition, which reactivates the symptoms of chemical dependency (Gorski, 1986, 1989). In this context, taking a drink is the endpoint of the relapse process. An alcoholic or addict is in the process of relapse when there has been a return to the thinking, feeling, and behaving which have previously had a drinking outcome.

Marlatt and Gordon's (1985) review of the research found that the three most common relapse determinants were the presence of negative emotional states, interpersonal conflicts, and social pressure. Relapse can be a time of learning. If the individual explores the personal determinants for relapse, this process may be identified, coping may be increased, and the individual's expectations of successful recovery may be enhanced.

A number of relapse prevention programs have been developed (Gorski, 1986, 1989; Krippenstapel, 1987; Marlatt & Gordon, 1985; Teichman, 1986). Marlatt and Gordon's program appears to be the most thoroughly presented approach, incorporating a strong cognitive-behavioral emphasis. The three major aspects of this prevention effort are: (a) identifying situational determinants for relapse; (b) addressing cognitive factors; and (c) promoting lifestyle modification. MHCs have the skills required to develop and implement effective relapse prevention programs, facilitating long-term sobriety.

THE CHANGING PERSONNEL IN AODA TREATMENT

Treatment providers in the alcohol and other drug field have often been recovering alcoholics and addicts. As chemical dependency treatment has evolved, more master's level professionals have entered the field. A survey of AODA counselors in New England revealed that 45 percent of respondents had a master's or doctoral degree (Mulligan, McCarty, Potter, & Krakow, 1989), while a similar survey in Pennsylvania reported 58 percent had received graduate training (Blane, 1985). Counselors with graduate degrees are less likely to be recovering, are more likely to be working in outpatient settings, spend more time providing individual counseling, and are more likely to attribute the cause of alcoholism to learned behavior (Kolpack, 1992). The MHC's skills and knowledge of the counseling process can promote personal growth and learning. In order to individualize treatment, the counselor must (1) recognize the personal concerns of the client, (2) design a treatment plan addressing the chemical dependency, and (3) facilitate the development of life skills which will enable the client to cope without chemicals. The MHC must have the skills to recognize the personal dynamics of the abuser, the knowledge and ability to facilitate change, and the willingness to focus on the chemicals in order to be an effective treatment provider.

AFFECTED FAMILY MEMBERS

Children of alcoholics (COAs) are at high-risk for developing chemical dependency. Heredity and environment contribute to the ongoing cycle of dependency. Children of alcoholics have higher rates of delinquency than those from nonchemically-dependent families (Whitfield, 1979). Lawson (1983) reports that they may have emotional problems (suicidal tendencies, depression, lack of self-confidence, fear of abandonment) and social and interpersonal problems (family relationship problems, adjustment problems, overresponsibility, inability to trust). A vital aspect of prevention and treatment of chemical dependency is the necessity of addressing these issues of children of alcoholics or children of chemically-dependent families. Fifty to 60 percent of the alcoholics (Black, 1986) and up to 80 percent of cocaine addicts (Shulman, 1987) are children of alcoholics.

COAs have lower levels of self-awareness and a tendency to be externally-focused in terms of self-evaluation (Sheridan & Green, 1993). Unpredictability and inconsistency are common characteristics in homes where there is chemical dependency (Wallace, 1987). Compared with children of nonalcoholic families, children of alcoholics describe their families as more dysfunctional and report less guidance from significant adults in their lives (Clair & Genest, 1986). Children of alcoholics are more likely to adopt unhealthy roles in an attempt to cope than are those from healthy families (Jenkins, Fisher, & Harrison, 1993). Clinicians have identified clear roles that children of alcoholics utilize to cope with familial alcoholism (Black, 1979; Wegscheider, 1981). Some research appears to support the development of these roles (Mucowski and Hayden, 1992), while others suggest that multiple roles may be developed (Jenkins, Fisher, & Harrison, 1993). Often these roles do not create problem behaviors in the family of origin (Black, 1986), but may be less functional when leaving the chemical dependency system. Children of alcoholics are seen as a special at-risk population, with many exhibiting psychological, medical, and social problems and being at risk for substance abuse and dependence (Wallace, 1987).

Children of alcoholics may enter counseling for a variety of reasons, but may not recognize the connection between these reasons and their family experiences. It is up to the MHC to explore family history and examine the impact of alcoholism and other chemical dependency. Education may play a significant part in the early counseling process, thus helping the client to understand the development of chemical dependency and its effect on others. Examining the coping mechanisms utilized and opening up feelings which have long been repressed become important parts of the recovery process. Many affected family members live their lives feeling inadequate and playing the role of victim. Counselors who understand the affective and cognitive processes and the impact of the dysfunctional family on early development are able to be significant caregivers in this area.

CONCLUSION

The alcohol and other drug treatment field continues to develop as new approaches to prevention, assessment, intervention, treatment, and relapse prevention evolve. The MHC should be aware of these approaches in order to effectively serve as a core provider for this population of chemically-dependent clients and others affected by their chemical dependency. Knowledge of chemical abuse/dependence and the treatment process is essential for all MHCs. This knowledge base, along with an understanding of mental health disorders and their treatment, provides a solid background for a chemical dependency professional. MHCs can then serve as active facilitators of the recovery process and avoid being enablers of chemical dependency. Chemical dependency treatment must continue to focus on the role of the chemical, while also incorporating this multifaceted, holistic perspective on recovery.

REFERENCES

Black, C. (1979). Children of alcoholics. *Alcohol, Health, and Research World, 4*(1), 23–27, 1979.

Black, C. (1986). Children of alcoholics. In R. J. Ackerman (Ed.) *Growing in the shadow: Children of alcoholics.* Pompano Beach, FL: Health Communications.

Blane, H. T. (1985). Short-term training needs among alcohol counselors: A survey. *Journal of Alcohol and Drug Education, 30*(3), 15–20.

Clair, D., & Genest, M. (1986). Variables associated with the adjustment of offspring of alcoholic fathers. *Journal of Studies on Alcohol, 48*(4), 345–355.

Gorski, T. T. (1986). Relapse prevention planning: A new recovery tool. *Alcohol Health and Research World, 63,* 6–11.

Gorski, T. T. (1989). The CENAPS model of relapse prevention planning. In D. C. Daley (Ed.), *Relapse: Conceptual, research, and clinical perspectives* (pp. 153–169). New York: Haworth.

Helzer, J. E.; Burnham, A., & McEvoy, L. T. (1991). Alcohol abuse and dependence. In L. N. Robins and D. A. Regier (Eds.) *Psychiatric Disorders in America.* New York: Macmillan.

Helzer, J. E., & Pryzbeck, T. R. (1988). The co-occurrence of alcoholism with other psychiatric disorders in the general population and its impact on treatment. *Journal of Studies on Alcohol, 49,* 219–224.

Jenkins, S. J., Fisher, G. L., & Harrison, T. C. (1993). Adult children of dysfunctional families: Childhood roles. *Journal of Mental Health Counseling, 15*(3), 310–319.

Kaplan, H. I., & Sadock, B. J. (1988). *Synopsis of psychiatry* (5th ed.). Baltimore: Williams & Wilkins.

Kolpack, R. M. (1992). Credentialing alcoholism counselors. *Alcoholism Treatment Quarterly, 9*(3/4), 97–112.

Krippenstapel, P. (1987). A fresh look at relapse. *Alcoholism and Treatment Quarterly, 4,* 1–17.

Lawson, G., Peterson, J., & Lawson, A. (1983). *Alcoholism and the family: A guide to treatment and prevention.* Rockville, MD: Aspen Publications.

Marlatt, G. A., & Gordon, J. R. (1985). *Relapse prevention: Maintenance strategies in the treatment of addictive behaviors.* New York: Guilford.

Mucowski, R. J., & Hayden, R. (1992). Adult children of alcoholics: Verification of a role typology. *Alcoholism Treatment Quarterly, 9*(3/4), 127–140.

Mulligan, D. H., McCarty, D., Potter, D., & Krakow, M. (1989). Counselors in public and private alcoholism and drug abuse treatment programs. *Alcoholism Treatment Quarterly, 6*(3/4), 75–89.

Peluso, E., & Peluso, L. S. (1988). *Women and drugs.* Minneapolis, Compcare Publishers.

Royce, J. E. (1989). *Alcohol problems and alcoholism: A comprehensive survey* (2nd ed.). New York: Free Press.

Schuckit, M. A. (1989). *Drug and alcohol abuse: A clinical guide to diagnosis and treatment* (3rd ed.). New York: Plenum.

Sheridan, M. J., & Green, R. G. (1993). Family dynamics and individual characteristics of adult children of alcoholics: An empirical analysis. *Journal of Social Service Research, 17*(1/2), 73–97.

Shulman, G. (1987). Alcoholism, and cocaine addiction: Similarities, differences, treatment implications. Alcoholism Treatment Quarterly, 4(3), 31–46.

Teichman, M. (1986). A relapse inoculation training for recovering alcoholics. *Alcoholism Treatment Quarterly, 3,* 222–226.

United States Department of Health and Human Services. (1990). *National survey on drug abuse: Population estimates 1990.* Rockville, MD, U. S. Government Printing Office.

Wallace, J. (1987). Children of alcoholics: A population at risk. *Alcoholism Treatment Quarterly, 4*(3), 13–30.

Wegscheider, S. (1981). *Another chance: Hope and health for the alcoholic family.* New York, Science and Behavior Books.

Whitfield, C. L. (1979). Children of alcoholics: Treatment issues. *Services for children of alcoholics.* Research monograph #4, National Institute of Alcohol Abuse and Alcoholism, 66–80.

SECTION IV
LICENSURE, CREDENTIALING AND LEGISLATION RELATED TO MENTAL HEALTH COUNSELING

Chapter 12

THE IMPACT OF CREDENTIALING ON MENTAL HEALTH COUNSELING

DAVID K. BROOKS, JR.

At the time of the writing of this chapter, 41 states and the District of Columbia had passed counselor licensure laws. That only nine states remain in which the practice of professional counseling remains unregulated may seem unremarkable, but the first of these statutes was not enacted until 1976. The last 20 years have witnessed an unprecedented surge in political and credentialing activity by the counseling profession. Prior to 1976, there was no state law that defined or regulated the profession of counseling. Counseling was in a state of legal limbo, not expressly forbidden (except where the activities of professional counselors were perceived as trespassing in the province of psychology), but not legally recognized, either.

Licensure, important as it is, is only one dimension of the larger picture of credentialing. Credentialing is the process by which a profession:

1. defines itself in terms of a body of scientific knowledge;
2. identifies societal needs to which its services are directed;
3. describes skills and competencies that address the identified needs;
4. establishes standards for professional preparation and training;
5. accredits training programs that meet the standards;
6. endorses individuals demonstrating requisite professional skills as being competent to practice the profession; and
7. acts to ensure professional competence by monitoring ethical behavior and requiring periodic evidence of ongoing professional growth (APGA Credentialing Brochure, 1983).

Put another way, credentialing is the process by which a profession demonstrates that its practitioners can do what they say they can do. In order to understand credentialing more fully, it is helpful to view the

259

process as a system of three independent and interrelated components. These components are standards, accreditation, and endorsement.

A Credentialing System

As is the case with most systems explanations, the credentialing system depends upon and interacts with elements that are external to the system itself. Among these elements are the assumption of a body of scientific knowledge upon which professional counseling is based, the assumption that there are societal needs to which counseling services are addressed, and the existence of governmental and nongovernmental institutions that have an interest (both moral and statutory) in regulating the practice of counseling. These elements will be dealt with only tangentially in this discussion. The discussion will begin with an overview of professional standards for training and ethical practice.

Standards of Professional Practice

The development of standards for preparation and practice is a task almost always undertaken by professional associations. As a general rule, the profession itself has existed for some time prior to the promulgation of standards. The impetus for standards development is usually the result of increasing diversity among the ranks of the profession and a concomitant desire to define the limits to which professional activity extends.

Standards for professional preparation usually begin with a statement of the profession's knowledge base, followed by guidelines detailing how this knowledge base is to be imparted to students, apprentices, and other neophytes seeking the skills and competencies necessary for entry into the profession. Criteria for evaluating how well the skills are learned are frequently included as well. There may also be portions of the document that point to development of procedures for accrediting preparation programs.

Standards for ethical practice tend to be based on broad philosophical principles related to the public good. Ethical standards are based on the assumption that the practitioner has received adequate professional preparation. It is further assumed that he/she will attempt no professional activity for which he/she cannot demonstrate competence. There are usually specific guidelines related to the idiosyncratic arts of the profession, such as testing, use of human and animal subjects in research, referral, and so forth. Also included are specific forbidden acts, such as sexual relations with clients. Most ethical standards conclude with procedures for investigating and disciplining those professionals who violate the standards.

Accreditation or Program Approval

The purpose of the accreditation or program approval component of a credentialing system is to ensure that practitioners to-be receive appropriate professional preparation. Accreditation activities are carried out by agencies of state and federal government, by regional accrediting associations composed of educational institutions, by professional associations, and by independent boards. All of these groups have as their purpose the assurance of minimal quality control in preparation programs.

Accreditation is always based on standards, but not always on standards that are relevant to a particular program. For example, a university can be accredited by the Southern Association of Colleges and Schools based on its overall budget, its physical plant, its faculty-student ratio, and its library holdings, but with no attention at all paid to whether its counselor education program adheres to professional standards. Similarly, a school of education, in which most counselor education programs are administratively housed, can be accredited by the National Council for the Accreditation of Teacher Education (NCATE) with total disregard for the standards of the Council for Accreditation of Counseling and Related Educational Programs (CACREP). Thus, statements of accreditation should be viewed skeptically. The questions "of what program?" and "by whose standards?" should always be asked.

Although accreditation procedures usually apply to preparation programs housed in academic departments, this is not always the case. Off-campus sites for internships such as hospitals, community mental health centers, and university counseling centers, may also be subject to accreditation by various governmental and professional bodies.

Licensure and Professional Certification

The endorsement component of a credentialing system ensures that individual practitioners meet minimal standards of professional competence. The two major types of endorsement are licensure and professional certification.

Licensure is a statutory form of endorsement involving an agency of state government. A licensing board established by an act of the state legislature is usually empowered to regulate both the use of the professional title and the scope of practice of members of a particular occupational group. Standards for education and supervised experience are adopted by these boards based on the preparation standards set forth by professional organizations. Individuals who meet these standards are administered a standardized written examination. Successful candidates often then sit for an oral examination by the board. Those who pass are granted a license to practice the profession in that state. The board may or may not require evidence of continuing professional education in order for the license to be periodically renewed.

State licensure boards are charged by law with the responsibility of overseeing the practice of the profession they regulate. In implementing this mandate, they adopt codes of ethics based on those of the relevant professional organization. When charges of unethical conduct are lodged against practitioners under their jurisdiction, they investigate the charges and if they find the practitioner at fault, administer the appropriate discipline, which may range from reprimand to revocation of license. One of the complaints frequently levied against state licensure boards is that they take action against only the most flagrant violations.

State boards are also responsible for investigating and, if necessary, prosecuting individuals who practice a regulated profession without a license. The underlying principle governing their activity is that the public must be protected against unscrupulous practitioners, whether they are licensed or not. Unfortunately, this principle has often been ignored in practice. The actions of professional boards in numerous jurisdictions and professions has had at least the appearance of serving the interest of the profession rather than the public. It is for this reason that legislators are sometimes skeptical of new groups seeking passage of a licensure statute.

Statutory certification and registration are less stringent forms of professional endorsement sometimes adopted by state governments. These procedures establish minimal educational and experience requirements and usually require satisfactory performance on an examination but they restrict only the use of the professional title. Other practitioners who engage in the practice of the profession but who do not use the professional title are not regulated by certification statutes.

Professional certification is an endorsement process administered by boards established by professional organizations. The mechanics of professional certification are similar to those of licensure, except that the procedure is voluntary rather than mandatory. Members of a profession seeking certification must demonstrate that they have met prescribed educational and supervised experience requirements, pass an examination, and pursue continuing professional education in order to keep their certificates current. Advantages of professional certification over licensure are that certification does not require the lengthy process of passing a state law, that the profession itself maintains more control over the credential, and that standards are frequently higher than is the case with licensure. Disadvantages include the inability of the certification board to enforce legal sanctions in cases of unethical conduct, inability to control the actions of those engaged in similar pursuits who are not certified, and lack of legal recognition of the profession.

Having set forth a general framework of credentialing, it is appropriate to look at historical developments in the counseling profession's efforts to achieve fully credentialed status.

Historical Developments in Counselor Credentialing

Almost all activities in the area of counselor credentialing have been the direct result of policies and actions taken by the American Counseling Association (formerly the American Personnel and Guidance Association), its national divisions, and its state branches. There are virtually no instances of any intentional activity in credentialing resulting from any other source. The divisions that have been most active in this area are the American Mental Health Counselors Association (AMHCA), the Association for Counselor Education and Supervision (ACES), the American Rehabilitation Counseling Association (ARCA), the American School Counselor Association (ASCA), and the National Career Development Association (NCDA, formerly the National Vocational Guidance Association [NVGA]).

Standards

The counseling profession first began to address standards for preparation and practice in the late 1950s. After several years of committee work, APGA adopted its first Ethical Standards in 1961. These guidelines have been revised several times since then, most recently in 1995, accounting for changes in the settings which counselors practice, especially in the private sector. The Ethical Standards are the basis for several other ethics statements, including those of state counselor licensure

boards and several professional certification bodies. Without such adop-
tions by other groups, the ACA Ethical Standards would have no
enforcement mechanism, save penalties determined by the ACA Ethics
Committee, the most extreme of which is expulsion from the association.

Preparation standards also received initial attention by the profession
in the late 1950s and early 1960s. A preliminary statement of training
standards for secondary school counselors was adopted by 1964 after
several years' work by an ACES committee. Following a period of
experimental implementation these standards were officially adopted by
ACES in 1967. Standards for the preparation of elementary school
counselors and of college student personnel specialists were adopted by
ACES in 1968 and 1969, respectively. Foreseeing the possibility of
further proliferation of setting specific standards, ACES leadership in the
early 1970s sought to combine these three standards statements into a
single document. This task was completed and *Standards for Preparation
of Counselors and Other Personnel Services Specialists* was adopted by the
ACES membership in 1973. This document anticipated the possibility
of preparation programs needing to provide appropriate experiences for
counselors whose career objectives and professional interests lay outside
educational settings by specifying the need for "environmental and
specialized studies" to be included in counselor education programs.

The 1973 Standards are directed at programs preparing counselors at
the master's degree or entry level. In 1977, ACES adopted standards for
preparation at the doctoral level. At that time, however, there was no
mechanism or procedure for evaluating programs to determine their
degree of compliance with the standards at either the master's or doctoral levels. What was needed was a set of procedures by which counselor
education programs could be evaluated in light of the standards and
those programs meeting the criteria could be so designated.

Accreditation

As was the case with standards development, most of the early leadership in the area of accreditation was assumed by ACES. The ACES
Accreditation Committee developed an accreditation procedures manual and conducted five regional workshops in the fall of 1978 to train site
visitors to conduct evaluations of counselor education programs. The
next year, five institutions were involved in a pilot program approval
study. Modifications were made to the accreditation procedures based
on this study, but there was growing pressure to make counseling

program approval the province of the entire profession, rather than an operation of only one of APGA's divisions.

The APGA Accreditation Committee, working collaboratively with ACES, but representing the interests of all of APGA's divisions, explored the development of a structure that would independently accredit counselor education programs. Such an independent body was believed to be necessary in order to avoid a conflict of interest between the professional organization and the academic integrity of training institutions. It was also believed to be highly desirable for this body to be accepted for membership in the Council on Postsecondary Accreditation (COPA), which was at that time the "accreditor" of accrediting bodies. Accordingly, the Council for Accreditation of Counseling and Related Educational Programs (CACREP) was established by APGA in 1981 to be an independent, legally incorporated accreditation body. All programs previously accredited by ACES and by a separate procedure administered by the California Association for Counselor Education and Supervision were accepted by CACREP. By 1995, counselor education programs at over 100 universities had been accredited by CACREP. These programs have been evaluated at the master's degree level according to specialty preparation in school counseling, student affairs practice in higher education, mental health counseling, marriage and family counseling/therapy, and community counseling (gerontological and career subspecialties), and at the doctoral level in counselor education and supervision. Considering that there are over 500 programs nationwide that prepare counselors, at least at the master's level, accreditation under the CACREP aegis has had considerable impact in terms of identifying preparation programs based on quality and professional standards.

An area that has not been addressed thus far is the accreditation of internship sites. The standards call for certain requirements to be met for both practicum and internship experiences, but there is no provision for the sites in which these experiences take place to be accredited. These sites are usually outside of university departments and, although many of them provide high quality experiences for trainees, there is no systematic vehicle for assuring quality control.

Endorsement

The counseling profession's efforts to put endorsement procedures into effect began around 1970. Prior to that time, most master's graduates of counselor education programs were employed in public elementary and secondary schools in which certification was a subcomponent of the same procedure of state departments of education that certified classroom teachers. Many doctoral graduates were routinely licensed as psychologists in most states by psychology licensing boards. At the beginning of the 1970s, three unrelated elements combined to focus attention and to direct action toward putting new endorsement structures for professional counselors into effect.

The first of these was occasioned by action of a growing number of state psychology boards. The same bodies that only a few years earlier had accepted counselor education doctoral graduates as candidates for psychology licensure, were now refusing to permit such persons to sit for the examination. The principal reason for this guild-oriented behavior was the expectation that national health insurance eligibility would require stricter professional standards that the boards could demonstrate were within the control of the discipline of psychology. There were also pressures from within professional psychology to restrict entry because of the market forces of supply and demand. More and more clinical psychologists were engaging in private practice on a full or part-time basis. The gradual removal of requirements that such activities be supervised by psychiatrists and the increasing availability of insurance reimbursement from private carriers made the private practice option more attractive, but only if the number of practitioners could be controlled. Those persons most adversely affected were new doctoral graduates from counselor education programs. Adding to these difficulties was the shrinking number of university level counselor educator positions available to new doctoral graduates.

The second element affecting the profession's interest in new endorsement structures also related to manpower supply and demand. The previous decade had been a time of tremendous growth in school counseling positions. With budget cutbacks and a declining birthrate beginning to be felt in the 1970s, increasing numbers of new counseling graduates were finding school counseling positions difficult to obtain. These persons began to be employed in a variety of community settings, for example, mental health centers, hospitals, and private clinics. Added to these recent graduates were counselors previously employed in school settings who were seeking new challenges in community settings. The effect was twofold: the identity of the mental health counselor began to emerge and an increasingly larger pool of professionals trained as counselors and identifying with the counseling profession were becoming employed in settings for which no credentialing options were available.

The third element leading to a concern about credentialing arose within the profession itself. This dimension can best be described as a new awareness of professional identity. In school settings, counselors increasingly saw themselves as different from teachers and administrators. In community settings, counselors were aware of the positive aspects (as well as the negative ones such as the lack of credentialing) of the differences between themselves and allied professionals such as psychologists and social workers. The effects of market demands on counselor education programs caused counselor educators to realize that they were preparing individuals to assume new roles and responsibilities that were different enough from those of the previous decade that a new mental health profession was emerging and that they were having to change their focus to accommodate these needs. The composite effect of all this was a sense of pride in the profession and a need to define what the profession was about in new and unique terms. The exclusion of doctoral graduates from psychology licensure, the new settings in which master's level practitioners were working, and the growing sense of professional identity led to the establishment by the APGA Board of Directors of a Special Commission on Counselor Licensure in 1974.

Licensure. It is instructive here to reproduce the charge given to the licensure committee by the APGA Board in 1974:

1. To formulate and disseminate model legislation on licensure for counselors.
2. To establish procedures for state and regional leadership workshops on licensure.
3. To help initiate and maintain liaison and dialogue with associations in the counseling related professions (e.g., psychology, psychiatry, social work, marriage and family).
4. To testify on federal legislation having implications for professionals trained in counselor education programs.
5. To identify for the membership nonlegislative activities having implications for the counseling profession (e.g., importance of liaison with related state professional groups in psychology and social work and with mental health insurance companies, when appropriate).
6. To consider other alternatives or avenues to earning recognition

for counseling as a profession (e.g., academy of diplomates and/or national registry of persons qualified to offer specialized counseling services to the public for a fee).

7. To encourage cooperative efforts between the various divisions, state branches, affiliates, and subgroups of APGA in the area of licensure.

8. To encourage research and innovations on traditional methods of licensure including possible use of more performance-based criteria and unified administrative boards for all counseling-related professions.

9. To identify test cases where evidence of discrimination against qualified members takes place by boards of related professions (APGA Board, 1974).

More than two decades have passed since the APGA Licensure Committee was given this charge. Six of the nine items of the charge remained at the center of the committee's activity until the early 1990s. Federal testimony (number 4) has been largely assumed by the ACA Public Policy and Legislation Committee, administrative staff, and lobbyists. Research and innovations in licensing methods (number 8) is an area still in the early developmental stages.

In addition to the three elements identified in the previous section as contributing to the initiation of concerted counselor licensure efforts, two specific events focused the profession's attention on the licensure issue. The first of these was a lawsuit in which John I. Weldon was charged by the Virginia Board of Psychologist Examiners with practicing psychology without a license. Weldon, an APGA member, did not hold himself out as a psychologist, but rather as a professional counselor in private practice. The court recognized counseling as a profession separate from psychology, but stated that since counseling used the tools of psychology and there was no statutory regulation of the practice of counseling, Weldon was to be enjoined from practicing as a counselor. The effect of this decision was to galvanize the Virginia Counselors Association (then the Virginia Personnel and Guidance Association) into a political force seeking passage of a statute to license counselors.

The second event that focused attention on licensure was the publication of the first article dealing with the issue in the *Personnel and Guidance Journal* (now the *Journal of Counseling and Development*) (Sweeney & Sturdevant, 1974). The authors eloquently depicted the plight of doctoral graduates and called for professional counselors to seek their own licensure.

Under the leadership first of Thomas J. Sweeney of Ohio and then of Carl D. Swanson of Virginia, the licensure committee produced several drafts of model state licensure legislation. During the tenure of the late Harold F. Cottingham as chair, the committee published the first edition of the Counselor Licensure Action Packet, which served as a guide for state committees working on the issue and went through five editions (McFadden & Brooks, 1983). Beginning with Richard W. Warner's leadership in 1977, the committee finally put in place a national network comprised of contact persons in every state. By the time David K. Brooks, Jr., assumed the chair in 1980, the committee was conducting regular training sessions at regional meetings and at the national convention. "Target States" were also identified for legislative grants and special consultation each year. The committee assumed a leadership role in facilitating communication among the growing number of state licensure boards, leading to the founding of the American Association of State Counseling Boards in 1986. Under Lawrence H. Gerstein's leadership, the committee initiated a comprehensive revision of the model legislation, the most recent version of which was adopted by the ACA Governing Council in 1995. Throughout its history the committee engaged in ongoing membership education activities resulting in the publication of more than a dozen informational brochures on licensure. The functions of the licensure committee were consolidated under the ACA Public Policy and Legislation Committee around 1990.

Legislative successes were distressingly slow in the years following 1974. Virginia was the first state to achieve passage of a licensure law in 1976, followed by Arkansas and Alabama in 1979. The first half of the 1980s were tremendously productive as years of frustration and near-misses began to pay off. By midsummer, 1985, 13 more states had passed licensure laws: Texas and Florida (1981), Idaho (1982), North Carolina (1983), Georgia, Ohio, and Tennessee (1984), and Mississippi, Montana, Maryland, Oklahoma, South Carolina, and Missouri (1985). The legislature of West Virginia also passed a statute in 1985, but it was vetoed by the governor in the first instance of executive opposition to counselor licensure. The decade since has seen passage of licensure statutes in all but nine states.

What the Licensure Laws Do. The stated purpose of all counselor licensure laws is to protect the public by regulating the practice of professional counseling. To implement this mandate, most of the laws establish licensing boards that vary in size and composition. Exceptions to this structure include Florida, in which the licensing authority is vested in the State Department of Professional Regulation and Tennessee where a committee was established under the Board of Healing Arts.

The licensing authorities in most states license or certify professional counselors only. Examples of so-called omnibus boards include Georgia, where the board licenses professional counselors, marriage and family therapists, and social workers; Ohio, where the board licenses professional counselors and social workers; Tennessee, where the committee certifies professional counselors and marriage and family therapists; and South Carolina, where the board licenses professional counselors and marriage and family therapists.

In each of the states, the enabling legislation or the rules of the board or other authority establishes the minimum education and experience requirements for licensure. The education requirements vary from a master's degree with no specified number of credit hours to a master's degree of 60 semester hours. Supervised experience requirements vary as well, ranging from one to three years. All states require a written examination and many states require that an oral examination by the board be conducted.

There is only slightly greater uniformity among state laws in the official professional title. "Licensed Professional Counselor" is the title used by most states, but "Certified Professional Counselor," "Licensed Mental Health Counselor," and "Licensed Clinical Mental Health Counselor" are also among the titles found in various state laws. Almost all of the laws provide for generic licensure of counselors, that is, all applicants are issued the same license, regardless of their academic training or years of experience. Exceptions to this rule are Ohio, New Mexico, and Illinois, all of which provide for both generic and clinical levels of licensure.

All of the laws provide for penalties to be imposed by the boards in the event of ethical violations. They also provide for exemptions for members of related professional groups who also provide counseling services (e.g., psychologists, psychiatrists, and members of the clergy). All but one of the laws (Ohio) are private practice acts, exempting professionals in public and private agencies from the requirements of the law. All of the laws contain provisions for license renewal and most of them require evidence of continuing professional education as part of the renewal process.

Professional Certification. There are at present one generic and five specialty certification procedures that pertain to professional counselors. The oldest of these is administered by the Commission on Rehabilitation Counselor Certification (CRCC), founded in 1973 by representatives of seven professional rehabilitation associations. The CRCC administered its first national examination in 1976. By 1993 more than 13,000 Certified Rehabilitation Counselors were practicing in the United States and overseas (Leahy & Holt, 1993).

The National Academy of Certified Clinical Mental Health Counselors (NACCMHC) was established by AMHCA in 1979 and administered its first national examination to 50 prospective certificants in that year. Because there was no "grandfathering" and because of the stiff requirements (including a clinical work sample) the growth in the number of Certified Clinical Mental Health Counselors (CCMHC) has been slower than has been the case with the other national certification procedures. By late 1994 nearly 1,800 practitioners had been certified as CCMHCs (Bradley, 1995).

Joining these two specialty certification bodies in 1982, the National Board of Certified Counselors (NBCC) was founded by APGA to provide a generic counseling certificate. The NBCC, like CACREP, is an independent, legally incorporated body. Its initiation occurred after several years' study and planning by the APGA Special Committee on Registry. More than 2,200 counselors took the first NBCC national examination in January, 1983. This striking number, combined with the 700 CRCs, and licensed professional counselors who chose to be certified through reciprocity and were thus exempt from the examination, constituted the first group of National Certified Counselors (NCC). By July, 1994, the ranks of NCCs had grown to more than 19,000 (Bradley, 1995).

The National Council for the Credentialing of Career Counselors (NCCCC) was established by the National Career Development Association (formerly the National Vocational Guidance Association [NVGA], ACA's oldest division) in 1983 and administered its first examination in 1984. The NCCCC in 1985 became a corporate affiliate of NBCC, the first specialty certification body to establish this relationship. By late 1994, 819 National Certified Career Counselors (NCCC) held this specialty credential (Bradley, 1995).

During the next decade, NBCC worked with several ACA divisions to establish new specialty certifications in gerontological counseling (Myers, 1995), school counseling (Paisley & Borders, 1995), and addictions counseling (Page & Bailey, 1995). In 1993, after several years of negotiations, NBCC absorbed the NACCMHC and its credentialing functions into its organizational structure (Smith & Robinson, 1995). The NBCC thus became both the generic and the specialty certification body for the counseling profession, with only the rehabilitation counseling certification operating outside of the NBCC umbrella.

As mentioned previously in this chapter, there are relative advantages and disadvantages to both licensure and professional certification. Licensure provides a legal definition for the profession in a given state and assures licensed professionals in that state of the right to practice. It also entails legal sanctions, including suspension, revocation, fines, and imprisonment, for violating the law. Greater public protection from unscrupulous practitioners is thereby assured. Professional certification boards can and usually do set higher standards for credentialing than is the case with licensing boards because they are much less subject to political repercussions. Certification is a less arduous process to institute because it does not depend upon the whim of state legislators.

Is one type of endorsement preferable to the other? Not really, because both are necessary to assure quality mental health care to the public. The combination of the legal sanctions and public protection afforded by state licensure together with the higher standards of professional certification provide a credentialing structure unequaled by any other mental health profession.

AMHCA and Credentialing

This is a book about mental health counseling. This chapter is entitled "The Impact of Credentialing on Mental Health Counseling." Thus far we have dealt with counselor credentialing almost entirely in a generic sense, rather than focusing on the professional specialty of mental health counseling. Why? Because the interests of mental health counselors are virtually inseparable from those of professional counselors in other settings as far as credentialing issues are concerned.

The identity of mental health counselors as embodied in the American Mental Health Counselors Association did not emerge until the licensure movement was already under way. AMHCA was not actively involved in the passage of a state licensure statute until the enactment of the Florida law in 1981, even though "war chest" grants to state AMHCA divisions to assist them in their lobbying efforts began in 1980. In every state effort since Florida, however, AMHCA members have been in the forefront and AMHCA funds have assisted in underwriting lobbyists' fees and other legislative expenses.

It is also interesting to note that what became the National Academy of Certified Clinical Mental Health Counselors was originally conceived as a generic rather than a specialty certification body. The Academy's working title prior to its incorporation was "Board of Certified Professional Counselors" (Messina, 1979), which is remarkably similar to the name of the generic certification body initiated by APGA three years later, the National Board for Certified Counselors.

The point here is twofold: (1) efforts toward counselor credentialing anticipated the emerging identity of mental health counselors and the founding of AMHCA; (2) the credentialing movement since 1980 has become more and more an endeavor in which AMHCA officers and AMHCA members have assumed the leadership role. The goals of counselor credentialing are far more crucial for mental health counselors than for any other counseling specialty. It is therefore appropriate that AMHCA should be in the forefront of this activity.

In addition to its political leadership at the state level, AMHCA during the 1980s moved the credentialing agenda to the congressional arena. The AMHCA National Legislative/Government Relations Committee caused several bills to be introduced to grant federal recognition to CCMHCs and licensed professional counselors as core service providers under the Medicare provisions of the Social Security Act and other federal programs. AMHCA also initiated efforts for recognition of mental health counselors as eligible service providers under programs administered by the Office of Civilian Health and Medical Programs of the Uniformed Services (OCHAMPUS) in 1984. OCHAMPUS recognition was finally extended in 1987.

Credentialing Interface with Allied Professions

Even after two decades, mental health counselors are still the "new kids on the block" among established professional mental health organizations. Mental health counselors' efforts at achieving our credentialing goals have met with reactions from these groups that ranged from close cooperation to wary neutrality to contemptuous sneers to virulent opposition. As our legislative successes have mounted, mental health counselors have witnessed significant changes in these reactions. In 1978, Georgia was a battleground between mental health counselors and marriage and family therapists of such a magnitude that the American Association of Marriage and Family Therapists (AAMFT) adopted a national policy of noncooperation with ACA in the area of licensure. Six years later Georgia and Tennessee adopted credentialing statutes that licensed or certified members of both professions under the same regulatory authority, the result of three years of intense collaboration by members of both professions.

There are several instances in which state divisions of the American Psychological Association (APA) have modified their stances toward counselor licensure from outright opposition to official neutrality. The APA's state affiliates remained among the more formidable adversaries to counselor licensure efforts, but as the 1980s ended there was evidence of greater collaboration.

The Future of Counselor Credentialing

Mental health counselors have achieved a momentum in credentialing efforts in the last few years that makes it appear only a matter of time before the remaining nine states pass counselor licensure laws. Emboldened by successes at the state level, mental health counselors have reached the threshold of core provider recognition at the federal level, with such validation possible in the very near future.

Mental health counseling is a profession and an ideal whose time has come. Counselor education programs have changed dramatically in the last two decades, influenced by the CACREP mental health counseling standards and by the increasingly clinical emphasis of the newer state licensure laws. The emergence of managed care as a force in insurance-supported mental health services has dramatically changed the landscape in terms of eligible provider status, but mental health counselors should be well positioned to compete in such an environment. The credentialing activities of the last 20 years have changed the face of the counseling profession in ways that would have been unimaginable only a few years earlier. While parity with other nonmedical providers remains to be achieved, the changes wrought by mental health counselors' licensure and other credentialing initiatives have literally created a new counseling profession, one that is poised for significant influence in the 21st century.

REFERENCES

American Association for Counseling and Development Licensure Committee (1983). Suggested legislative language for counselor licensure laws. In J. McFadden & D. K. Brooks, Jr. (Eds.), *Counselor licensure action packet* (pp. 55–77). Alexandria, VA: AACD Press.

American Personnel and Guidance Association (1974, July). Licensure in the helping professions. Minutes of the APGA Board of Directors Meeting. Washington, DC: Author.

American Personnel and Guidance Association (1983). APGA credentialing brochure. Falls Church, VA: Author.

Association for Counselor Education and Supervision (1973). *Standards for the preparation of counselors and other personnel services specialists.* Washington, DC: American Personnel and Guidance Association.

Bradley, L. J. (1995). Certification and licensure issues. *Journal of Counseling and Development, 74,* 185–186.

Leahy, M. J., & Holt, E. (1993). Certification in rehabilitation counseling: History and process. *Rehabilitation Counseling Bulletin, 37,* 71–80.

McFadden, J., & Brooks, D. K., Jr. (Eds.) (1983). *Counselor licensure action packet.* Alexandria, VA: AACD Press.

Messina, J. J. (1979). Why establish a certification system for professional counselors? A rationale. *American Mental Health Counselors Association Journal, 1,* 9–22.

Myers, J. E. (1995). From "forgotten and ignored" to standards and certification: Gerontological counseling comes of age. *Journal of Counseling and Development, 74,* 143–149.

Page, R. C., & Bailey, J. B. (1995). Addictions counseling certification: An emerging counseling specialty. *Journal of Counseling and Development, 74,* 167–171.

Paisley, P. O., & Borders, L. D. (1995). School counseling: An evolving specialty. *Journal of Counseling and Development, 74,* 150–153.

Smith, H. B., & Robinson, G. P. (1995). Mental health counseling: Past, present, and future. *Journal of Counseling and Development, 74,* 158–162.

Sweeney, T. J., & Sturdevant, A. D. (1974). Licensure in the helping professions: Anatomy of an issue. *Personnel and Guidance Journal, 52,* 575–580.

Chapter 13

THE MENTAL HEALTH COUNSELOR
AS POLITICAL ACTIVIST

WILLIAM J. WEIKEL

As recently as twenty years ago, there was no lobbying effort at the state or national level by or for mental health counseling professionals. The profession was in the infancy stage, addressing the developmental concerns of a new profession, with little awareness of the future need for effective lobbying. There was not the time, money, or organizational maturity that is needed to effect governmental changes at the state or national level that could benefit the members of the emerging profession or their clients.

Ten years ago, the neophyte mental health profession had matured to the point where it had hired a part-time lobbyist to provide a presence in Washington, D.C., along with developing a government relations program to select and train mental health counselors (MHC) at the grass roots level to serve as lobbyists and advocates in their states. Thanks to recent efforts by the American Mental Health Counselors Association, and their parent organization, the American Counseling Association, MHCs are finally placing their political agenda before the power brokers at the local and national levels.

It has taken AMHCA over 20 years to develop a nationwide system of MHCs who are trained as government relations experts who can be called upon to respond via letters, phone calls, and visitations to legislators regarding any governmental concern at the state and federal level. Typically, AMHCA and ACA have been strong advocates of credentialing and licensing of professional counselors at the state level; however, the associations have directed the majority of their financial support and programming toward federal legislation. Since MHCs are now recognized through licensure legislation in forty-one states and the District of Columbia, the legislative push for federal recognition of the profession will continue to gain momentum. Concurrently with the push for recognition by the government agencies controlling the programming for mental health in the United States, MHCs must continue to work with private third-party payers, health maintenance groups, and other "managed care" providers to achieve full recognition as a profession.

The late Harley M. Dirks wrote in an earlier edition of this book (1986), "Over the years, Congress has created a massive Federal government . . . national health programs, including Medicare, have flourished . . . but now the legislative climate is changing . . . it is time to reexamine the pulse of the nation regarding social programs . . . the watchword for the forseeable future in all health-related legislation is cost containment . . . " It is no secret that the Republican-controlled 104th Congress of 1995–1996 is taking a close look at the social and entitlement programs that consume such a large portion of the federal budget. In all areas, health care costs continue to outpace otherwise modest inflation, so it is highly unlikely that there will be any new health-related legislation that does not attempt to contain or reduce delivery costs.

MHC Recognition

In the early 1980s, MHCs scored a major victory in receiving recognition for counseling services by the Civilian Health and Medical Program for the Uniformed Services (CHAMPUS). Other attempts to include MHCs in federal legislation or to recognize MHCs as the fifth core service providers along with psychiatrists, psychologists, clinical social workers, and psychiatric nurses have failed. These failures have been attributed to a variety of causes, including the lack of universal licensure/certification of MHCs, objections from the other politically powerful professions, and a fear by legislators of opening the flood gates to new and vaguely defined groups. Thanks to the efforts of AMHCA and ACA, many of the issues are now being addressed in the political and health care arena.

With the onset of managed care over the past five years, professional recognition of MHCs by the state and federal government has become of paramount importance. The typical managed care contractor recognizes the licensed core mental health providers (psychiatrists, psychologists, social workers, and psychiatric nurses) while only rarely accepting licensed counselors. Unfortunately, at this time, MHCs are not specifically recognized as providers under most managed care contracts, with the typical contractor possibly recognizing the general title of licensed professional counselor or marriage and family counselor.

For MHCs, there is much work to be done before the profession is fully recognized by the "powers that be," in this instance, government bodies and health insurance companies. Over the next five years, it is imperative for MHCs to become involved with lobbying and political activities. Without political activity, MHCs will be left behind by the other core providers.

The Legislative Process

The legislative process is quite complex. Proposed bills are written by various groups to make their ideas or causes into law at either the state or federal level. Before a bill is introduced into a legislative body, it must have a sponsor or several cosponsors to have any chance of being passed by the full legislative body. Several common questions are usually asked by any group attempting to introduce a bill:

"What is the best strategy to guarantee successful passage of the proposed bill?"

"Should the bill be submitted to the House, Senate, or both?"

"Is there a legislative individual who can be a champion for the cause?"

"Is the legislative champion willing to introduce the bill as well as write letters to his/her colleagues to promote the bill?"

"Are there special interest group members ready to write and call legislators once the bill has been introduced?"

"Are there lobbyists who can relate with key congressional committee members to make sure the bill moves through committee intact and then successfully to the floor?"

The development and passing of a bill is a very long and complex process, with many proposed bills never making it out of committee.

If a bill makes it through the committee process and passes the full vote of a legislature, it is then sent to the executive branch for to be signed into law. Because the President or a governor must sign the bill, lobbying of the executive branch is also a necessity. All of this is not an easy process, with passing of successful legislation requiring enormous amounts of time, energy, and money.

How to Lobby. Lobbying is simply an attempt to influence the outcome of legislation through contacting the important people responsible for the legislative process. To be a successful nonpaid lobbyist, several important points must be taken into account:

Establish a relationship — Before any successful lobbying can take place, an MHC must establish and nurture a relationship with his/her legislators. Usually, the relationship is with the legislator's aides, and not directly with the legislator. Establishing a relationship means making frequent contacts through letters and phone calls keeping the legislators' office informed of your interest and willingness to maintain involvement with their office.

Campaign Contribution — Although many mental health professionals are put off by having to give money in order to get an "audience" with a legislator, this is frequently the fastest way to get the legislator's attention. Giving a donation to his/her political fund shows him/her that you are interested in his/her career and welfare. Unfortunately, money is often the only way to have an influence or get the "ear" of the legislator.

Face-to-face Contact — Taking the time to visit legislators while they are in their home district is a key to successful input. Often, while at their home offices, they are more willing to take the time to listen and exchange ideas about legislation. At home, legislators are less involved with the day-to-day politics of Washington or their state capitol. Taking the time to know your legislators before approaching with a lobbying agenda can be quite helpful and may guarantee legislative successes at a later time.

Long-Term Relationships — Stay in touch with the legislators during the times that you have no agenda. In this way, the legislator can learn to know you and will possibly seek your opinion on other matters affecting his/her home district. Most elected officials like to hear from their constituents; therefore, staying in contact over the long term can mean a great deal to both the legislator and the MHC.

Numbers Talk — Most politicians begin to run for re-election the day after they take office and keeping in contact with their constituents is of utmost importance to them. If they hear from 100 or 200 MHCs in their district asking them to support a potential law, they see this as the opportunity to have 100 or 200 votes in the next election. Numbers talk, and direct contact from voters "back home" always gets a lawmaker's attention.

PACs and Lobbyists — Political Action Committees and paid lobbyists can significantly assist the movement of legislation and influence the process. All of this takes financial funding, meaning the professional associations have to push the memberships to contribute. However, it should be remembered that grassroots support is vital to any legislation. The voters back home keep the legislator in office, not the PAC or lobbyists!

Grassroots Efforts — Grassroots efforts typically include the development of phone trees to all members of a state association. When it is time to activate a piece of legislation, the state association begins the phone tree and asks members to write or phone the legislators asking them to support their effort. As a part of the grassroots effort, the members are taught how to write appropriate letters and make successful phone calls. The involvement of all members of the association is needed to guarantee success in the legislature, and a phone tree can activate a large number of MHCs in a very short period of time.

Communicating an Issue — When speaking with a legislator, a nonpaid lobbyist has to learn to be brief and to the point. A quick phone call, brief telegram, or short handwritten note on letterhead are ways to successfully let the lawmaker know your point of view. Most importantly, when presenting your point of view, you must stress how the bill will positively effect the consumers. Keeping the MHCs clients in mind when lobbying is most helpful. As mentioned above, maintaining constant contact with the legislative aides is very important in this process. Be informed and be ready to answer questions about the legislation.

Timing — Timing is crucial to any successful legislation. When the bill is being voted upon in committee, activate the MHCs. When it passes from the committee, activate the MHCs. When it is voted upon in the legislature, activate the MHCs. Do not stop the involvement until it is signed by the executive branch officer.

ACA Public Policy and Legislative Agenda for the 104th Congress

ACA actively lobbies on behalf of all professional counselors throughout the United States. Although the lobbying efforts are primarily directed at federal legislation, other items of concern support state initiatives through the state chapters and branches. Many of the divisions of ACA, such as AMHCA, also maintain committees actively involved in lobbying for their members' political agendas. The ACA Legislative Agenda for the 104th Congress includes the following:

I. Health Care/Core Providers
    A. Impact of Managed Care Organizations on Counselors
    B. Impact of Legislation on Mental Health Rehabilitation, Substance Abuse, and Treatment Benefits
    C. Recognition of Professional Counselors as Qualified Providers

II. Education Reform
    A. Implementation of the Elementary-Secondary Reauthorization Act
    B. Implementation of Elementary School Counseling Act
    C. Comprehensive Counseling Legislation
    D. Vocational Education Legislation and Rewrites

III. State Counselor Legislation
    A. Technical Assistance for Uniform Licensure Legislation
    B. Freedom of Choice/Third Party Reimbursement
    C. Technical Assistance for Uniform School Counselor Certification
    D. Medicaid Waiver Advocacy for Counselors

IV. Budget and Appropriation
    A. Financing of Legislative Efforts Supporting Counseling
    B. Broader Legislative Activity for Counseling in Education, Hospitals, and Community

Recap

Obviously, MHCs and professional counselors everywhere have a full plate of legislative activities as they approach the 21st century. Attaining these goals will require a coordinated, well-funded lobbying effort over the next 10 years for sure, and maybe even longer. If MHCs are to prosper, they must continually work with state and federal legislators, private insurers, and managed care organizations to assure core provider status for the profession.

The legislative battles will be long and hard. With each single battle, and each victory, the next battle will become easier. MHCs must stress education, training, and ability to perform the job in a cost-efficient manner, if they are to break the barriers put forth by the older, established core professions. The entire health care system in the United States is coming under more and more scrutiny by legislators, as well as the consumers. For sure, health service providers of the 21st century will be more efficient, well-organized, and more cost-effective than their 20th century counterparts. As Dirks wrote in 1986,

> The future for MHCs growth and recognition as bona fide core providers of mental health services, and overall recognition as a significant professional group lies within the membership of the profession. Many of the doors are closed now, but the keys are there to be found. None of these doors open quickly. Persistent, steady effort is necessary to provide the means to propel the professional mental health counselor into the future. Dedicated, thoughtful leadership must continue. Counselors must take responsibility and be accountable for their professional endeavors, recognize a real challenge is ahead, and commit themselves to meeting the challenge. Recognition and professional identity was once, and still is, a goal of the other core providers. Time and monumental effort was responsible for their success, and will continue to be for the MHCs success (p. 269).

This chapter is dedicated to the memory of Harley M. Dirks, AMHCA Lobbyist, 1982–1985.

REFERENCES

American Counseling Association (1995). *ACA public policy and legislative agenda for the 104th Congress 1995–1996.* Alexandria, VA: Author.

Dirks, H.M. (1986). Legislative recognition of the mental health counselor: The profession shapes its destiny. In A.J. Palmo & W.J. Weikel. *Foundations of mental health counseling* (pp. 263–269). Springfield, IL. Charles C Thomas.

Chapter 14

MENTAL HEALTH COUNSELORS AND THIRD PARTY REIMBURSEMENT

WARREN THROCKMORTON

Since Rudolph's (1986) examination of third party reimbursement for the services of mental health counselors (MHCs), a revolution has occurred in health care. Discussions concerning the delivery and financing of mental health care have preoccupied practitioners, payers, and policy makers alike. Due to concerns about inconsistent quality and rising costs of mental health services, employer scrutiny of mental health benefits—and the professionals who provide them—has never been greater (Geisel, 1990b). In response to the plight of the uninsured and the economic burden of rising health costs, state and federal lawmakers have elevated the cost of mental health care to public debate (Castro, 1993; Hilzenrath, 1994). Despite the failure of the 103rd Congress to enact comprehensive health care reform, market forces continue to bring change in the reimbursement and delivery of health care services (Geisel, 1995).

Concurrent with the changes in health care delivery and financing has been the expansion of the profession of mental health counseling. For instance, counseling is currently regulated by statute in 41 states and the District of Columbia. Within the last decade, MHCs have made significant progress in establishing reimbursement eligibility in both private and government health plans. Often, MHCs have been viewed by payers and employers as an asset in the struggle to provide high quality care with cost effective service delivery (Kelley, 1986; Throckmorton, 1992b). This chapter will survey the current marketplace for mental health counseling services, examine the extent to which MHCs are recognized by public and private benefits programs, and then discuss the work that remains to be done.

Third Party Reimbursement: An Overview

Mental health services are available to most people by virtue of an employment benefits plan or via one of many government agencies which subsidize or directly provide them. Consequently, there are many methods of delivery and reimbursement for mental health services. Employers and government entities act as third party payers when they provide an arrangement for the provision and financing of health care. Third party reimbursement refers to procedures and policies used by private and public sector payers to compensate health care providers for their independent professional work.

Frequently, MHCs have viewed success in third party reimbursement as both a business issue and an evidence of professional recognition (Rudolph, 1986). Thus, the extent of voluntary reimbursement by third party payers can be viewed as a means of assessing the viability of the profession (Madden, 1988; Zimpfer, 1995). This section will describe private sector methods of financing mental health care, provide data concerning the extent of MHC reimbursement and discuss criteria used by payers to make reimbursement decisions.

Health Insurance

In essence, insurance is a method to provide protection against financial loss. An insurance policy is "a private contractual arrangement allocating the burden of individual losses to members of a selected group who are exposed to similar losses" (Mehr & Cammack, 1976, p. 5). Insurance allows the sharing of risk.

Group health insurance requires the employer to pay a fee (premium) to the insurer to be "at risk" for expenses related to the employees' health. The cost of insurance is generally proportional to the probability and severity of loss. Premiums elevate as the likelihood and severity of a loss increases. As applied to health, insurance is a guard against financial loss due to accident or sickness (Mehr & Cammack, 1976). In the event of sickness or accident, the insurer will indemnify (reimburse) the employee or the provider of health services directly. Disability, specific disease insurance (e.g., cancer insurance), hospitalization, and medical expense insurance are all forms of health insurance.

Mental health professionals often think of health insurance as a means of securing optimal health. This notion does not fit the traditional concept of insurance (Feezor, 1987). While the use of health insurance benefits may enhance health, the actual benefit is an arrangement to prevent financial loss due to health related problems. This mismatch of expectations is often at the root of controversy between providers and traditional health insurers.

Due to the relationship of reimbursement eligibility to professional viability, researchers have attempted to estimate the extent of voluntary coverage by insurers. Such estimates are difficult due to the large number of insurers and variations in plan language from employer to employer. However, investigators have approached this issue from the perspective of the provider (Covin, 1988; Covin, Wright & Preston, 1990; Gillen, 1988; Seligman & Whitley, 1983; Zimpfer, 1995) and the payer (Carlson, 1988; Texas Department of Insurance, 1992; Throckmorton, 1992c).

The first reported survey of counselors was Seligman and Whitley's (1983) survey of licensed professional counselors (LPCs) in Virginia. They found that 43 percent of respondents were successful in collecting reimbursement from 26 different payers. In a 1984 survey of Alabama LPCs, Covin (1985) reported that 84 percent of respondents who sought reimbursement had some success in achieving it.

Covin (1988) surveyed MHCs in Arkansas, Florida, Virginia and Texas early in 1986. For MHCs in surveyed states, rates of reimbursement without benefit of physician supervision were: Arkansas, 34 percent; Florida, 64 percent; Virginia, 33 percent; and Texas, 40 percent. While the number of counselors receiving payment in some states was small (e.g., two in the Arkansas study), Covin concluded that a "large percentage" of MHCs were receiving reimbursement. In Alabama, Covin, Wright, and Preston (1990) determined via a survey of LPCs that 88 percent of respondents had collected third party payments when filing claims using only the counseling license. He also listed 175 companies which have reimbursed counselors. However, no attempt was made to determine what percentage of claims had been reimbursed or to verify eligibility status with the payers.

Gillen (1988) surveyed 100 randomly selected licensed professional clinical counselors (LPCCs) in Ohio to determine reimbursement experience. Of the 58 respondents licensed only as a counselor, only 3 respondents (5%) considered themselves eligible to submit claims for third party reimbursement. The remaining respondents either did not believe such reimbursement was possible or thought that supervision was required to receive it. Despite the few counselors filing claims, 6 out of 14 (43%) insurance companies were listed as paying for MHC's services. Interestingly, three of the companies in Covin et al's (1990) list of reimbursing companies were listed by Gillen's respondents as rejecting the claims of Ohio's LPCCs.

Zimpfer (1995), in 1992, surveyed all LPCCs in Ohio to determine their success in receiving insurance reimbursement. Out of 970 licensees contacted, 387 (40%) returned the survey. Zimpfer further limited his sample to those clinical counselors who were seeking reimbursement solely on the basis of their clinical counseling license, yielding a sample of 61. Each of these 61 was instructed to randomly select and report the reimbursement records of up to 10 clients. Zimpfer reported that 78 percent of claims disclosed by respondents were approved for reimbursement by insurance carriers, a significant advance compared to Gillen's respondents.

These studies of provider reported reimbursement provide evidence that independent reimbursement for MHCs has occurred at least since the early 1980s. However, the results do not shed light on the extent of such recognition. Studies which simply ask MHCs if they have received reimbursement do not assess the frequency of claims payments. If a MHC had received reimbursement from one insurer, the MHC would be included in the percentage of successful reimbursement recipients. While Zimpfer (1995) attempts to estimate degree of reimbursement success, some important controls are absent. For instance, respondents were asked to pull 10 cases from their files. Although they were asked to do so at random, no controls existed to insure that the reimbursement reported was representative of all cases. Another problem is that insurance companies (e.g., Aetna) were not distinguished from managed care companies (e.g., Biodyne), confounding the voluntary reimbursement of insurers with the contractual reimbursement of network managed care arrangements.

In addition to the problems noted above, results of provider reported reimbursement could be confounded by claims paid in error. For instance, Throckmorton (1992c) noted that one major insurer reimbursed his practice improperly in 68 percent of the claims submitted. Some clients have reported that insurers will claim that benefits were paid in error due to the insured seeing a "non-covered provider." Occasionally, the insurer will demand reimbursement from the client. Since no efforts were made to verify the reimbursement policies of the insurers, the rates reported should be interpreted with caution.

Three studies have reported results of surveys of employers and payers.

Carlson's (1988) survey of 193 corporate employee benefits specialists reported the extent of coverage for a variety of mental health providers. Respondents indicated that 27 percent of benefits plans covered counselors, in contrast to 99 percent which cover the services of psychiatrists, 84 percent for clinical psychologists, and 45 percent for social workers (Carlson, 1988).

The Texas Department of Insurance (TDI) (1992) began surveying health insurers in Texas concerning provider reimbursement policies in 1991. Texas requires insurers to reimburse licensed professional counselors (LPCs) for clinical services. The Department also asked insurers if LPCs were available to 50 percent or more of their insured lives prior to the passage of the mandate law. Seven out of 20 companies responding (35%) reported that they voluntarily reimbursed the charges of LPCs prior to the law requiring such payment. Concerning contracts outside of Texas, the survey asked, "is this benefit commonly included in your policies sold in states where the benefit is not mandated?" Sixty-five percent of the insurers responded that LPCs are not included in policies written in other states (TDI, 1992).

Throckmorton (1992c) surveyed 228 insurers and 32 HMOs doing business in Ohio concerning their mental health provider eligibility policies. The 65 percent insurance company response rate included many insurers which no longer sold health insurance. Of the remaining 28 companies which marketed group health insurance, 25 percent covered Ohio's licensed professional clinical counselors (LPCCs) in their best selling insurance plan, while 46 percent considered LPCCs eligible in at least one plan (Throckmorton, 1992c).

Examining these studies together, provider reported reimbursement is considerably higher than would be suggested by the surveys of payers. Provider reported reimbursement probably overestimates the actual extent of MHC eligibility in traditional health insurance. The aim of each survey methodology has been to estimate the success of MHCs in the marketplace. However, each perspective tells a different tale. Provider reported reimbursement probably says more about the business acumen and practice management skills of the respondents. Providers with high reimbursement rates have apparently learned to seek reimbursement from insurers where the probability of success is high and/or have developed contractual arrangements which guarantee reimbursement (e.g., managed care contracts). On the other hand, payer reported eligibility rates probably give a truer picture of the extent of MHC insurance recognition through the 1980s and early 1990s. Thus, although a minority of insurers surveyed have purposely reimbursed MHCs, MHC practitioners have been reasonably successful in finding them.

In the current marketplace, research attempting to estimate the eligibility of MHCs in insurance contracts would be inadequate. With the advent of self-insurance and managed care, traditional health insurance plans cover much less of the employed population than a decade ago, as little as 33.3 percent by one estimate ("Practice issues," 1994). Thus, MHCs have begun to focus private sector advocacy efforts on self-insured companies and managed care organizations.

Self-Insurance

Employers who assume responsibility for employees' health care instead of purchasing insurance are referred to as "self-insured." Employers may choose to be completely at risk for all health claims or they may opt to purchase "stop-loss" insurance, i.e., insurance against catastrophic claims which might be more than the employer can handle. Such coverage can be either for large claims generated by individual employees or significant health costs accrued by an entire group, often 125 percent of annual group health costs (Cowans, 1995a).

Employers often choose to self-fund to avoid taxes on health care premiums, to provide a consistent health benefits plan in multistate operations, and to avoid state mandates (Geisel, 1990a; Schachner, 1995). The Employee Retirement Income Security Act (ERISA, PL 93-406) preempts state laws which relate to employee benefits plans, including health insurance (Feezor, 1987; Schachner, 1995). Employers who self-insure are not subject to state mandate laws which require insurers to reimburse for mental health benefits or the services of certain providers.

Self-insured companies often use the services of third party administrators (TPA). A TPA is a company which administrates the claims for a self-insuring company. Sometimes called administrative services only (ASO), this arrangement is often confusing to providers. Since insurance companies also provide the administration services, providers and clients often believe they are dealing with an indemnity insurance plan.

The market impact of self-insurance is significant. In 1994, 77 percent of employers with between 1000 and 4999 employees self-funded their health plans, while an estimated 84 to 89 percent of companies with over 5,000 employees self-insured (Schachner, 1995). In 1994, 69 percent of companies with 500 to 999 workers self-funded, while only 18 percent of smaller companies (100 to 499 employees) did so (Cowans, 1995b).

As with traditional insurance, determining the extent of MHC recognition is a task beyond the scope of this chapter. There are no directories of self-funded companies that are readily accessible for use in survey research and benefits offerings change frequently. Since the respondents of Carlson's (1988) survey included some benefit specialists of self-insured employers, MHC eligibility at that time may be approximated by those results.

Blue Cross/Blue Shield

Blue Cross and Blue Shield (BC/BS) are independent, nonprofit membership organizations providing health insurance by arranging for the care to be provided by participating providers within a specified geographic area (Health Insurance Association of America [HIAA], 1990). Often called a hospital service association in state legislation, Blue Cross typically covers the hospital services with Blue Shield (medical service association) responsible for the services of health care practitioners. BC/BS plans sell only health coverage and are actually service arrangements whereby employers purchase access to a group of participating providers for their employees. Covered employees seeing nonparticipating providers will often face higher costs or denied claims.

Both BC/BS are trademarks controlled by the Blue Cross/Blue Shield Association (BCBSA) (Eilers, 1963). Each BC/BS plan is independent with the national organization providing research support, coordination of benefits and lobbying support services (G. Babcock, personal communication, March, 1991). There are currently 69 BC/BS plans operating nationally (Woolsey, 1994). Enrollment in all private plans is an estimated 66 million lives with an additional 34 million enrolled in plans underwritten by the government (P. Kelch, personal communication, March 8, 1995).

Currently, at least one BS plan (Idaho BS) voluntarily accepts MHCs as participating providers (J. Dignan, personal communication, March 3, 1995). BC/BS plans are also subject to the mandates requiring insurers to offer or provide reimbursement for MHCs (see Appendix). BC/BS is opposed to new mandates of any kind (Woolsey, 1992) and has been potent opposition to such legislation in a number of states (e.g., Arkansas) (R. Gerst, personal communication, January, 1995).

Managed Care

Managed care is a term for a wide ranging set of activities which are designed to provide oversight to the delivery of health services. Managed care has been described as "a system that integrates the financing and delivery of appropriate health care services to covered individuals . . . " (HIAA, 1990, p. 19). A managed care organization (MCO) may provide some or all of the following elements: networks of selected providers to furnish a preselected group of health care services, explicit standards for the selection of health care providers, formal programs of quality assurance and utilization review and financial incentives for clients to use the network of providers (Harden, 1994; HIAA, 1990).

Familiar forms of managed care include Health Maintenance Organizations (HMOs), Preferred Provider Organization (PPOs), Exclusive Provider Organizations (EPOs) and more recently Point-of-Service Plans (POS) (Harden, 1994). An HMO is a system of doctors, health care providers and hospitals which deliver health care services to a group of subscribers. Members of the HMO pay an annual fee in advance for all health services rather than paying for each procedure. High utilizers of care do not pay more than low utilizers which is the rationale for HMOs seeking healthier individuals. Approximately 550 HMOs are regulated nationwide with approximately 50 million members (Harden, 1994; "Managed Care," 1994). In Ohio, Throckmorton (1992c) found that three out nine responding HMOs contracted with LPCCs, with another two considering inclusion at the time of the survey.

Most MHCs are familiar with PPOs. Managed care networks are often types of PPOs involving a group of providers selected by a MCO to deliver health care to employer groups which have contracted with the MCO. The savings in costs comes via the MCO negotiating reduced rates from the network providers in exchange for a steady stream of referrals. Members can go to out-of-network providers but are usually penalized by higher deductibles and co-payments (Harden, 1994). An EPO is a more exclusive form of PPO. With some exceptions for emergency care, EPO contracts provide health benefits only if services are secured from network providers (Coopers & Lybrand, 1990).

In a POS plan, the subscriber decides at the time of service whether to secure care from within the network or from an outside provider. The POS plan allows the client to go off network but with significant reduction in reimbursement (HIAA, 1990). Out-of-network services can be self-funded by the employer or underwritten by an insurance company.

The spread of managed mental health care has been nothing short of breathtaking. According to Sipkoff and Oss (1995), 102 million people are enrolled in managed care plans, representing approximately 46 percent of the nation's 222 million insured individuals. Employers using a managed care arrangement for group health coverage jumped from 52 percent in 1993 to 63 percent in 1994 (Geisel, 1995). Employers attribute recent declines in per employee costs for health coverage (1.1% nation-wide from 1993 to 1994) to this large shift of employers away from indemnity health insurance plans and into managed care plans (Geisel, 1995).

MHCs have found increasing acceptance into managed care provider networks. For instance, of the 74 companies reporting provider selection data in a 1994 *Business Insurance* survey of MCOs, 80 percent either employ or contract with licensed professional/mental health counselors ("Directory of Managed," 1994). This is a significant increase from 1992 when only 44 percent of directory respondents listed professional/mental health counselors as network providers (Throckmorton, 1992a). However, among the largest managed care companies, the share of these networks is not great. In that same survey, MHC participation in large managed care networks (3 million+ covered individuals) ranged from 2 percent (Green Springs Health Services) to 9.1 percent (MCC Behavioral Care) of total mental health network providers.

Bistline, Sheridan and Winegar (1991) have identified skills which are vital for competence in managed care practice. They include: orientation to brief psychotherapy, an understanding of the relationship between substance abuse and mental disorders, crisis intervention skills, an understanding of changes in health care delivery and a willingness to use self-help groups. In response to managed care, Foos, Ottens, and Hill (1991) recommend MHCs upgrade credentials, improve marketing strategies, collaborate with primary care physicians and consider forming or joining a group practice.

Employee Assistance Programs (EAPs)

EAPs are offered by many employers to provide confidential problem identification and resolution. Historically developed as resources for employees with substance abuse problems, EAPs have evolved into more comprehensive tools to identify any issue which may impact job performance (Caldwell, 1994). EAPs may offer referral to another mental health practitioner once the assessment phase is complete. Employers may contract with an outside agency or vendor for EAP services or they may create an internal EAP to service only the company employees. Nearly 80 percent of *Fortune 500* companies had initiated EAPs by the late 1980s (Pope, 1990).

In a 1988 survey of EAPs, Hosie, West, and Mackay (1993) reported that 38 percent of employers with in-house EAPs employed masters level counselors. Counselors were employed by 51 percent of external agencies (e.g., community mental health agencies, hospitals) providing EAP services to employers. Finally, 69 percent of external vendors which provide only EAP services employed counselors. Comparatively, Hosie, West, and Mackay found that 67 percent of the external EAP-only respondents employed social workers and 42 percent used doctoral level psychologists. More recently, in a 1994 *Business Insurance* survey of EAPs, 66 percent of the 50 EAPs reporting provider data either employ or contract with professional/mental health counselors ("Directory of Employee," 1994). Thus, MHCs appear to be finding broad acceptance and reimbursement opportunities in EAPs.

Nursing Homes

Despite the exclusion from Medicare eligibility, nursing homes are employing and reimbursing MHCs for their services. In their survey of 124 nursing home administrators in Indiana, Crose and Kixmiller (1994) report that 7 percent of respondents employ counselors and 20 percent contract with counselors as consultants. One large managed care firm, First Mental Health, contracts with MHCs to provide nursing home preadmission screenings and resident reviews where allowed by state law (M. Joyce, personal communication, February 16, 1995).

Common Factors in Eligibility Decisions

Throckmorton (1992c) sought to clarify criteria by which third party payers determine eligibility of counselors. Using qualitative methodology, Throckmorton examined four reimbursement and delivery systems in Ohio, i.e., managed care (American Biodyne, Preferred HealthCare, United Behavioral Systems, Humana HMO), self-insured benefits plans (a local school system, Coresource, British Petroleum, Health Risk Management), traditional health insurance indemnity plans (Aetna Health

Plans, Travelers), and Blue Cross/Blue Shield (Community Mutual Insurance Company).

Eleven different payers were studied in depth. The principal method was to interview those who determined provider eligibility and examine the rationale behind the payer's eligibility decisions concerning MHCs. Complementing the interviews was a mail survey of 228 health insurance companies and 32 Ohio HMOs concerning mental health reimbursement practices.

Throckmorton (1992c) delineated seven factors common to eligibility decisions across delivery systems. The remainder of this section describes these factors and their impact upon the reimbursement eligibility of MHCs in private reimbursement systems.

Employer Preference

Across all reimbursement systems, the most common rationale for payer eligibility decisions was the approval of the purchaser of the health plan. If an employer requests the inclusion of MHCs, most payers will comply. As Hight and Hight (1986) noted, "it is basically the employer's dollar we are all running after" (p. 80).

The current environment of reform increasingly places the employer in the role of determining provider eligibility. For instance, a recent issue of *Practice Strategies* noted that some large employers are requiring managed care companies to alter the provider composition of their networks ("Addictions first", 1995). IBM has established a mental health advisory board to help establish policies relating to provider eligibility ("Select Medco," 1995). As employers have shouldered an increased portion of the risk for coverage of health costs, their role in determining health care policy has increased.

Cost Impact

Companies that reimburse MHCs often noted the positive impact of lower fees. This issue seemed to cut both ways for counselors. Some payers, notably managed care and HMO respondents, believed the lower fees agreed to by masters level providers gave them a competitive edge in selling a network. However, some insurers believed that making MHCs eligible for reimbursement inflates expenditures for mental health services (Feezor, 1986).

Despite the expressed cost concerns of insurers, Throckmorton (1992c) found that many insurers do not collect the data which would allow them to determine the costs of adding MHCs. When asked if costs increased due to the addition of counselors to eligibility status, no insurer responded that adding counselors would raise costs. One responded that adding counselors had not raised costs and the remaining 14 indicated that they were uncertain about the cost consequences. However, half of these unsure respondents disclosed that their company did not track the charges of individual provider groups and thus did not know if adding a provider group to an existing benefit would elevate costs. Apparently, insurer estimates of cost increases due to expanded provider eligibility policies are based on something other than data. Indeed, the available data suggests that expanding provider eligibility has little impact on costs in an indemnity insurance market (Fairbank, 1989; Health Data Institute, 1985; Texas Department of Insurance, 1992).

Licensing Status

By law, some payers in some states, notably Blue Cross/Blue Shield (e.g., Pennsylvania Statutes 40-6322(c)) and HMOs (e.g., Indiana Code 27-13-1-28) must use licensed providers. In addition, Throckmorton (1992c) found that many payers and employers with interstate operations are interested in the national licensing status of a profession. On this dimension, licensing has been a boon and a bane. Positively, MHC licensing has increased the visibility of the profession to consumers and the general public. On the downside, a *Psychotherapy Finances* article noted that managed care companies did not consider counselors "*a uniformly qualified profession* (article emphasis), largely because licensing varies greatly from state to state. Descriptions of services that counselors are qualified to provide under law are as varied as their titles" ("Feedback," 1991, p. 7).

As Throckmorton (1992c) notes, "similar concerns over lack of uniformity of licensing standards has been noted by national Blue Shield organizations, insurers and managed care vendors . . . Payers seem to use the license as a guide to assess the status of a profession. In the case of counselors, a repeated finding is that the profession is not defined consistently by its regulatory laws" (p. 256).

Recently, there is evidence that this perception has found its way into the public sector as well. For instance, when lobbying to include counselors as "essential community providers" in health reform legislation in the 103rd Congress, this author was told by Representative Ted Strickland's (D–OH) health care policy aide that, according to her sources, there were inconsistencies in the training and licensing of counselors. In addition, some of her legislative contacts in the mental health community believed counseling licensing laws were not customarily clinical, i.e., they did not uniformly authorize the practice of diagnosis and treatment of mental and emotional disorders (S. Zettler, personal communication, June 9, 1994). Despite research suggesting that the vast majority of counseling licensing boards consider such clinical practices within the scope of MHC practice (Throckmorton, 1992d, 1994a) and inconsistencies within the statutes regulating colleague professions (e.g., psychology, social work) (Graddy, 1991; Morrissey, 1994), the perception of undue variability continues to hinder full recognition from public and private payers.

Qualifications to Practice

Closely related to the licensing issue is the payer's perception of qualifications. American Biodyne (now Medco Behavioral Care) representatives suggested that some employers have expressed reluctance to purchase services from managed care companies using masters level providers (Throckmorton, 1992c). However, according to the Biodyne respondent, "there have been fewer of these requests as the quality of subdoctoral providers is demonstrated and increased freedom of choice is requested" (p. 214). For most payers, the masters degree with between two to five years of postmasters experience and a license authorizing independent clinical practice were basic qualifications for reimbursement eligibility.

Interestingly, despite the existence of voluntary, national specialty certifications (e.g., CCMHC) available to MHCs, only one payer (Preferred Health Care, now Value Behavioral Health) mentioned the CCMHC as impacting reimbursement. Even in this case, the payer used the educational and experience criteria, not membership in the Academy, to provide a standard. None of the other payers were familiar with this credential.

Statutory Mandates

Currently, 14 states require insurers to provide or offer coverage for the services of MHCs (see Appendix). Ten states require insurers to reimburse for MHC services (mandated coverage legislation), while four states only require insurers to offer such coverage to employers contracting for insurance (mandated offering). Some states include counselors by virtue of an insurance requirement to cover any licensed health or mental health provider. Once counseling became a regulated profession via licensing, those licensed became eligible for reimbursement. Two states, Colorado and Ohio, require insurers and BC/BS plans to reimburse licensed counselors if a physician or psychologist reviews and approves a treatment plan once every three months.

Despite the fact that self-insured companies are not regulated by mandates, such laws may function as a form of payer education. Throckmorton (1992c) found that many payers only recognize a profession as able to practice independently when a mandate requires direct reimbursement. The Aetna Health Plan respondent indicated that one reason Aetna began directly reimbursing social workers in all contracts was the recognition that reimbursement was already mandated in 24 jurisdictions. The increasing prevalence of these requirements caused an heightened awareness of the profession.

Typically, insurers argue that mandates add unnecessarily to the costs of health care (Woolsey, 1992). Further, they argue that adding a new class of providers is cost-prohibitive (Feezor, 1987). Contrary to such fears, the available evidence suggests mandating reimbursement for MHCs does not add significant costs to benefits plans. For instance, the Texas Department of Insurance has monitored the costs of requiring insurers to cover the services of licensed professional counselors (LPCs). Combining 1991 and 1992 costs, the aggregate charges of Texas' LPCs amounted to .07 percent of health care claims paid by companies reporting (Texas Department of Insurance, 1992, 1995). In other words, for every $100 of health costs in Texas, MHCs accounted for seven cents! These data are consistent with the work of Fairbank (1989) and the Health Data Institute (1985) who reported insignificant changes in mental health costs due to the addition of clinical social workers to the list of Massachusetts mandated mental health providers.

A more current form of statutory reimbursement requirement is "any willing provider" legislation. Any willing provider laws regulate managed care networks by permitting any provider willing to meet the conditions and credentialing criteria of a health network to be admitted to that network (Babcock, Laudicina & Oakley, 1994). Limited provider laws regulate a certain profession (e.g., pharmacists) while broader laws require MCOs to contract with providers from any licensed profession. Currently, AR, ID, IN, KY, UT, VA, WA and WY have laws which require HMOs and/or PPOs to contract with any licensed health provider (Babcock et al., 1994). Many of these laws are recent and the application to MHCs is unclear.

Accessibility

Reimbursement eligibility is enhanced by a provider's willingness to adapt to the needs of the payer and by a high level of payer awareness of the provider's profession. This factor responds to the question, does the payer understand the scope of the profession's practice? This factor has worked against MHCs. Nearly 29 percent of insurers responding to Throckmorton's (1992c) survey concerning mental health benefits had not heard of licensed counselors before receiving the survey. Counselors were the least known of all the mental health professions. Only 21 percent of insurers knew that the Ohio license permitted the independent practice of psychotherapy. Individual MHCs may be quite willing to adapt to the needs of payers but find payers have little awareness of the profession.

Inconsistencies in professional titles regulated by state laws and the inability of counseling professional associations to educate payers may have some impact on payer information deficiencies. For instance, when Throckmorton (1992c) asked an Aetna Health Plan policy maker in which states were counselors reimbursed by Aetna, the respondent asked, "which kind of counselor do you want to know about?" (p. 262). The respondent then listed "professional counselors" separately from "mental health counselors." The perception of the insurer was that the different titles represented separate professions.

Organization Specific Factors

Despite the general criteria developed above, some factors were more important for some payers than others. For instance, some BC/BS organizations use Medicare provider eligibility criteria as guidelines whereas most insurers, self-insured companies, managed care organizations and even other Blue Cross/Blue Shield organizations do not.

For most payers, the determination concerning MHC eligibility is a business decision. Payers may defer to the employer, some promote the expanded access and lower costs which comes from including MHCs, whereas others limit provider choice in fear of overutilization or to capitalize on the greater name recognition of other professions. Of course, each of the above factors is not operative in all reimbursement decisions, but knowing that payers evaluate mental health counseling according to these criteria should give focus to the advocacy efforts of MHC professional associations.

Government Programs

The inclusion of mental health counseling in enabling federal legislation is a relatively recent phenomena. Due to regulations allowing federal employees in medically underserved areas (MUAs) to choose LPCs, MHCs have been available to beneficiaries of the Federal Employees Health Benefits Plan (FEHBP) since 1980 (Covin, 1995). The initial inclusion of mental health counseling by title was in the CHAMPUS program in 1988 ("CHAMPUS includes," 1988). In 1992, the Public Policy and Legislation Committee (PPLC) of the American Mental Health Counselors Association (AMHCA) made inclusion in the Public Health Services Act its prime objective. This initiative came agonizingly close to realization, but failed in the waning hours of the 103rd Congress. Inclusion was supported by both parties, but the bill which contained the amendment was not voted on due to concerns about other elements of the legislation (Picard, 1994).

Perhaps the most visible public policy issue in the history of mental health counseling was the effort to insure recognition of MHCs in each health reform bill during the 103rd Congress. The American Counseling Association (ACA) had representation on the Mental Health Liaison Group which lobbied for an expanded mental health benefit in any health care reform legislation. On April 12, 1993, AMHCA and ACA presidents, executive directors and government relations staff persons met with the Mental Health Working Group concerning the inclusion of counselors as eligible providers in the President Clinton's Health Security Act (Hacker, 1993). While all of the major health reform initiatives failed, the efforts of ACA, AMHCA and thousands of MHCs who wrote and called were not in vain. Due to lessons learned during the twin efforts of health care reform and inclusion in the Public Health Services Act, MHCs have taken great steps in increasing legislator's awareness of the profession (Nestor, 1995). The remainder of this section examines each of the major government programs and the role of MHCs in each one.

Public Health Service Corps

As noted above, a prime objective of ACA/AMHCA is to amend article 303(d)(1) of the Public Health Service Act (PHSA). This amendment would place counseling in what is commonly called the list of "core providers." Being so listed would enable counselor education programs to apply for clinical training funds from the Substance Abuse and Mental Health Services Administration (SAMSA). As stated by Senator Mark Hatfield (R–OR), such training grants might encourage "these professionals to serve rural and other underserved populations." (U.S. Senate, 1993, p. S12662). Some MHCs mistakenly believe enumeration in the PHSA is synonymous with inclusion in such programs as Medicare and Medicaid. However, due to the clinical training funds authorized by the PHSA, policy makers for these programs may be more inclined to recognize the professions listed as "clinical" professions. ACA/AMHCA have planned to attempt this legislative change again in the 104th Congress (Nestor, 1995).

Despite absence from the core provider list, MHCs may find employment and internship placements in the Public Health Service Corps (PHSC). Currently, requirements for appointment to the PHSC include a "masters degree in a professional health-related specialty . . . a determination that there is a long-term need within PHS for the person in the specialty concerned" (Department of Health and Human Services [DHHS], 1991, p. 52). Recently, ACA has been informed that the PHS will soon declare that a need exists for MHCs in such underserved areas as corrections, native American reservations and community health centers (H. Stidham, personal communication, March 3, 1995).

Medicare

Medicare insures approximately 30 million people, mostly elderly and totally disabled. There are two Medicare programs. Part A provides inpatient, hospital, and home care benefits while Part B covers outpatient benefits, including mental health treatment. Part B is optional, although most Part A recipients pay a small premium and enroll in the outpatient program.

In 1990, psychologists and clinical social workers were included as eligible providers of mental health services within the Medicare, Part B program (Cummings, 1990). Administered by the Health Care Financing Administration (HCFA) within the Department of Health and

Human Services (DHHS), Medicare claims are paid by insurance companies contracted by HCFA. These companies, known as "fiscal intermediaries" (Part A) and "carriers" (Part B) administer the federal guidelines but make no provider eligibility decisions.

Currently, MHCs may be reimbursed for services performed in partial hospitalization program's furnished by community mental health centers. The MHC may be an employee of the partial program or in private practice and maintain a subcontractual relationship with the program ("Coverage," 1994). However, MHCs are not eligible for direct reimbursement of outpatient services performed in independent practice.

Efforts by MHCs to amend Medicare provider eligibility rules date to at least 1982. Richard Wilmarth, then Chair of AMHCA's Government Relations Committee provided testimony before the House Ways and Means Committee in support of including MHCs in House Bill 6092 (Wilmarth, 1982). Much correspondence between AMHCA and the Ways and Means Committee was conducted but with no eligibility change. In the 1992–93 Congress, MHCs, psychiatric nurses and marriage & family therapists were the subject of HR 4457, a bill that would have made these providers eligible for reimbursement. This bill was not reported out of committee.

While currently ineligible for direct reimbursement, MHCs can be covered for services "incident to" a physician's or clinical psychologist's (but not a clinical social worker's) professional services. Ironically, "incident to" services often receive a higher per unit rate of reimbursement than if billed independently. To be reimbursable, the following conditions must be met: (1) The physician must initially render a covered personal, professional service for which the services of the nonphysician can be considered integral, although incidental; (2) the service must be appropriate, rather than a procedure which would be reserved for the physician; (3) the service must be rendered under the direct supervision of a physician or clinical psychologist; (4) the physician or clinical psychologist must be physically present in the office suite and available to render assistance if necessary; (5) the physician's professional responsibility for the patient's care should be documented in the patient's medical record; (6) evidence of collaborative development of a treatment plan must be documented; (7) the nonphysician must be an employee of the physician, physician directed facility or an employee of the clinical psychologist or the organization that employs the psychologist; and (8) incidental services must represent an expense incurred by the physician, clinic, or clinical psychologist (Nationwide Insurance Company, 1993). Consequently, MHCs working in a group practice or community agency may be able to provide services to Medicare eligible individuals.

Medicaid

Initiated in 1965, Medicaid was initially conceived as a safety net for the "deserving poor" (Maloy, 1990). Initially, the recipients were poor women and children and the elderly, blind and disabled receiving Social Security benefits. Eligibility requirements have been expanded somewhat, but Medicaid remains a program of basic insurance for individuals below the poverty line. Medicaid is funded with a complex combination of federal and state money. While federal law determines the services covered, the states determine the provider eligibility requirements. Outpatient mental health services are optional but, as of 1990, were included in some form in 40 states (Maloy, 1990).

Traditionally, outpatient psychotherapy reimbursement is limited to psychiatrists and community mental health centers (CMHC). However, as a means of improving mental health services while attempting to contain cost increases, states are increasingly seeking federal permission (waivers) to serve Medicaid eligible citizens via community-based and managed care approaches ("Medicaid," 1995). As of 1993, 36 states were implementing at least one managed care program for Medicaid recipients (General Accounting Office, 1993). Waivers allow states flexibility in the location (e.g., schools) and the model (e.g., managed care) of service delivery. Given the increasing willingness of managed care organizations to include MHCs, these changes may be advantageous for counselors who are currently involved in managed care networks (Cohen & O'Brien, 1994).

Counselors direct reimbursement eligibility is sparse nationally. Counselors in independent practice are required to be reimbursed by Medicaid in Montana. Oregon LPCs can be directly reimbursed if under contract with the county mental health authority (D. Steinke, personal communication, March 10, 1995). Frequently due to Medicaid waivers, program specific Medicaid reimbursement is available for preventive health services in Alabama (Covin & Jackson, 1993), nursing home resident screening in Georgia (M. Joyce, personal communication, February 16, 1995), school based mental health services in Oregon and Ohio (F. Blazewicz, personal communication, January 25, 1995), crisis intervention services in Tennessee (Cohen & O'Brien, 1994) and physician-referred mental health services to children 18 and under in Texas (R. Dubois, personal communication, March 2, 1995). Medicaid provider eligibility is expected to become more flexible with the increased use of waivers and state willingness to attempt service innovations.

CHAMPUS

The Civilian Health and Medical Program of the Uniformed Services (CHAMPUS) is an insurance program for military families, retirees and their families, and some former spouses and survivors of deceased military members (CHAMPUS, 1990). A comparable program—CHAMPVA—exists for families of veterans with a 100 percent service-connected disability. Mental health treatments are covered in this program but are subject to utilization review. CHAMPUS will only cover medically necessary services in the treatment of disorders listed in the DSM-IV (CHAMPUS, 1990).

MHCs were recognized by CHAMPUS as a separate professional classification in 1988 ("CHAMPUS includes," 1988). Clients must be referred to the MHC by a physician. Furthermore, CHAMPUS requires that services be performed under the supervision of a physician. "Physician referral" means that the "physician must actually see the patient, perform an evaluation and arrive at an initial diagnostic impression prior to referring the patient" (CHAMPUS, 1990, p. 46). Documentation is required and communication must occur between the MHC and physician. These requirements only apply to MHCs or pastoral counselors.

To be eligible for CHAMPUS reimbursement, MHCs must have a masters degree, two years postmasters experience consisting of 3000 hours experience and 100 hours supervision and a state license authorizing mental health counseling. If the MHC practices in a state without licensing, the MHC must possess certification from the Academy of Certified Clinical Mental Health Counselors, or be eligible for such certification (CHAMPUS, 1990).

Currently, AMHCA's Public Policy and Legislation Committee has identified the removal of the physician referral requirement as a legislative objective (Picard, 1994). CHAMPUS policy makers have suggested that a change in federal statute may be required in order to remove the physician referral requirement (R. Sabo, personal communication, February 1, 1995).

Vocational Rehabilitation

Vocational rehabilitation (P.L. 102-52) is a program in the Department of Education which supports state effort to retrain disabled workers. Vocational rehabilitation reimburses for evaluations of rehabilitation potential and other rehabilitation services. The reauthorization of the Rehabilitation Act Amendments of 1993 removed the requirement that a physician or psychologist must be consulted to diagnose and treat mental and emotional disorders. This change allows diagnostic and restorative services to be provided by any professional with a license authorizing diagnosis and treatment. For instance, Ohio's Bureau of Vocational Rehabilitation specifically designated licensed professional clinical counselors as eligible service providers due to the change in federal law (Throckmorton, 1994b).

Head Start

A DHHS program to provide comprehensive child development and family support services to needy families, Head Start has a mental health component. Qualified mental health professionals (state licensed providers) may provide consultation and direct service to Head Start grantees. The Head Start Health Performance Standards (45-CFR. 1304, 3–8) note that "the mental health part of the (health) plan shall provide that a mental health professional shall be available, at least on a consultation basis, to the Head Start Program and to the children." (DHHS, 1984, p. 34). Head Start grantees require classroom observation, consultation, staff-in-service training, direct service to parents and children and community referral. MHCs with appropriate education and experience with children are eligible to serve in this capacity.

Veteran's Administration

The Veteran's Administration provides a variety of services to veterans of all wars. One outpatient program open to MHCs in some regions is the Readjustment Counseling program (P.L. 98-160). Veterans serving during war time from August 5, 1964 to the present may be eligible for counseling services specifically to assist the veteran to adjust successfully to civilian life. Expertise in treating Post-traumatic Stress Disorder is important. Woman veterans who suffered sexual assault or abuse during military service were given additional access to services by Public Law

102-585, passed in 1992. To gain authorization to treat such clients, one should contact the nearest VA hospital or VET Center.

MHCs with licenses permitting independent clinical practice are generally eligible, although some regional differences exist. Application is once per year (usually August-September) and is a competitive bidding process. Since the VA Hospitals also provide this treatment, the most desired providers are those operating at great distances from these facilities.

Federal Employees Health Benefits Program (FEHBP)

The Federal Employees Health Benefits Program (FEHBP) insures more than 10 million federal employees. Although the Office of Personnel Management (OPM) has federal oversight of the program, a variety of private insurers, HMOs and managed care companies administrate this program throughout the country. Mental health services are covered, but MHCs are not required to be reimbursed. In 1980, MHCs became eligible for reimbursement in Medically Underserved Areas (MUAs) due to Public Law 96-179 (Covin, 1985). Current states considered MUAs are AL, GA, LA, MS, NM, ND, SC, SD, WV & WY (Covin, 1995).

Since in the author's experience, intermediaries have some flexibility in reimbursement decisions, MHCs should contact the claims office designated on the client's claim form to preauthorize payment. Individual carriers may selectively authorize treatment based upon availability of providers and type of service required.

ACA/AMHCA conducted a major initiative to include MHCs in FEHBP during 1994. However, OPM's response to numerous subscriber requests for MHC eligibility was negative. In a letter to Helen Stidham, ACA Assistant Executive Director, OPM's Lucretia Myers, Assistant Director for Insurance Programs wrote, "During the recent negotiation cycle, OPM did not require that all plans include LPCs in their definition of a 'covered provider'... Although we did not include LPC services in our benefit initiatives this year, we will reconsider our position when we develop our strategy for the next negotiation cycle." (H. Stidham, personal communication, March 2, 1995).

State Employees Benefits Plans

Comparable to the FEHBP, states provide medical benefits to state employees. States typically self-fund these plans and have considerable involvement in the provider eligibility policies. Some states contract the administration of the mental health benefits to an outside managed care vendor ("Green Spring," 1995). At present, at least 18 states (AR, AL, CA, CO, FL, ID, IL, LA, MI, MT, OH, OK, OR, SC, TX, VT, VA, WV) involve MHCs as eligible providers of mental health care to state workers (AMHCA, 1995).

Reimbursement for MHCs: Summary and Outlook

Hopefully, this chapter will be incomplete by publication. As these words are being written, MHCs are involved in licensing efforts, negotiations with third party payers and innovations in service delivery. Rapid changes in the health care marketplace, legislative changes due to MHC lobbying and state and federal initiatives in health reform all make predicting the future of MHC reimbursement difficult. This chapter was designed to give the reader a current summary of MHC reimbursement experience in private and public sector markets.

Looking back, MHCs over the last decade have taken some of the steps necessary to achieve broad recognition and reimbursement eligibility. For instance, to address a variety of credentialing issues which hindered MHCs' development as a profession, ACA's Professionalization Committee convened a meeting of ACA and division leaders in January, 1993. One purpose of this meeting was to examine the usefulness of ACA's model licensing law. The participants of this meeting recommended that the model licensing law be revised to include clinical language. A task force of Harriet Glosoff, James Benshoff and Thomas Hosie headed the revisions of the model licensing bill to include language which, when adopted by a state, would permit the diagnosis and treatment of a full range of mental and emotional disorders (ACA, 1994). Taking ACA/AMHCA's lead, state associations have found legislative success in modifying definitions of counseling to insure the authorization of clinical activities ("Counselors," 1994; Throckmorton, 1994a).

Along with statutory success, the last decade has seen a significant increase in the reimbursement opportunities for MHCs. Contrary to the warning of Asher (1979) that counselors may find themselves eliminated from reimbursement systems, MHCs are making strides toward parity with their colleague professions. As evidenced by the increased managed care presence, MHCs are demonstrating resilience in a changing marketplace. Given the continuing focus on cost containment, preventive care and care provided in the least restrictive environment, the future has brightened for the involvement of MHCs in mental health care delivery.

Despite the positive tone of this reflection on MHC progress, counseling professional associations have much work to do in order to make the profession accessible to payers and employers. Employers, legislators and government payers continue to display information deficiencies of the kind which surfaced during the health reform debate. For example, in a recent point paper released by the Department of the Navy, counselor professional preparation was incorrectly described as primarily a one-year masters degree with an emphasis on educational issues (A. Harris, personal communication, February 17, 1995). ACA and AMHCA should expend additional resources toward a comprehensive educational program targeted toward large employers, business trade groups and each office of government which impacts mental health care delivery. The establishment of a registry identifying "clinical service providers in counseling" may assist payers to identify individual MHCs who have met state licensing and professional standards.

Research concerning third party reimbursement should take on a more collaborative approach (Throckmorton, 1992c). For instance, additional use of qualitative methods in studies of private employers and government reimbursement sources might serve twin functions of understanding the evolving criteria for reimbursement decisions and gaining additional eligibility successes. Replicating the surveys of payers in various jurisdictions would allow for a more complete understanding of MHC acceptance in the marketplace.

While the licensing successes have been impressive, nine states are without any form of credentialing. Existing laws without clinical scope of practice should be brought in line with current professional standards. Licensing has become a basic requirement for independent practice and direct third party compensation. Completing the credentialing process should be a high priority for state and national counseling associations.

Health care reform and legislation to regulate payers will continue to be a focus of political activity. State and national MHC associations will continue to lobby for appropriate inclusion of MHC services. Faced with exclusionary policies which bar consumers from MHCs, state MHC associations likely will collaborate with other professional groups to support mandate and/or any willing provider bills. Such laws may be subject to interpretation and court challenge (Babcock et al., 1994).

State and national associations will probably be required to support legal initiatives to maintain legislative gains.

Despite the priority of legal regulation for MHCs, market forces are likely to make demonstrated areas of competence more important to payers than professional identification. The decision of the American Psychological Association to certify psychologists in proficiency areas, such as substance abuse treatment and hospital practice is portrayed as a response to requests from private and government payers ("APA to credential," 1995). Weikel (1986) anticipated that payers might opt for voluntary certification as one means of quality assurance. However, the credentials desired seem to be in addition to licensing and related to expertise in a clinical specialization rather than designating a professional identity. Perhaps, MHC organizations will need to adapt credentialing initiatives away from those which define professional "turf" and toward an in-service, competency based approach.

While MHCs can point to a number of significant policy gains, Rudolph's (1986) warning should be heeded today, "the favorable legislation previously mentioned should not and must not lull MHCs into an unfortunate and ill-founded complacency." (p. 282). Without vigilance and flexibility from MHC leaders and grassroots involvement from all MHCs, the gains could be quickly marginalized by a rapidly changing practice environment.

REFERENCES

Addictions first; therapy later. (1995, February). *Practice Strategies*, pp. 4–6.

American Counseling Association. (1994, April). *Model legislation for licensed professional counselors*. Alexandria, VA: Author.

American Mental Health Counselors Association. (1995, February 10). *MHCs in state employees health benefits plans*. (Unpublished chart available from AMHCA, P.O. Drawer 22370, Alexandria, VA, 22304.

APA to credential proficiencies. (1995, February). *Behavioral Health Practice Advisor*, pp. 8–9.

Asher, J.K. (1979). The coming exclusion of counselors from the mental health system. *American Mental Health Counselors Journal, 1*, 53–60.

Babcock, G., Laudicina, S.S., & Oakley, B.C. (1994, December). *State legislative health care and insurance issues: 1994 Survey of plans*. Washington, DC: Blue Cross Blue Shield Association.

Bistline, J.L., Sheridan, S.M., & Winegar, N. (1991). Five critical skills for mental health counselors in managed health care. *Journal of mental health counseling, 13*, 147–152.

Caldwell, B. (1994, December). EAPs: Survey identifies uses and administration. *Employee Benefit Plan Review,* pp. 36–38.

Carlson, B. (1988, May). *Growing uncertainties—Mandated benefits and long term care: Commentary. Census results of certified employee benefits specialists.* Brookfield, WI: International Society of Certified Employee Benefits Specialists.

Castro, J. (1993, May 31). What price mental health? *Time,* pp. 59–60.

CHAMPUS includes mental health counselors as authorized providers. (1988, April). *AMHCA News,* pp. 1, 10.

Civilian Health and Medical Program of the Uniformed Services (1990, May 24). *CHAMPUS Provider Handbook.* Aurora, CO: Author.

Cohen, M. & O'Brien, J. (1994, November 15). *OhioCare special mental health related service: A report to the Ohio Department of Mental Health on the design of its Medicaid managed care program—Final Report,* Technical Assistance Collaborative & KPMG Peat Marwick (Available from the Ohio Department of Mental Health, 30 East Broad St., Columbus, OH, 43266.

Coopers & Lybrand. (1990). *Managed health care: A reference guide.* Chicago: Author.

Counselors battle for legal recognition. (1994, July). *Psychotherapy finances,* p. 3.

Coverage for partial hospitalization services furnished by community mental health centers. (1994, April). *Medicare, Part B Update,* p. 43.

Covin, T.M. (1985). *How to collect third party payments: The professional counselor's guide to successful third party reimbursement.* Ozark, AL: Center for Counseling and Human Development.

Covin, T.M. (1988). Trends in third-party reimbursement among non-medical mental health providers in the United States. Unpublished manuscript, Center for Counseling and Human Development, Inc., Ozark, AL.

Covin, T.M. (1995, January). Freedom of choice and the Federal Employees Health Benefits Plan—1995 update. *Advocate,* p. 4.

Covin, T.M., & Jackson, R.M. (1993, February). Alabama MHCs are pioneers in primary health care services. *Advocate,* p. 6.

Covin, T.M., Wright, K., & Preston, F. (1990). Current trends in third party reimbursement among licensed professional counselors in Alabama. *Alabama Association for Counseling and Development Journal, 16*(2), 35–42.

Cowans, D.S. (1995a, February 6). An explanation of stop-loss insurance. *Business Insurance,* p. 19.

Cowans, D.S. (1995b, February 6). Insurers eager to stop loss of business. *Business Insurance,* pp. 18–19.

Crose, R. & Kixmiller, J.S. (1994). Counseling psychologists as nursing home consultants: What do administrators want? *The Counseling Psychologist, 22,* 104–114.

Cummings, N.A. (1990). Collaboration or internecine warfare: The choice is obvious but elusive. *Journal of Counseling and Development, 68,* 503–504.

Department of Health and Human Services. (1984, November). *Head Start performance standards, (45-CFR 1304).* (DHHS Publication No. OHDS-86-31131). Washington, DC: U.S. Government Printing Office.

Department of Health and Human Services. (1991, January 2). *Personnel instruction 4: Appointment standards and appointment boards, Public Health Service Corps.* (DHHS

Publication No. PHS–CC 533). Washington, DC: U.S. Government Printing Office.

Directory of employee assistance program vendors. (1994, June 27). *Business Insurance,* pp. 22–37.

Directory of managed mental health care networks. (1994, June 27). *Business Insurance,* pp. 38–51.

Eilers, R.D. (1963). *Regulation of Blue Cross and BlueShield plans.* Homewood: Richard D. Irwin.

Fairbank, A. (1989). Expanding insurance coverage to alternative types of psychotherapists: Demand and substitution effects of direct reimbursement to social workers. *Inquiry, 26,* 170–181.

Feedback: Answers to your questions. (1991). *Psychotherapy Finances,* p. 7.

Feezor, A. (1986). Private third party payment as a source for mental health care. In M.M. Hastings, *Financing Mental Health Services: Perspectives for the 1980's* (pp. 16–22). Washington, D.C.: U.S. Department of Health and Human Services.

Feezor, A. (1987, April). No future guarantees for self-insured plans. *Business and Health, 4*(6), 16–19.

Foos, J.A., Ottens, A.J., & Hill, L.K. (1991). Managed mental health: A primer for counselors. *Journal of Counseling and Development, 69,* 332–336.

Geisel, J. (1990a, December 3). ERISA pre-emption upheld. *Business Insurance,* pp. 2, 66.

Geisel, J. (1990b, December 3). Mental health costs: Large employers see 50% increase: Study. *Business Insurance,* p. 64.

Geisel, J. (February 13, 1995). Health market changes spur 1% drop in costs. *Business Insurance.* pp. 1, 10.

General Accounting Office. (1993, March 17). *Medicaid: States turn to managed care to improve access and control costs.* (GAO/HRD-93-46), Washington, DC: Author.

Gillen II, V.L. (1988). *Licensed professional clinical counselors and third party reimbursement: An Ohio study.* Master's thesis. Ohio University, Athens, Ohio.

Graddy, E. (1991). Interest groups or the public interest: Why do we regulate health occupations? *Journal of Health Politics, Policy and Law, 16,* 25–49.

Green Spring to serve VA state employees. (1995, March). *Practice Strategies,* p. 10.

Hacker, C. (1993, April). Robinson meets with the Clinton health care task force. *Advocate,* p. 16.

Harden, S.L. (1994). *What legislators need to know about managed care.* Denver, CO: National Conference of State Legislatures.

Health Data Institute. (1985). *The impact of vendorship for social workers on the use and cost of ambulatory mental health services.* Lexington, MA: Author.

Health Insurance Association of America. (1990). *Source book of health insurance data — 1990.* Washington, D.C.: Author.

Hight, E.S. & Hight, R.G. (1986). Third party financing for family therapists: Views of an insurance executive and a family therapist. *Journal of Independent SocialWork, 1*(2), 79–87.

Hilzenrath, D.S. (1994, July 25). The quandary over mental health care costs. *The Washington Post,* p. A6.

Hosie, T.W., West, J.D., & Mackay, J.A. (1993). Employment and roles of counselors in Employee Assistance Programs. *Journal of Counseling and Development, 72,* 355–359.

Kelley, M. (1986). Mental health services and insurance in California. In M.M. Hastings, *Financing Mental Health Services: Perspectives for the 1980s* (pp. 23–26). Washington, D.C.: U.S. Dept. Health & Human Services.

Madden, R.B. (1988). The relationship between degree level and credentialing with four professional descriptors of mental health counselors. (Doctoral dissertation, Northern Arizona University) *Dissertation Abstracts International, 49,* 2157A.

Maloy, K. (1990, November). Medicaid financing for mental health services: Intertwined in the health care policy Gordian Knot. *Policy in Perspective,* pp. 1–4.

Managed care: The industry is preparing for rapid growth in 1995. (1994, December). *Psychotherapy Finances,* pp. 3–4.

Medicaid waivers. (1995). *Practice Strategies,* p. 3.

Mehr, R.I., & Cammack, E. (1976). *Principles of insurance—Sixth Ed.* Homewood, IL: Richard D. Irwin.

Morrissey, M. (1994, September). State licensing regulations vary for many professionals. *Counseling Today,* p. 11.

Nationwide Insurance Company. (1993, August). *Medicare, Part B, handbook.* Columbus, OH: Author.

Nestor, J. (1995, January). AMHCA prepares for the 104th Congress. *Advocate,* p. 1.

Picard, R. (1994, November/December). Public policy and legislative issues. *Advocate,* p. 7.

Pope, T. (1990, August). EAPs: Good idea, but what's the cost? *Management Review,* pp. 50–53.

Practice issues: Do freedom-of-choice laws still matter? (1994, December). *Psychotherapy Finances,* pp. 6–7.

Rudolph, J. (1986). Third-party reimbursement and mental health counselors. In A.J. Palmo & W.J. Weikel (Eds.). *Foundations of Mental Health Counseling,* (pp. 271–284). Springfield, IL: Charles C Thomas Publisher.

Schachner, M. (1995, February 6). Self-insurers rally to defend favored benefit funding tool. *Business Insurance,* pp. 3–4.

Select Medco provider groups, staff will treat IBM and FedEx employees. (1995, February). *Practice Strategies,* pp. 1–2.

Seligman, L., & Whitely, N. (1983). AMHCA and VMHCA members in private practice in Virginia. *AMHCA Journal, 5,* 179–183.

Sipkoff, M.Z. & Oss, M.E. (1995, January). I need to sign a managed care contract: Who are these people anyway? *Behavioral Health Practice Advisor,* pp. 4–5.

Texas Department of Insurance. (1992). *1991 group health insurance survey report.* Austin, TX: Author.

Texas Department of Insurance. (1995, March). *1992 group accident and health insurance survey report.* Austin, TX: Author.

Throckmorton, E.W. (1992a, Spring/Summer). Forty-four percent of managed care companies include professional counselors in networks. *Access,* p. 4.

Throckmorton, E.W. (1992b, Spring/Summer). J.W. Didion & Associates covers the services of LPCCs. *Access,* p. 3.

Throckmorton, E.W. (1992c). *Mental health counselors and reimbursement decisions: How do third party payers of mental health benefits decide which mental health providers to pay?* (Doctoral dissertation, Ohio University, Athens, OH, 1992).

Throckmorton, E.W. (1992d, March 29). *State licensure and third party reimbursement: Which states permit professional counselors to provide reimburseable clinical services?* Paper presented at the national convention of the American Association of Counseling and Development, Baltimore, MD.

Throckmorton, E.W. (1994a). *Clinical scope of practice and state licensure.* Presentation given at the Winter Workshop of the Ohio Association for Counselor Education and Supervision, February 25, 1994, Columbus, OH.

Throckmorton, E.W. (1994b). Ohio Rehabilitation Services Commission recognizes LPCCs. *Access,* pp. 1, 3.

U.S. Senate. (1993, September 29). Mental health counselors. *Congressional Record-Senate,* p. S12662.

Weikel, W.J. (1986). Future trends in mental health counseling. In A.J. Palmo & W.J. Weikel (Eds.). *Foundations of Mental Health Counseling* (pp. 271–284). Springfield, IL: Charles C Thomas Publisher.

Wilmarth, R. (1982, December 14). *Testimony before the Subcommittee on Health of the Committee on Ways and Means, House of Representatives, on H.R. 6092.* Washington, D.C.: U.S. Government Printing Office.

Woolsey, C. (1992, April 6). 41 benefit mandates added by states in '91. *Business Insurance,* pp. 2, 10.

Woolsey, C. (1994, August 15). Blues switching to managed care to be competitive. *Business Insurance,* pp. 1, 25.

Zimpfer, D.G. (1995). Third party reimbursement experience of licensed clinical counselors in Ohio. *Journal of Mental Health Counseling, 17,* 105–113.

Appendix

States with Insurance Vendorship
for Professional Counselors

State	Date Enacted	License Required	Additional Requirements	Type of Mandate[1]	Extra-territoriality[2]
Arkansas	1991, 1995	LPC	willing to accept insurers' conditions	coverage	yes
California	1981	MFCC	physician referral if required by policy	coverage	yes
Florida	1992	LMHC	none	offering	no
Mississippi	1992	LPC	none	coverage	no
Missouri	1993	LPC	none	offering	no
Montana	1987	LPC, LCC, LCPC	none	coverage	yes
Nebraska	1994	any licensed mental health provider	none	coverage	yes
Rhode Island	1994	CCMH	none	coverage[3]	yes
South Dakota	1987,1994	any qualified mental health professional	none	coverage	yes
Texas	1989	LPC	none	coverage	yes
Utah	1986,1994	any licensed health care provider	none	coverage	yes
Vermont	1976,1988	any licensed or certified mental health professional	none	offering	no
Virginia	1987	LPC	none	coverage	no
Wyoming	1971,1987	any licensed health care professional	none	coverage	no

Compiled by Warren Throckmorton, PhD
AMHCA, PP&L Committee, 3/95

---

[1] A **mandated coverage** law requires an insurer to reimburse a mental health professional when the policy includes benefits for mental health servi which are within the professional's scope of practice. A **mandated offering** law only requires the insurer to offer to the employer the coverage for ; benefit or a provider group and the employer has the option to refuse to include the benefit or provider group in the employee benefits plan.

[2] **Extraterritoriality** refers to a requirement to reimburse a provider no matter where the insurance policy was written or delivered. If a law requir all policies, whether written in state or out of state, to reimburse, then the law provides for extraterritorial coverage. Some laws only regulate policie written in the state. This provision is often unclear in law and is subject to varying interpretations by insurers and providers.

[3] Although insurers must reimburse all CCMHs, Blue Cross/Blue Shield plans and HMOs do not have to reimburse all licensed providers, just those with whom they have a contract. BC/BS and HMOs can limit coverage to services provided in conjunction with a related medical illness.

SECTION V
ASSESSMENT, RESEARCH, ETHICS, CURRICULUM, AND TRENDS IN MENTAL HEALTH COUNSELING

Chapter 15

THE ROLE OF ASSESSMENT IN MENTAL HEALTH COUNSELING

DEAN W. OWEN, JR.

A central idea which lies at the heart of mental health counseling, both in theory and in practice, is the process of individual assessment. A fundamental belief held by mental health counselors is that each client, regardless of presenting problem or circumstance, brings to counseling a unique pattern of traits, characteristics, and qualities which have evolved as a combination of genetic endowment and life experience. It can be argued that, through counseling, a client becomes more aware of and in tune with these many facets. This self knowledge forms the basis for effective decision making and enhanced coping.

It often falls on the mental health counselor to assist the client in the acquisition of this self knowledge and this awareness of the unique constellation of traits, qualities, abilities, and characteristics which defines each individual as unique in all the world. The initial phase of virtually any branch of counseling then is probably best described as one of information gathering or appraisal and provides the mental health counselor "stuff" with which to begin work. Despite the fact that counselors quite routinely gather large amounts of subjective information about their clients, many seem to view systematic and objective appraisal and testing not as an integral part of the counseling process but as an infrequently used adjunct to their work (Loesch & Vacc, 1991). Since information with, for, and about a client is gathered anyway as an integral part of the counseling process, the formal and objective collection of relevant data through the use of psychometric instruments and techniques should be a central and fundamental component of the work of a mental health counselor. Shertzer & Linden (1979) argued that a primary reason for assessment is to assist in understanding an individual and, perhaps more importantly, to foster an individual's understanding of him or herself.

Before going any further, it would be helpful to define a number of basic terms which are central to any discussion of psychometrics. The first of these is the term "measurement." Since ours is a society which tends to value science, this term has a rather precise meaning. That meaning is grounded in the concept of quantification or the process of assigning a numeric value to a trait, quality, or characteristic. To describe an individual as being "very tall" obviously implies that some sort of value judgement has been made. That value judgement can vary among individuals. To say that a person is six feet seven inches tall has a very different meaning which is consistent from one person to another provided, of course, that the units of measurement, in this case feet and inches, are known.

The term "test" is the second term which requires some comment. Some of the traits and qualities possessed by an individual are more or less directly observable. One's height or weight can be measured quite directly using a tape measure or scale. Even one's ability to run can be assessed by using a stopwatch. But the problem becomes somewhat more difficult if the task is to measure something other than a physical characteristic or a psychomotor behavior, both of which are directly observable. Since behavior in the cognitive or affective domain is not directly observable, something else must be done to elicit some sort of psychomotor activity which can be observed. That something else is called a test. Generally, a test will represent a task or series of tasks designed to elicit a psychomotor behavior which permits one to infer the existence of an internal cognitive or affective state.

Finally, the term "evaluation" may be best defined as a process of collecting as much information as is practical for the purpose of enhancing the quality and confidence of a decision. Generally, the more important the decision, the more carefully information is gathered and considered. Evaluation will usually involve some sort of interpretation and value judgement.

Assessment Techniques

There are a great many techniques and procedures which can be utilized by mental health counselors to assist in the gathering of needed information with, for, and about a client. These procedures can generally be divided into two major categories.

Nonstandardized Procedures: This category of assessment techniques may be regarded as somewhat less rigorous but is absolutely essential to the work of a counselor. These procedures are idiosyncratic and may be specifically tailored to a given client or situation. Chief among the nonstandardized assessment procedures is the direct observation of a client. Gibson and Mitchell (1981) identified three levels of observation:

First Level: Casual Informational Observation. The daily unstructured and usually unplanned observations that provide casual impressions. Nearly everyone engages in this type of activity. No training or instrumentation is expected or required.

Second Level: Guided Observation. Planned, directed observations for a purpose. Observation at this level is usually facilitated by simple instruments such as checklists or rating scales. This is the highest level used in most counseling programs. Some training is usually desirable.

Third Level: Clinical Level. Observations, often prolonged, and frequently under controlled conditions. Sophisticated techniques and instruments are utilized with training usually at a doctoral level (Gibson & Mitchell, 1981, p. 111).

Observational instruments have been utilized for many years to structure and organize the process of collecting observational information during counseling and therapy. Peterson and Nisenholtz (1987) describe a number of these instruments including:

Checklists: A simple checklist may include whether or not a particular characteristic was observed. For example, characteristics may include: __1. Is Punctual; __2. Is able to carry on a sustained conversation.

Rating Scales. A rating scale is, in reality, a special form of checklist on which a rater can indicate not only the presence or absence of a characteristic but an estimation of strength, frequency, or the degree to which it is apparent. Frequently a Likert type scale is used as is the case in the following example. 1. Client initiates conversation spontaneously __1. never __2. rarely __3. sometimes __4. usually __5. always.

Anecdotal Reports. These reports are often nothing more than subjective descriptions of a client's behavior at a specific time or place. Often case notes, completed at the conclusion of a counseling session, may include anecdotal reports which can be evaluated periodically to determine the existence of themes or patterns of behavior.

Structured Interview: The structured interview is quite literally a questionnaire which is read to a client by a counselor who carefully records the client's responses. They can be developed by the counselor or, as in many cases, may be a standard interview utilized by an agency as part of the case management system.

Questionnaires: This type of instrument is often used to collect information directly from the client and the responses collected often form the basis for initial discussions with the client to investigate areas of concern.

Personal Essays/Journals: These instruments can be a rich source of information which can be requested directly from the client and which can often be quite helpful in clarifying patterns of thought and behavior.

Standardized Assessment Techniques

The techniques described above all have a common characteristic in that they can be modified or changed to suit the client or situation. The use or administration of any of these techniques could vary from one counselor to another. The category of standardized assessment techniques differs from those above in that they are usually developed and published by commercial test publishers, have years of development and research supporting them, and are administered and scored in strict accordance with published procedures. In this way, such a test is given and evaluated in the same fashion for each client.

Nearly any test which can be administered can be categorized into one of the following five general domains, all of which represent an area of interest for mental health counselors and their clients.

Achievement: These are tests which purport to measure what has been learned in the recent past and usually represents the change in ability as the result of formal training or life experience.

Aptitude: This is a test which purports to predict the degree to which an individual can learn and master some skill or body of information in the future. As Hills (1981) has suggested, the distinction between achievement and aptitude tests lies more in the purpose for testing than in what is tested. Both tests measure what has already been learned, but in the case of the aptitude test, the purpose is to predict future performance rather than to measure the effects past learning or life experience.

Intelligence: These tests purport to measure a highly specialized and differentiated form of aptitude and they seek to predict the extent to which an individual can succeed in school. In this sense they are often regarded as scholastic or academic aptitude tests if for no other reason than the fact that they have been validated against measures of academic performance (Anastasi, 1988). These tests are frequently used during initial evaluations conducted for occupational and educational counseling and in personnel selection.

Vocational Preference. This type of test is, in reality, not a test in the usual sense of the word since there are usually no "right" or "wrong" answers. These instruments usually rely on a self-report format in which an individual is asked to indicate from among groups of activities his or her preferences. These preferences are then later grouped and categorized into related areas and the results generate a pattern which is assumed to be characteristic of the individual.

Personality: This group of tests purport to measure a large group of traits, preferences, and values which conspire to make each person a unique individual. While each of us has a personality, each of us is unique because our particular constellation of behaviors, attitudes, beliefs, and values has been molded by a lifetime of experience. This group of tests can be further subdivided into two large categories. The first of these is a group of tests which purport to assess the degree of mental health or the existence of psychopathology. Tests of psychopathology are typically used for diagnostic purposes and typically have as their central theme a theoretical base of what constitutes a healthy or unhealthy, adaptive or maladaptive pattern of behavior. The second category represents tests which seek only to categorize the traits and patterns of normal behavior which may predispose an individual to success or happiness in particular occupations, work settings, or leisure activities, for example. These tests are frequently used to assist clients in making decisions regarding education and work but may also be used in providing insight into other patterns of human interaction such as in marriage and family counseling, for example.

Assessment Functions in Mental Health Counseling

As mental health counselors seek to work effectively with their clients, there are those occasions where the necessary information cannot be obtained through conversation or observation and the use of tests or some structured psychometric technique is considered desirable. These situations are usually tied to the need for the client and/or the counselor to make a decision. Generally, these decisions are based upon some information which can often be most objectively and efficiently collected through the use of a test. These decisions, and therefore, reasons for testing can be categorized as follows:

Selection: Tests are frequently administered to detect differences among individuals which may make them more or less suitable for some future activity. Tests like the Graduate Record Exam (GRE) or the Law

School Admissions Test (LSAT) are quite well known for their use in selection. There are many other situations, however, when a mental health counselor may suggest the use of a personality or vocational preference test to assist a client with a personal selection decision regarding educational or career choices.

Placement: Tests are frequently utilized to assist in determining the best possible placement for training, treatment, or effective functioning. It should be emphasized that placement is not necessarily something which is done to a client. For many clients, placement is a personal decision often related to selecting a college major or making a career choice, for example. For such clients, the information provided through the use of psychometric techniques can be invaluable in assisting with such decisions.

Diagnosis: Tests and psychometric techniques are often employed by mental health counselors to assist in identifying specific strengths and weaknesses in a variety of areas of human performance. While often thought of in a medical sense or for the purpose of generating a DSM IV diagnostic label, this area of testing may include much more. The systematic use of diagnostic tests in reading, mathematics, and language development, for example, often provides clients and counselors with the necessary information to plan programs of remediation deemed necessary to achieve the desired counseling goal. Also, third party payers such as insurance carriers typically require a DSM IV diagnosis before reimbursement for services can be made.

Individual Progress: Perhaps one of the most frequent uses of tests in counseling is to assess the client's individual progress toward a stated goal. Working with a group of adolescent clients with the goal of enhancing self-esteem and self-acceptance may be facilitated by periodically assessing changes in the clients' behavior. The use of psychometric instruments provides both client and counselor with objective and recordable evidence of change and progress which can be used to document rate of change and achievement of outcomes. Clearly, a counselor who sought to lead a weight control program with a group of clients would logically rely on periodic measures of body weight using a scale. Why then should it be so different to use a well-accepted, valid, and reliable measure of social skills development to assess the degree of change for a group of clients seeking to enhance their social skills.

While there are numerous other reasons for using tests such as motivation, program evaluation, and research, the areas listed above provide the basic foundation for test usage among mental health counselors.

Classification of Assessment Instruments

Psychometric instruments can be classified according to a variety of categories on the basis of qualities or attributes, and an awareness of these categories is essential in the proper selection and use of assessment tools. The classifications appearing below represent only a few of the many possible.

Group vs Individual: Although the distinction between these categories would appear to be obvious, a bit more is usually implied through the use of these terms. Instruments designed for group administration may be used with one or more than one client at a time and usually permit administration by individuals who do not have extensive training or experience in testing. Additionally, group-administered instruments usually take the form of a paper and pencil test in which a client is presented a test booklet, an answer sheet, and a pencil with which to mark responses. These materials are relatively inexpensive and add to the economical nature of the group test.

On the other hand, individual tests must only be administered to one individual at a time and usually require that the administrator be highly skilled, experienced, and often, specially certified for a valid and ethical administration. Because of the fact that only one individual can be assessed at a time and the administrator must have much more than a general familiarity with the test administration, scoring, and interpretation, such instruments are correspondingly more expensive and time consuming to use.

Paper & Pencil vs Performance Tests. These classifications generally refer to the means for collecting the behavior sample to be evaluated. Paper and pencil tests generally take the form of a prepared test booklet with a separate answer sheet on which the client marks responses. These tests have formed the backbone of group assessment for they possess a number of highly desirable characteristics. The materials, a test booklet and answer sheet, are generally quite inexpensive and permit the collection of information from potentially large numbers of individuals at the same time. Additionally, this form of testing lends itself to quick and objective scoring. Such tests generally are developed by test publishers and come with excellent supporting documentation. Administration, in most cases, requires little more than distributing materials, reading aloud a set of directions, keeping accurate track of the elapsed time provided for the test, and finally the collection of the materials.

Among the limitations of this class of tests is the requirement for reading. A valid administration of a paper and pencil test demands that the client possess the ability to read at a certain level. Although many tests have been intentionally designed to require relatively low levels of reading ability, the practicing mental health counselor is likely to encounter far more illiterate and functionally illiterate clients than one might suppose. For this reason, such well known paper and pencil tests as the Minnesota Multiphasic Personality Test (MMPI) have been adapted for use with poor or nonreaders and for those with visual disabilities through the use of audiocassette presentations (Anastasi, 1988).

Performance tests generally elicit a behavior sample which is quite different and, in some ways, is more authentic. In response to verbal instructions, the client performs a task. A common example is represented by the Goodenough-Harris Drawing Test (Harris, 1963). This instrument is frequently used to assess intellectual functioning and is administered by simply asking the client to "make a picture of a man; make the very best picture that you can." While removing the need for reading, such tests elicit more complex behaviors such as drawing a person, which must be evaluated by an administrator, and the results cannot be run through an optical scanning machine for grading. Such tests generally demand higher levels of training and experience and present more complicated grading and evaluation issues than does the paper and pencil format.

Norm vs Criterion-Related Tests. The principle means for distinguishing between these two groups of test forms rests with the way in which a single score is evaluated. Typically, after an administration, a test is scored and a raw score is generated. This raw score generally represents the number of correct responses or, in the case of a self-report survey, a pattern of responses is recorded. This raw score in and of itself has very little meaning until it is compared with something. If the score is compared with the scores obtained from a large and hopefully representative sample of others in a norm group, the relative position of the raw score can be determined. It can be said, for example, that a score might represent the 89th percentile, which would be interpreted as being equal to or better than 89 percent of the scores from the norm group. The question such tests answer is one of relative position. Does the raw score place the individual near the top, in the middle, or near the bottom compared to others who have taken the same test.

A more recent development, which is becoming more widely utilized in a variety of tests, is the application of criterion-related scoring. In this process, the obtained score is not compared with a norm group but with a criterion score or measure. The difference is that a norm-referenced score provides an indication of relative performance within the norm group, while criterion-related scoring provides a measure of absolute performance. Such scoring has become increasingly popular particularly with the publishers and users of diagnostic tests where the achievement of a particular score may be indicative or diagnostic of a particular attribute. Such scoring methods are increasingly being utilized on diagnostic tests of reading or mathematics where scoring below a particular criterion may be indicative of a failure to achieve mastery or to demonstrate minimum competency.

Structured vs Unstructured. The distinction here is not dichotomous. These terms are best thought of as the ends of a continuum with some tests being considered highly structured and others relatively unstructured. The basis upon which the classification may be made revolves around the degree of response freedom offered to the client. A vocational preference test, like the Strong Interest Inventory, may present clients with a series of activities to which they are permitted only three options: like, indifferent, or dislike. The client is given a very limited array of options from which to choose a response. Such a test is regarded as highly structured. Among the principle advantages of such a test are the fact that quick and objective scoring is possible.

At the other end of the spectrum are tests like the Rorschach inkblot test developed by the Swiss psychiatrist Hermann Rorschach, which was first described in 1921. Quite literally, the test is composed of a standardized series of 10 cards on which are printed bilaterally symmetrical inkblots. The client is asked to tell the examiner what each of the blots could represent. Unlike a highly structured test with very limited response freedom, the Rorschach elicits responses which are not limited in any fashion. Because of the virtually unlimited response freedom given to the client scoring of such a test is neither quick nor easy and demands a very high level of clinical skill and competence.

The Selection of Tests for Use in Counseling

The process of choosing the best or correct test for a given client and a given situation will depend upon a variety of factors. These include client-related factors, counselor-related factors, and finally test-related factors. Each of these must be weighed and balanced. If reasonable care is exercised in determining each of these factors, appropriate and useful testing information can be obtained.

Client-Related Factors. First of all it should be emphasized that not only from an ethical standpoint but from a very practical standpoint, the needs, wishes, and desires of the client should heavily influence the decision to utilize tests or other psychometric techniques. As a general rule, testing should be considered if the information needed can be obtained no other way. Obviously, if a client is bright, insightful, and possesses a large fund of personal information, testing may not be required. On the other hand, if the client and counselor both agree that additional information would be helpful in enhancing the counseling process, the idea of testing should be introduced as a relative quick and easy means of obtaining that information. The nature of the client's information deficit or interest should be the determining factor in offering the opportunity for testing. Within the counseling relationship, testing should be regarded as an offered service rather than an obligation or requirement. In many instances, unless the client is eager, willing, and enthusiastic about the opportunity to learn about himself/herself, testing will not yield useful information. If testing is considered, it should be offered as an opportunity to obtain information that cannot be easily obtained in other ways. The client's willingness to participate will depend upon the degree to which the testing situation is perceived as a threat or manipulation. If the client objects, these objections should be explored, if possible, with the intent of reassuring the client of the utility of the process. Testing should be something that is done with someone rather than to someone. Unfortunately, previous experience in schools and elsewhere may make many clients inherently suspicious of testing as an unwarranted intrusion or means of grading, classifying, or valuing. If clients are convinced that testing is being offered for their benefit, information, and use and that information can be of help in addressing the counseling issues, most will not only agree but will take an active and interested part in the assessment process.

Counselor-Related Factors. One of the most important of the counselor-related factors is the counselor's competence in the field of testing. It should be emphasized that testing is a tool and the effective application or use of any tool presumes a high degree of skill in the use of the tool. For the practicing mental health counselor, this means that not only does he/she possess a basic familiarity with testing theory, the technical aspects of testing, and the specific instruments to be used, but that the counselor is comfortable and confident in the selection, administration, scoring, and interpretation of the instruments. Simply having completed a graduate course or two in testing does not necessarily provide the necessary clinical skills to utilize tests effectively with clients. Not only must the counselor be technically competent but equally important is the requirement to know and to work within the limits of that competence. From a legal and ethical standpoint, each counselor must recognize the limits of her/his competence and limit the scope of practice to those areas for which training, experience, and legal authority permit professional service. The laws regulating the scope of practice with regard to testing vary widely among those states with counselor licensure laws. The counselor is then guided by both ethical and legal factors in the selection and use of psychometric techniques appropriate for use with clients. The limiting factors are personal training, experience, and competence as well as legal authorization.

Test-Related Factors. The third basic group of factors which guide the selection of tests revolve around the technical qualities and limitations of the instruments themselves. Among these technical factors are validity, reliability, and the existence of appropriate and representative norms. For the practicing counselor, the most important of these is validity. The counselor must have a clear idea of what it is that the test measures. An understanding of the validity of a test presumes that the counselor has a working understanding of the evidence for validity presented by the publisher of the test and others. It should be borne in mind that a standardized test is a commercial product and claims for validity made by the publisher may at times be somewhat overstated. One of the values of using psychometric instruments which have been in use for some time is the fact that their validity will likely have been independently verified through their use in multiple research studies with a wide variety of subjects and situations. Any test to be considered for use in counseling should have considerable evidence establishing that it possesses acceptable levels of face, construct, criterion-related (including predictive and concurrent) or content validity depending upon the purpose for which the test is designed.

The second major area which determines the utility of a test for a given purpose is the reliability of the test's results. Again, the counselor has an ethical obligation to insure that instruments chosen for use with clients possess the ability to provide scores which are relatively precise and stable over time. The counselor's ability to interpret the meaning of a reliability coefficient and its associated standard error of measurement for the test as a whole as well as any component scores is essential in selecting from among related tests as well as meaningfully interpreting the results. Among the various forms of reliability with which the mental health counselor should be familiar are test-retest reliability which measures stability over time, alternate forms reliability which assesses the equivalence among various forms of the same instrument, and split-half reliability which measures internal consistency.

The final area to be considered is the recency and representativeness of the test norms. A counselor who fails to recognize the effect that age, sex, ethnic origin, cultural background, and socioeconomic status have in influencing test performance may grossly underestimate or overestimate the significance of a test score. A working knowledge of the characteristics of the normative sample and the recency of that sample is absolutely essential in deriving meaningful information from a test score for a client.

Communicating Test Results

The selection and administration of psychometric instruments is only half of the responsibility which falls on the practitioner. Equally important is the ability to first interpret the results in a technically competent fashion and then to present these findings to the client in a way that is both meaningful and accurate. Since one of the primary purposes for the use of tests in counseling is to enhance the client's self-knowledge, little is gained by using a test the results of which create confusion, self-doubt, or defensiveness. It should be emphasized that, for most clients, their past experience with testing has often been primarily associated with school or employment and was judgemental or evaluational in nature. The testing done in counseling is quite different and seeks to assist in providing needed information which the client may need or want.

The two essentials for communicating test results in a meaningful and compassionate fashion are an awareness of the client and his or her needs or wants and the ability to organize the test results in a clear, understandable, and coherent fashion. The job of interpreting the results of a test should begin early in the counseling process when initial discussions with a client result in a joint determination of the need for additional information. The entire process of testing is obviously for the benefit of the client and not the counselor. When testing is offered as an option to the client, information should be given to describe what needed information the test results will provide. In this way, the client has a general understanding of the purpose and rationale for the test and therefore can have a preexisting framework into which the final results will comfortably fit. A second essential in effectively communicating results is the need to organize the results in such a fashion that the client is not provided with what may seem to be a huge amount of quantitative data. There is virtually nothing to be gained by simply presenting a client with a basket full of numbers and then expecting her or him to first understand and then to incorporate that information into some meaningful construct. Instead, it is generally useful to return the test results and then to review with a client the basic reasons which prompted the use of the test. This provides a basis for a discussion of the results in such a way that the client begins to understand what the scores mean in light of those original questions. With clients who possess a reasonable intelligence and insight, it is sometimes a wise technique to explain the meaning of the scores but to refrain from providing any interpretation or ascribe any meaning to them. Instead, one may gently suggest that the client offer his or her own interpretation or meaning once the score is understood. Asking a client to offer his or her own interpretation of a score engenders a cooperative relationship and helps avoid a passive acceptance or defensive rejection of a test result on the part of the client.

A final word of caution is appropriate. It is sometimes very difficult to give information without also giving advice. This is frequently much more easily said than done, especially with regard to testing. For many clients, the presentation of test results suggests that the counselor has all of the necessary information with which to deal with a particular problem. Clients may frequently ask the counselor's opinion or advice but are more likely to do so if they perceive that the counselor has all of the information and they have very little or what they have is of poor quality. By communicating the test results in a way that the client can understand, and by affirming the value of the client's perceptions, interpretations, and understandings, the results of tests can be effectively communicated to those most in need of them . . . the client.

Ethical Issues in Testing

There is little doubt that the practicing mental health counselor will be faced with a multitude of ethical and value dilemmas throughout his or her career, both in counseling-related situations in general and in testing as well. Perhaps the best source of guidance in effectively confronting these ethical dilemmas is a clear and current knowledge of an appropriate code of ethics. A working knowledge of a code of ethics is essential in first recognizing the existence of a potential ethical problem and in providing options for the successful resolution of such problems.

Mental health counselors come into the field from an amazing variety of academic backgrounds and there seems to be no single professional affiliation which speaks for the entire profession. Perhaps the two most comprehensive statements of standards for ethical and professional conduct which address issues in testing are provided by the American Psychological Association's *Ethical Principles of Psychologists and Code of Conduct* (APA, 1981) and *Code of Ethical Standards*, currently undergoing revision by the American Counseling Association (1995). Both of these professional associations address many of the same fundamental ethical issues associated with the use of psychometric instruments. It is of particular note that both of these organizations, in revising their codes of ethics, has begun to address issues which previously were largely unknown. Perhaps the best example of this is the inclusion of tenants which address the issue of computer applications in the construction, administration, scoring, and interpretation of psychometric instruments. Two of the issues to have arisen relate the comparability of computer and paper/pencil versions of the same instrument and the dramatically increased use of computerized interpretations of test results (Anastasi, 1988). Another area which is again receiving increased attention in statements of ethical practice relates to ability testing, particularly with regard to the validity of many instruments in assessing cognitive development of minority students. These, and many other issues will continue to pose questions as the use of tests to assess human performance and characteristics collide with technology and the values of a rapidly changing society. There are a few basic components, however, which form the foundation of ethical conduct in testing and each of these is briefly described below.

Professional Competence and Qualification. Professional conduct demands that the user of a test first be technically qualified to do so. This typically requires one or more graduate level courses in testing to establish minimal competency. Many psychometric instruments such as individually administered tests of intellectual development, more specialized diagnostic and projective tests of psychopathology, and neuropsychology assessment require much more specialized training including supervised clinical internship. A second issue relates to the legal authorization to administer such specialized instruments. The licensure laws of each state are somewhat different, but nearly all states limit the scope of practice of licensed practitioners. Ethical conduct would require that not only should the practicing counselor be appropriately trained and licensed but should limit his or her practice to the use of those instruments for which qualifications have been established. An additional safeguard in this area is the increasing scrutiny test publishers are using to determine who may purchase, and presumably use, their tests. Many test publishers now restrict the purchase of some or all of their testing products to those individuals who have established their qualifications through some mechanism.

Protection of Privacy. This area of concern has arisen particularly during the past two decades as the mechanism for information transmission and storage has undergone massive change with the increased use of computers. Practitioners are expected to obtain consent from every client before testing and this often requires the provision of information relating to the possible storage and use of the information following the termination of counseling. The use of tests makes gathering of information with, for, and about a client relatively easy. Because it is so easy to gather this information the ethical practitioner is conscious of potential abuse and offers testing only when it is appropriate and necessary. The unwarranted and unnecessary gathering of testing information should be regarded as a clear invasion of privacy and when such information is gathered, it should be guarded and used in ways fully consistent with the good ethical practice. Protecting such information and releasing it only with the client's approval and when it is in the best interest of the client should be foremost in the mind of the counselor.

Conclusion

Of the many roles played out in offices, schools, and agencies each day by mental health counselors, the process of assisting clients acquire a clear and objective view of their unique pattern of traits and abilities is likely to continue to be one of the most important. Unlike clinical psychologists who may often use assessment as a tool to enhance diagnosis of psychopathology, the mental health counselor's focus is often quite different. The ability to identify areas of concern for a client and then to select, administer, score, and interpret the results to promote effective personal and social functioning is essential. It should be emphasized that these skills in assessment are nothing but tools with which to make a difficult task easier, more objective, and efficient.

The future of mental health counseling is sure to include advances in assessment technology and increased use of interactive and computer-based assessment models. Together with a humane, ethical, and compassionate attitude toward service to clients, these advances do much to ensure that counseling services will become even more effective and efficient.

REFERENCES

Anastasi, A. (1988). *Psychological testing* (6th ed.). New York: Macmillan.

American Counseling Association. (1995). *Ethical standards.* Alexandria, VA: Author.

American Psychological Association. (1981). *Ethical principles for psychologists.* Washington, DC: Author.

Gibson, R., & Mitchell, M. (1981). *Introduction to guidance.* New York: MacMillan.

Harris, D.B. (1963). Childrens drawings as measures of intellectual maturity: A revision and extension of the Goodenough Draw-a-man test. New York: Harcourt, Brace & World.

Hills, J.R., (1981). Measurement and evaluation in the classroom. Columbus: Charles E. Merrill.

Loesch, L., & Vacc, N. (1991). Testing and counseling. In D. Capuzzi & D. Gross (Eds.). *Introduction to counseling* (pp. 158–180). Boston: Allyn and Bacon.

Peterson, J., & Nisenholtz, B. (1987). *Orientation to counseling.* Boston: Allyn and Bacon.

Shertzer, B., & Linden, J. (1979). *Fundamentals of individual appraisal.* Boston: Houghton Mifflin.

Chapter 16

THE ROLES OF SCIENCE AND RESEARCH IN THE COUNSELOR'S WORK

RODNEY K. GOODYEAR AND STEPHEN L. BENTON

Counselors share a tradition with psychologists of being trained as scientist-practitioners. This, called the Boulder model after the location of the 1949 Conference on Graduate Training in Clinical Psychology (Raimy, 1950) at which it was articulated, has been affirmed as a model for counseling psychology (Thompson & Super, 1964) and has been incorporated into AACD's Standards for the Preparation of Counselors and Other Personnel Services Specialists (1977). These standards list **Research and Evaluation** (including such areas as statistics, research design, and the development of research and demonstration proposals) as one of the core areas "considered to be necessary in the preparation of all counselors . . . " (p. 598).

Training as scientists is one dimension distinguishing counselors and psychologists from such other mental health professionals as social workers, psychiatrists, and psychiatric nurses. Garfield (1983), in fact, argues that the reason rigorous research on psychotherapy dates only from about World War II is that psychologists—with their training as scientists— were allowed to enter the psychotherapy arena at that time.

But despite this tradition of training counselors to be competent both as scientists **and** as practitioners, very few seem to adopt this ideal balance. Counselors in practice tend to give primary emphasis to one or the other of these roles. Faculty, particularly in doctoral programs, tend to stress the research role. In fact, Goldfried (1984) notes that

> students who end up in academic/research positions are spoken of with great pride, in comparison to the disappointed if not disparaging references made to those offspring who are 'lost' to straight clinical work. . . . and those graduates who **do** end up in academic/research settings are likely to be confronted with the message that it is indeed unfortunate that the pure gold of their research activities must be diluted with the copper of clinical work" (p. 477).

331

Most counselors, however, enter professional training to become practitioners. Marwit (1983), for example, recently found that only 2 percent of a national sample of clinical psychology students aspired to academic/research careers and Stapp and Fulcher (1982) report that only 14 percent of 1980 counseling psychology doctorates were in university positions (for which research is a significant demand) one year later. Krauskopf, Thoreson, and McAleer (1973) found that only 58 percent of counseling psychologists published anything after getting their doctoral degree and that the modal number of publications for this group of doctorates was one.

Because this pattern of professional priorities has existed for decades, it is unlikely to change. In fact, the development of Doctor of Psychology (Psy.D.) degree programs as alternatives to the Ph.D. was a response to the many psychology practitioners who wanted students to spend proportionally more of their graduate training in clinical rather than in research courses; in education, the Doctor of Education (Ed.D.) degree is a parallel that has been supported for similar reasons. It is true that Gelso, Raphael, Black, Rardin, and Skalkos (1983) found that counseling psychology students became increasingly more interested in research as they progressed through their programs. These students, however, were in a very research-oriented program in which faculty with national reputations modeled active research involvement. The typical counseling doctoral program would have a very different environmental press; it is safe to assert that few faculty in masters-only institutions serve students as scientist role-models.

Emulation of faculty and other professional role models no doubt accounts for some portion of counselor role behavior. However, it is probable that counselor's general preference for practice over research is heavily influenced by the very needs and interests that influenced their vocational choice. For example, recent data from Betz and Taylor (1982) reaffirm earlier findings that counseling students have very strong social/interpersonal needs. In a particularly interesting study, Royalty (1982) demonstrated that counseling faculty who are active in publishing their research manifest different interests and personality characteristics than those who do not publish. In drawing from a nationwide sample of counseling psychology faculty, she found that producers of research were typified more by Investigative and less by Social personality traits (Holland, 1966) than were nonpublishers. Moreover, the nonpublishers expressed a great deal of interest in counseling and in classroom teaching, but little in conducting research, whereas the opposite pattern was true of the researchers. Walton (1982) obtained similar results with a national sample of counselor educators whom he broke into high and low producers of research, and Frank (1984) has summarized a number of studies supporting his argument that basic personality differences exist between researchers and practitioners. Beyond such personality differences, of course, employers of practitioners exert little pressure for the production of research, for it generates no revenue and is typically not perceived as directly related to agency purposes.

Too often, what the research counselors and psychologists do publish is, in Rogers' (1955) words, "small caliber." Although he attributed this primarily to behavioral science's overreliance on a Newtonian model of physics, he seemed also to imply a pervasive lack of creativity among psychological researchers. Marx (1976), in fact, has explicitly discussed this as a worrisome issue. In light of this concern, it is interesting to consider the work of Grater, Kell, and Morse (1961) as it might apply to counseling researchers. These authors speculated that because of the nature of counselors' early parental relationships, they have a need to nurture in order to obtain positive emotional reactions from others. This can be detrimental to creativity, for:

> creative thought in itself is anxiety-provoking, at least in part, because it involves departing from normal conforming channels. . . . If our hypothesis regarding nurturance is valid, the counseling psychologist is a conforming individual, because his past pattern of adjustment has been to meet his needs by conforming to the needs of a significant person in his early life . . . Creative thought brings the nurturant individual face to face with a primary threat which his nurturance is designed to control—the threat of separation from others (p. 11).

However, while research is an important component of science, the two terms are not synonymous. A primary purpose of this chapter is to argue that the counselor should function as a scientist regardless of his or her involvement in formal research. Also, counselors should be sufficiently sophisticated to function as informed consumers of research—only in this way can the knowledge base essential for a viable counseling profession be developed and maintained. Each of these issues will be addressed in turn in the remainder of the chapter.

Scientist as a Metaphor for Counselors

Art and science are metaphors that have been applied frequently to counseling. Typically they have been regarded as mutually exclusive, so it is not unusual to find arguments over whether counseling is an art or a science. The artist metaphor seems to connote warmth, creativity, and an openness to new experiences. The scientist metaphor often seems to connote coldness, intellectualization, and perhaps even manipulativeness.

This dichotomy, however, oversimplifies the situation and perhaps exists because of a misunderstanding of the scientist role. That is, scientists are too often confused with technicians, the people who apply the findings of science, but who tend to do so without theoretical understanding. It is therefore the **technician** who is more likely to be cold, mechanical, and so on. The best scientists overlap in many ways with the best artists in their capacity for alternative ways of perceiving, in their creativity, and in their openness to new experiences.

Counselors and psychotherapists from many diverse theoretical orientations have employed a scientist metaphor to describe their work. Not surprisingly, it has been the behaviorists—who have insisted on rigor in specifying exactly what measurable quality is the focus of intervention and on how change would be measured—who have been particularly adamant about their role as scientists. Thus, for example, Thoresen (1969) made an early call for counselors to become "applied behavioral scientists," a call Berdie (1972) later echoed in his now-classic article. Rational and cognitive therapists, too, have employed a scientist metaphor. For example, Mahoney (1976) has argued for a person-as-scientist model as has Albert Ellis, who contends clients should challenge their own irrational beliefs in a hypothesis-testing manner.

But therapists of other orientations have also employed the scientist metaphor. For example, it was almost incidental that Freud's work had a therapeutic effect: he preferred to consider himself a scientist or detective. Kelly's (1970) central premise was that each individual functions as a "personal scientist," forming hypotheses about and responding to his or her world. Even Carl Rogers (1955) supports the scientist role for therapists, apparently having arrived at his position only after careful deliberation. He concluded that "science will never depersonalize, or manipulate, or control individuals" (p. 277); only people could do that. His ideal is really a version of the scientist-practitioner model in "that each researcher would be a practitioner in some field and each practitioner would be doing some research" (Heppner, Rogers, & Lee, 1984, p. 19). The scientific method is valuable to him as a therapist in that it is

> a way of preventing me from deceiving myself in regard to my creativity formed subjective hunches which have developed out of the relationship between me and my material. . . . [Scientific tools] exist, not for themselves, but as servants in the attempt to check the subjective feelings or hunch or hypothesis of a person with the objective fact. (Rogers, 1955, p. 275)

Skinner has been quoted as saying something very similar—that "science is a willingness to accept facts even when they are opposed to our wishes" (Mahoney, 1976, p. 108).

There is ample evidence to suggest that all humans—counselors included— are selective in their perceptions. They attend to data that confirm beliefs they already hold and ignore data that disconfirm those beliefs (Lichtenberg, 1984). In fact, people will actively "pull for" data to support their existing world views. Data supporting this active construction of reality come from both clinicians (Berne, 1972) and researchers (Snyder & Swann, 1978). These tendencies can lead the counselor to at least two common pitfalls.

First, counselors tend to develop what might be called a "walk-through empiricism" with regard to their technique. That is, as the counselor has successes, he or she will form impressions of what techniques are proving useful. Although this walk-through empiricism can be valuable, it is also subjective and therefore unreliable if it is used as the sole source of data.

An analogy might be drawn from medicine where not so long ago a frequent remedy was to treat people by bleeding them of "bad blood." Physicians believed a cause-effect relationship—that the bleeding caused a cure—and continued to offer this as a common treatment for many years. Yet, the treatment was no doubt responsible for many patient deaths that might have been avoided if the procedure had been tested empirically.

Second, is a related tendency among counselors to maintain beliefs about a particular client despite evidence to the contrary. Research shows that experienced helpers typically form early, lasting impressions of clients (e.g., Bishop, Scharf, & Adkins, 1975; Brown, 1970). Snyder and Swann (1978) found that people tended to test their hypotheses about other individuals by asking questions that would confirm those hypotheses (e.g., by asking people they suspect of being extroverts "In what situations are you most likely to feel self-assured and confident in yourself?" or "What would you do if you wanted to liven things up at a party?"). Perhaps more counselors should receive training under professors such as T. Ernest Newland (University of Illinois) who used to bellow at students that unless they could develop **at least** two hypotheses to explain a given client's behavior, they had no business being in the profession!

Professor Newland's challenge correctly urges counselors to employ a scientific approach as a means of avoiding the two pitfalls discussed above. Pepinsky and Pepinsky (1954), in fact, went even farther in articulating a prescriptive model for counselors that is based on the scientific process. Strohmer and Newman (1983) summarize this model as follows:

> the counselor observes the client, makes inferences about his or her current status and the related causal factors, and then, based on these inferences, makes a tentative judgment about the client. The counselor then proceeds in an experimental fashion to state the judgment as a hypothesis and to test it against independent observations of the client. Through a series of such tentative judgments and tests based on these judgments, the counselor constructs a hypothetical model of the client. This model then serves as the basis for making predictions (e.g., which treatment approach is most appropriate) about the client. (p. 557)

To illustrate this, consider George Brown who works on an inpatient psychiatric ward. His new client is very guarded—indeed, suspicious—in his interactions with Mr. Brown and others. Based on these and other data, Mr. Brown concludes that the two most likely hypotheses about the client's behavior are that it (1) reflects underlying paranoid processes, or (2) is a consequence of the client's current, self-admitted abuse of amphetamines. Mr. Brown knows that after the client has been in the drug-free ward environment for a while, he will be able to rule out one of those hypotheses.

The counselor understands that paranoid clients typically fear intimacy and that they may even respond with explosive anger if the therapist tries to get too close. If drug abuse is not the cause of this client's behavior, Mr. Brown will then work from the hypothesis that he should adopt a cognitive style with the client and not push for self-disclosure. He will test this hypothesis by making small changes in his own behavior during counseling while carefully observing the client for changes in the extent of his suspicion and/or hostility.

This very brief vignette illustrates the general manner in which counselors might function as hypothesis-testers. It also provides the opportunity to introduce several essential concepts:

1. Any science must allow its adherents to describe and predict causal relationships, that is, how changes in A (e.g., turning the steering wheel of a moving car clockwise) will cause change in B (the car will veer right). Interestingly, this function of science responds to what seems to be an enduring human need to explain phenomena in causal terms. In the absence of sophisticated explanations, people will develop explanations that may seem quite naive. For example, primitive people will often describe natural events such as storms as having been caused by gods or spirits. And with phenomena associated with personal discomfort, **cause** and **blame** are closely related. If I believe that a devastating earthquake is caused by an angry god or that my spouse has caused me to experience a particular difficulty, then the god or my spouse is blamed for the particular situation. It is this tendency to ascribe causality that characterizes attribution theory, the model that has dominated social psychology for the past decade (Weiner, 1985).

   In the example of Mr. Brown's work, the first causal question concerned the basis for the client's behavior: drugs versus an underlying paranoid process. In research, a cause such as this would be called the **independent variable.** Changes in the client's suspicious behaviors would be the **criterion measure** or **dependent variable.** The point is that criterion measures or dependent variables are those that are monitored for changes that might be anticipated in response to particular differences in the independent variable. In true experimental research, independent variables are manipulated while the dependent variables are monitored; in correlational research the researcher observes the relationship between the independent and dependent variables as they occur in nature (Cronbach, 1957). Unfortunately, causality cannot be inferred from correlational data.

2. Dependent variables must be measurable, observable, and quantifiable. Behaviorists have made a valuable contribution with their demand that client outcomes be stipulated in such terms (e.g., after treatment, the shy adolescent will be able to call a girl for a date); although concepts such as "self-actualizing" may be useful as "ultimate goals" (Patterson, 1980), their nonspecificity limits clinical utility. In this case, the counselor is interested in the extent to which his client manifests suspicious behavior. It is important, then, that Mr. Brown's operational definition of paranoid behavior include specific, observable behaviors (or a set of behaviors) such as unwavering eye contact and frequent questions about what the counselor is trying to intimate about the client's behavior.

3. Such specificity can become particularly difficult when counselors and counseling researchers focus on **hypothetical constructs** (MacCorquodale & Meehl, 1976). These are entities that do not exist as tangible, observable phenomena, but as theoretical entities that are treated as if they exist. Paranoia and self-actualization are such entities; ego is another. Despite the tendency of many

psychoanalytic theorists to reify (i.e., to treat it as if it were real) the ego, no one has ever seen, touched or tasted an ego. It is simply a hypothetical construct that is treated as if it existed because it has clinical usefulness. Such constructs abound in counseling and, though they serve a useful purpose, they cause difficulties for both practitioners and researchers. Such problems can be minimized to the extent that the terms can be operationalized in concrete terms.

4. Kurt Lewin's comment that there is nothing so practical as a good theory is true in counseling both for practitioners and researchers. Marx (1976) defines theory as "a provisional explanatory proposition concerning natural phenomena . . . " (p. 280). It is propositional in that it is offered for acceptance or rejection and provisional in that it is subject to change. This is not to argue that theory is groundless as the creationists seem to imply when they contend that evolution is **only** a theory. Theory is built on observable data that are organized into generalizations. This process of building from the specific to general is an **inductive** process.

    It is imperative both that we build better theories and that we use our theories to attain better understanding of individual behavior. Theory, then, should be both a tool and a goal. It is a tool because it guides our practice and research (**deductive** reasoning) and a goal because we each strive to build and to refine our own models of human behavior based on our observations (**induction**). Although the vignette with Mr. Brown was too short to depict inductive processes, deduction guided him when he reasoned that if the client's suspiciousness were a function of paranoid processes, he should then adopt a cognitive style and not push for self-disclosure.

By utilizing a hypothesis-testing model, the counselor can more readily avoid the two pitfalls that have been discussed and will be enabled to continue to refine, challenge, and critically examine his or her work. Hill and Gronsky (1984) argue that this process of operationalizing terms, forming hypotheses, and testing them forces one to think in a critical fashion and to hone one's thinking; it also systematizes observations. It is interesting to note that counselors trained in individual testing have been exposed to this model even though it may not have been presented to them explicitly in these terms. That is, the individual test, whether an intelligence or projective test, is essentially a single-subject experiment in which the examiner provides a relatively standard environment across clients; the stimuli (test questions; TAT cards; etc.) constitute the independent variable; the client's response is the dependent variable—variance in the examinee's responses from those of a normative group can be attributed to individual differences.

Counselor as Research Consumer and Producer

In the counselor-as-scientist model, science provides the counselor with a model for practice, a way of thinking. The public record of psychological science, however, is manifest in published reports of research. This research literature ultimately provides the foundation for our profession itself, because practice must respond continually to refinements in knowledge that occur through research.

For the individual counselor, the reasons for staying abreast of research literature are more immediate and less abstract. Maletzky (1981) has commented, for example, that "It is a lonely and sometimes frightening task to face a patient and try to help; what a comfort it would be if our colleagues' experience could always accompany us!" (p. 287). Published research encapsulates our colleagues' experience in formal, systematized reports. Also, counselors who are conversant with current research findings are likely to (1) be more effective in their counseling, (2) speak more knowledgeably about their work to lay groups and/or to groups who affect funding for services, and (3) conduct meaningful research of their own.

Garvey and Griffith (1965) concluded that from survey data that only about one-half of psychology research reports in journals are read or skimmed, and these by no more than *1 percent* of psychologists. It is true that much published research does not seem to address directly the needs of practitioners. However, many counselors apparently use this as a rationale for not reading any research. Harmon (1978) has noted that "such reasoning is analogous to the thought processes of the man who decided to stop using ammunition in his gun because he never hit anything" (p. 29).

It is certainly necessary for counselors to have some preparation if they are to read research articles critically. Persell (1976) estimated that of all social science articles published in a single year, 43 percent are deficient in their contribution to theory, 35 percent are deficient in their contribution to practice, and 39 percent are deficient in their methodology. Gelso (1979), in fact, contends that all experiments are "highly imperfect." Counselors' should prepare to become informed consumers of research through graduate coursework. Harmon (1978) also has written a very useful guide to reading and utilizing counseling research.

Certainly it is important that counselors read individual research studies. However, reading reviews of research on particular topics is even more important. No single behavioral science study can ever be regarded as definitive; only when a number of related studies have been conducted and considered as a group can conclusions be entertained with any real confidence. The strength of review articles is that they provide the opportunity to begin drawing such conclusions.

The practicing counselor will find clinically relevant reviews in such journals as the *Journal of Counseling and Development* and *The Counseling Psychologist*. More concentrated information is available in several "handbooks," including the *Handbook of Counseling Psychology* (Brown & Lent, 1984), the *Handbook of Psychotherapy and Behavior Change* (Garfield & Bergin, 1978) and *Effective Psychotherapy: A Handbook of Research* (Gurman & Razin, 1977). *The Psychological Bulletin* is devoted entirely to review articles from the entire field of psychology. Although only a portion of those articles are directly clinical (e.g., the review of literature on bulimia by Schlesier-Stropp, 1984), there is considerable merit in the professional counselor remaining conversant with broad areas of psychological knowledge. Knowing what research tells us about the relationship between television and violence (Freedman, 1984), for example, is the type of knowledge that maintains the counselor's status as an applied behavioral *scientist*.

In a related vein, it is important that counselors also be willing to read occasional articles that may have limited external validity (external validity refers to the extent that findings can be generalized to real-life situations). Both Mook (1983) and Stone (1984) have cogently argued this point. In fact, Mook used the example of Harlow's well-known experiments with rhesus monkeys on the nature of mother love (in which, for example, baby monkeys were found to prefer terry-cloth covered "mothers" over wire "mothers"), pointing out that specific findings of these studies did not readily generalize to real-life settings. Those studies have been extremely important, however, for what they added to our knowledge of maternal love. In short, many studies with low external validity nevertheless make important contributions to theory. The counselor who does not use theory both as a tool and as a goal is little more than a technician.

Practitioners as Researchers: Philosophy and Practice

This chapter has so far discussed how science might provide counselors with a model for conceptualizing their work. It has also argued that practitioners need to operate as informed consumers of research. This last chapter section will discuss counselors as producers of research.

The substantial literature on personality differences between practitioners and researchers confirms that practitioners are unlikely to become the major source of published counseling research. This does not mean, however, that practitioners will not or should not conduct any research. Demands for accountability will require counselors increasingly to document the effectiveness of their work. But this is an external motivation. Counselors are curious enough about the effectiveness of their work that they would likely conduct a great number of studies if research were demystified (e.g., if there were greater recognition that research does not equal statistics) and if they did not feel constrained to emulate the research of their academically-housed colleagues.

Consider Roberta Shoop, a counselor working with married couples. She has read that having couples demonstrate a caring attitude toward each other is a first step toward reconciliation (Stuart, 1980). According to Stuart, each spouse can show caring by performing such nurturing behaviors as doing the dishes, fixing breakfast, giving a hug, or even taking out the garbage. However, Ms. Shoop finds that couples either are reluctant to follow through with her directives to demonstrate these behaviors or that they do so with no success. Perhaps the counselor has operationally defined success in terms of responses to a short, Likert-type scale to assess feelings that couples are to complete at the end of each day.

Let's assume that Ms. Shoop wishes to test her hypothesis that client couples have not received sufficient information to adequately implement her directives. To test this, she will randomly assign couples she treats to one of three conditions: one group will continue to receive the treatment as she has offered it in the past; a second group will receive the same treatment, but with bibliotherapy to provide them with additional instruction; a third group will receive the treatment and view a videotape of successfully treated couples discussing how they have used the technique in their own lives. Based on how couples in these three groups respond to treatment (as assessed by the Likert scale), Ms. Shoop can develop further, more specific hypotheses to test in her future work. In this manner, she is adopting a between-subjects (i.e., grouped data) research design such as is commonly used by her research-oriented academic colleagues.

This sort of research could be conducted rather easily and routinely by counselors. However, in a well-regarded book, Bergin and Strupp (1972) concluded that traditional group designs were simply not applicable to clinical research. Whether they overstated the case or not, practitioners are more likely to prefer research that has high external validity, is idiographic, and/or is phenomenological.

External Validity. Goldman (1978) has spoken for most practitioners with his argument that real-life settings rather than laboratories should be the source of data from which behavioral scientists draw their conclusions. The more closely research settings approximate real counseling situations, the greater the external validity of the results. To take just one example, "clients" in laboratory studies are typically introductory psychology students whose motives for participating likely differ from those of real clients. Even though Helms (1978) has provided evidence that results of laboratory studies will generalize to field settings, many counselors would regard generalizing from laboratory studies as similar to trying to understand human behavior by observing people on TV game shows: taken out of their natural context, people may respond differently to particular stimuli.

Idiographic. Another criticism of psychological research is that it is most often **nomothetic,** or directed at general laws. This kind of research is conducted using data pooled from groups of individuals; treatment effects are assessed by comparing the one group versus another. Allport (1937) is among those who have argued for more **idiographic** research—research tailored for the individual on the assumption that each person is unique. Because, as counselors, we are interested in practice rather than in general laws, an idiographic approach may be more germane to the field. It is a rare situation in which all clients will have the same needs.

Phenomenological. It is also important to acknowledge that different philosophical assumptions may underlay research. For example, Howard (in press) points out that while most researchers are deterministic and concerned with cause-effect relationships, practitioners are more often teleological, believing people's behavior is guided by free-will or volition. Academically-housed researchers are generally positivists, but this is not the sole philosophy on which research can be based.

Positivism, or Logical Positivism evolved during the late 19th century (Stevens, 1976). The positivist seeks facts and causes of behavioral phenomena that are directly observable. Any phenomenon as speculative as a person's subjective states, is considered inappropriate for consideration. Behaviorists are counseling's best representatives of the positivistic tradition. The contrasting philosophy is that of **phenomenology,** the adherents of which are concerned with understanding human behavior from the individual's own frame of reference (Colaizzi, 1978; McLeod, 1964). Phenomenological research differs in several important ways from that which is positivistic:

1. Research is conducted within the context of its behavioral setting rather than in the controlled setting that typifies the positivistic tradition.
2. This research does not limit itself to one or perhaps a few selected variables, but is open to a range of variables.
3. Qualitative description may be as important as quantitative description. For example, in a study by Hutt, Scott, and King (1983), the researchers asked supervisees to describe either the positive or the negative aspects of supervision they received, and reported the results in an impressionistic manner.

The day-to-day work of many counselors might therefore be regarded as a loose form of phenomenological research. The theories of Freud and Piaget evolved from what was essentially phenomenological research.

Counselors' generally greater affinity for idiographic and phenomenological approaches leads almost naturally to single subject research. In its least rigorous form, this is the case study. Its data are derived not only from interviews, but from such other sources as psychological testing, autobiographies, and cumulative records. This approach, common in medicine, dates back in our field to the beginnings of psychoanalysis. It is an approach ideally suited to the counselor's circumstances for as Thoresen (1978) notes, "it offers a flexible, person-centered approach to scientific research" (p. 282). Moreover, it provides a rich source of hypotheses. For example, Breuer's work with Anna O. (Breuer & Freud, 1957) led Freud to develop the concept of transference that is now so central in psychoanalytic treatment.

Unfortunately, the case study approach does not allow the counselor to confirm or disconfirm particular hypotheses. For example, Shlein (1984) has reexamined the "data" in the case of Anna O. and concluded that the strong positive feelings she experienced for Breuer were real feelings in response to a genuine human encounter rather than transference. It is the nature of case studies that there is no way to refute either his or Freud's hypothesis.

A form of single-subject research that can have both *rigor* (i.e., internal validity—the assurance that changes in the dependent variable are a function of changes in the independent variable) and *relevance* (i.e., external validity) is N = 1 research that may also go by such terms as "intensive designs," "multiple baselines methods," "same subject research," "empirical case studies," and "interrupted time series" (Anton, 1978). Rather than examining aggregate data, N = 1 research allows the counselor to examine what techniques work best for the individual client. Replication affords external validity for this design. That is, the results of one analysis performed on one client will need to be replicated with another client in another setting.

To illustrate, consider one counselor's application of a multiple-baseline procedure with a client, Fred. Fred is a salesman who is experiencing several distressing symptoms: heart palpitations, telling dirty jokes to his customers without discriminating appropriateness, and daydreaming to excess. In the multiple-baseline procedure, the counselor has Fred keep detailed records on the number of times per day each of these three symptoms occurs, but chooses to work on alleviating only one symptom at a time (in this fashion, the counselor avoids the ethical problem of providing **no** treatment while baselines for the client's behaviors are established).

After Fred has been examined by a physician to rule out physical problems, the counselor begins by employing a cognitive restructuring procedure, teaching Fred, for example, that although the heart palpitations are distressing, they are not dangerous and, further, that he is to regard these as "allies" that are cueing him about stressors in his life. As this symptom is brought under control, treatment for it is maintained while treatment for a second symptom is begun; the process is repeated later with the third symptom. Counseling continues until the client is able to bring all three symptoms under control. Throughout the process Fred continues to record his symptoms daily and these are graphed by the counselor. Fred's graph might look like that depicted in Figure 16.1.

One possible ambiguity in interpretation would arise, however, if all three symptoms decreased after the first phase of treatment. If this were to happen, it is possible that such nonspecific relationship factors as the counselor's warmth and empathy were responsible. It is also possible that there was response generalization: that is, the cognitive restructuring techniques (in this case) were applied by the client to all three areas with good effect.

A second type of multiple baseline design is the multiple baseline across situations. Here a particular behavior of an individual is monitored across several situations. For example, let's assume that Fred experiences heart palpitations not only at work with customers, but also at home when his children disobey and in his car when he is caught in heavy traffic. In this case, the counselor might decide to proceed as with the first example, but instead of tackling separate symptoms in turn, the counselor serially tackles the one symptom across situations.

These are but two examples of N = 1 research. There are other variations that are not possible to cover in this space. The interested counselor would find a recent book by Barlow, Hayes, and Nelson (1984) to be a particularly valuable source for learning more about the implementation of this important methodology.

Two aspects of N = 1 research are important to underscore:

1. This is a methodology that depends on replication for external validity. Until findings are obtained with two or more clients, it is difficult to generalize them meaningfully.
2. Barlow et al. (1984) recommend that single-subject researchers approach the task with an attitude of "investigative play." That is, they should find some intrinsic enjoyment in looking for patterns in their own and in the client's behavior and in seeking clues about how best to proceed. This also means the practitioner should not begin a particular N = 1 investigation with a rigid strategy. Doing so "virtually eliminates the applied environment as an appropriate place to do science" (p. 178). Because clients are unique, counselors should be flexible enough to abandon preexisting hypotheses if data from a particular client do not fit.

It would be important for any chapter such as this to at least mention program evaluation. Whereas the frequently discussed publish-or-perish environment provides a source of external motivation for academically-based researchers, demands for accountability are likely to provide analogous pressures on the practitioner. Like scientific inquiry, program evaluation "can be boiled down to three issues: What are the independent variables? What are the dependent variables? And how are the two related?" (Sechrest, 1982).

However, while the basic methodologies are essentially the same, the two forms of research differ in purpose. Whereas scientific inquiry is aimed at advancing knowledge, evaluative research has the purpose of

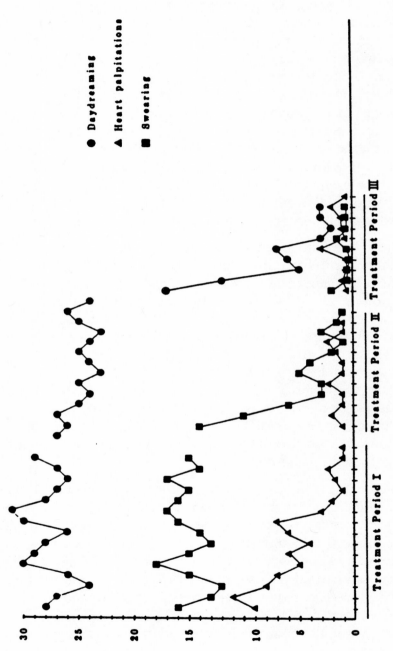

Figure 16.1. Hypothetical depiction of Fred's symptoms during phases of treatment. (Note: In the interest of space, every third day is plotted.)

obtaining practical knowledge that will be of immediate value in decisionmaking about a particular program or practice (Oetting, 1976, 1982). Oetting (1982) also makes the further point that science-oriented psychologists have been taught to look for the flaw or weakness in a study or design because their goal is to provide a rigorous test of theory. Practitioners, on the other hand, look for something of practical value to them in research. Because of their primary need to provide service and to develop new tools for that purpose, weaknesses in design or in data only raise questions for them rather than result in automatic rejection.

Ethical Considerations

As with any professional intervention, ethical principles exist to guide practice. Essentially, the principles may be summarized for counselors as:

1. The investigator bears primary responsibility for any violation of rights or harm that research participants endure.
2. The counselor-investigator must inform the client that he or she is participating in a study: the participant's informed consent is necessary for any data collected for research purposes unless those data are nonintrusive and based on observations of public behavior. Beauchamp and Childress (1979) note that nothing in biomedical research has received more attention than has the issue of informed consent.
3. If subjects are deceived, they must subsequently be informed why this was done. Although deception would be detrimental to the counseling relationship, it is much less likely to occur in clinical field setting research than in laboratory research. In laboratory settings, however, it is widespread: Menges (1973) concluded that in only about 3 percent of 1,000 psychology articles in 1971 were subjects provided complete information.
4. Client confidentiality must be protected. For research with the traditional, between-subjects design this is rarely a problem, for data are reported as group averages and it would be virtually impossible for the reader of the research report to identify individuals. With the use of N = 1 research, however, this issue becomes much more salient. The counselor reporting such research should be careful to take steps to ensure confidentiality. In the rare

situation where client identification must be made, it is essential that the client provide consent in writing.

Conclusions

Although the scientist-practitioner is the ostensible ideal for counselors, science has been too little evident in their work. There are many reasons for this, but a major one seems to be the failure of many counselors to differentiate science from technology, research, and statistics. The primary thesis of this chapter has been that science provides an approach to thinking about clients and about clinical intervention. Although research is also important for the scientist-practitioner, it is unrealistic and perhaps even inappropriate to demand that counseling practitioners emulate the formal, rigorous research of their academic-based colleagues. Counselors should, however, be informed consumers of research. Moreover, they should regularly conduct ongoing evaluations of their own work, using research designs appropriate to their settings.

These ideals do assume certain skills: skills in a certain way of thinking (e.g., hypothesis testing); skills in reading and understanding research reports; and, skills in conducting clinically-relevant research. Counselor training programs, however, do not typically foster these skills or the attitudes necessary to support them. For example, there is usually no attempt to integrate the material of research courses (often only **one** in masters programs) with that of clinical courses; research that students are taught typically does not include methodologies they are likely to use in their day-to-day practice; and, too few counseling faculty model the use of science in their own work.

Until training programs are modified to remedy these shortcomings, the scientist-practitioner model will remain only an ideal. It is a worthy ideal, however, for it is integral to counselors' professional identity. To give it up would be to remove one more distinction between mental health counselors and such other mental health practitioners as psychiatrists, social workers, and psychiatric nurses.

REFERENCES

Allport, G. W. (1937). *Personality: A psychological interpretation.* New York: Holt.

Anton, J. L. (1978). Intensive experimental designs: A model for the counselor/researcher. *Personnel and Guidance Journal, 56,* 273–278.

Barlow, D. H., Hayes, S. C., & Nelson, R. O. (1984). *The scientist practitioner.* New York: Pergamon Press.

Beauchamp, T. L., & Childress, J. F. (1979). *Principles of biomedical ethics.* New York: Oxford University Press.

Berdie, R. F. (1972). The 1980 counselor: Applied behavioral counselor. *Personnel and Guidance Journal, 50,* 451–456.

Bergin, A., & Strupp, H. (1972). *Changing frontiers in the science of psychotherapy.* Chicago: Aldine.

Berne, E. (1972). *What do you say after you say hello?* New York: Grove Press.

Betz, N., & Taylor, K. (1982). Concurrent validity of the Strong-Campbell Interest Inventory for graduate students in counseling. *Journal of Counseling Psychology, 29,* 626–635.

Bishop, J. B., Scharf, S. R., & Adkins, D. M. (1975). Counselor intake judgments, client characteristics, and number of sessions at a university counseling center. *Journal of Counseling Psychology, 22,* 557–559.

Breuer, J., & Freud, S. (1957). *Studies of hysteria.* New York: Basic Books.

Brown, R. D. (1970). Experienced and inexperienced counselors' first impressions of clients and case outcomes: Are first impressions lasting? *Journal of Counseling Psychology, 17,* 550–558.

Brown, S. D., & Lent, R. W. (Eds.) (1984). *Handbook of counseling psychology.* New York: Wiley.

Colaizzi, P. F. (1978). Psychological research as the phenomenologist views it. In R. Valle and M. King (Eds.), *Existential-phenomenological alternatives for psychology.* New York: Oxford University Press.

Cronbach, L. J. (1957). The two disciplines of scientific psychology. *American Psychologist, 12,* 671–684.

Frank, G. (1984). The Boulder model: History, rationale, and critique. *Professional psychology: Research and practice, 15,* 417–435.

Freedman, J. L. (1984). Effects of television on aggressiveness. *Psychological Bulletin, 96,* 227–246.

Garfield, S. L. (1983). Effectiveness of psychotherapy: The perennial controversy. *Professional psychology: Theory, research, and practice, 14,* 35–43.

Garfield, S. L., & Bergin, A. E. (Eds.) (1978). *Handbook of psychotherapy and behavior change,* (2nd ed.). New York: John Wiley.

Garvey, W., & Griffith, B. (1965). Scientific communication: The dissemination system in psychology and a theoretical framework for planning innovations. *American Psychologist, 20,* 157–164.

Gelso, C. J. (1979). Research in counseling: Methodological and professional issues. *The Counseling Psychologist, 8,* 7–36.

Gelso, C. J., Raphael, R., Black, S. M., Rardin, D., & Skalkos, O. (1983). Research training in counseling psychology: Some preliminary data. *Journal of Counseling Psychology, 30,* 611–613.

Goldfried, M. R. (1984). Training the clinician as scientist-professional. *Professional psychology: Research and practice, 15,* 477–482.

Goldman, L. (Ed.). (1978). *Research methods for counselors.* New York: Wiley.

Grater, H. A., Kell, B. L., & Morse, J. (1961). The social service interest: Roadblock and road to creativity. *Journal of Counseling Psychology, 8,* 9–13.

Gurman, A. S., & Razin, A. M. (Eds.) (1977). *Effective psychotherapy: A handbook of research.* New York: Pergamon Press.

Harmon, L. W. (1978). The counselor as consumer of research. In L. Goldman (Ed.), *Research methods for counselors.* New York: Wiley.

Helms, J. E. (1978). Counselor reactions to female clients: Generalizing from analogue research to a counseling setting. *Journal of Counseling Psychology, 25,* 193–199.

Heppner, P. P., Rogers, M. E., & Lee, L. A. (1984). Carl Rogers: Reflections on his life. *Journal of Counseling and Development, 63,* 14–20.

Hill, C. A., & Gronsky, B. R. (1984). Research: Why and how. In J. M. Whiteley, N. Kagan, L. W. Harmon, B. R. Fretz, and F. Tanney (Eds.), *The coming decade in counseling psychology.* (pp. 149–159). Schenectady, New York: Character Research Press.

Holland, J. L. (1966). A psychological classification scheme for vocations and major fields. *Journal of Counseling Psychology, 13,* 278–288.

Howard, G. S. (in press). Can research in counseling become more relevant to practice? *Journal of Counseling and Development.*

Hutt, C. H., Scott, J., & King, M. (1983). A phenomenological study of supervisees' positive and negative experiences in supervision. *Psychotherapy: Theory, Research, and Practice, 20,* 118–123.

Kelly, G. (1970). A brief introduction to personal construct theory. In D. Bannister (Ed.), *Perspectives in personal construct theory.* London: Academic Press.

Krauskopf, C. J., Thoreson, R. W., & McAleer, C. A. (1973). Counseling psychology: The who, what, and where of our profession. *Journal of Counseling Psychology, 20,* 370–374.

Lichtenberg, J. W. (1984). Believing when the facts don't fit. *Journal of Counseling and Development, 63,* 10–11.

MacCorquodale, K., & Meehl, P. E. (1976). The intervening variable. In M. H. Marx & F. E. Goodson (Eds.), *Theories in contemporary psychology* (2nd ed.; pp. 31–39). New York: Macmillan.

Mahoney, M. (1976). *Scientist as subject.* Cambridge, MA: Ballinger.

Maletzky, B. M. (1981). Clinical relevance and clinical research. *Behavioral assessment, 3,* 283–288.

Marwit, S. J. (1983). Doctoral candidates' attitudes toward models of professional training. *Professional Psychology: Research and Practice, 14,* 105–111.

Marx, M. H. (1976). Theorizing. In M. H. Marx & F. E. Goodson (Eds.), *Theorizing in contemporary psychology* (2nd ed.; pp. 261–286). New York: Macmillan.

McLeod, R. B. (1964). Phenomenology: A challenge to experimental psychology. In T. Wann (Ed.), *Behaviorism and phenomenology: Contrasting bases for modern psychology.* Chicago: University of Chicago Press.

Menges, R. J. (1973). Openness and honesty versus coercion and deception in psychological research. *American Psychologist, 28,* 1030–1034.

Mook, D. G. (1983). In defense of external invalidity. *American Psychologist, 38,* 379–387.

Oetting, E. R. (1976). Evaluative research and orthodox science. *Personnel and Guidance Journal, 55,* 11–15(a).

Oetting, E. R. (1982). Program evaluation, scientific inquiry, and counseling psychology. *The Counseling Psychologist, 10*(4), 61–70.

Patterson, C. H. (1980). *Theories of counseling and psychotherapy* (3rd ed.). New York: Harper and Row.

Pepinsky, H. B., & Pepinsky, P. N. (1954). *Counseling theory and practice.* New York: Ronald Press.

Persell, C. H. (1976). *Quality, careers, and training in educational and social research.* Bayside, NY: General Hall.

Raimy, V. C. (Ed.). (1950). *Training in clinical psychology.* New York: Prentice-Hall.

Rogers, C. R. (1955). Persons or science? A philosophical question. *American Psychologist, 10,* 267–278.

Royalty, G. (August, 1982). The research training of the counseling psychologist. Paper presented at the American Psychological Association convention, Washington, D.C.

Shlein, J. M. (1984). A countertheory of transference. In R. F. Levant & J. M. Shlein (Eds.), *Client-centered therapy and the person-centered approach: New directions in theory, research, and practice.* (pp. 153–181). New York: Praeger.

Schlesier-Stropp, B. (1984). Bulimia: A review of the literature. *Psychological Bulletin, 95,* 247–257.

Sechrest, L. (1982). Program evaluation: The independent and dependent variables. *The Counseling Psychologist, 10*(4), 73–74.

Snyder, M., & Swann, W. B. (1978). Hypothesis testing in social interaction. *Journal of Personality and Social Psychology, 36,* 1202–1212.

Stapp, J., & Fulcher, R. (1982). The employment of 1979 and 1980 doctoral recipients in psychology. *American Psychologist, 37,* 1159–1185.

Standards for the Preparation of Counselors and Other Personnel Services Specialists. (1977). *Personnel and Guidance Journal, 55,* 596–601.

Stevens, S. S. (1976). Operationism and logical positivism. In M. H. Marx and F. E. Goodson (Eds.), *Theories in contemporary psychology* (2nd ed.; pp. 2–31). New York: Macmillan.

Stone, G. L. (1984). Reaction: In defense of the "artificial." *Journal of Counseling Psychology, 31,* 108–110.

Strohmer, D. C., & Newman, L. J. (1983). Counselor hypothesis-testing strategies. *Journal of Counseling Psychology, 30,* 557–565.

Stuart, R. B. (1980). *Helping couples change: A social learning approach to marital therapy.* New York: Guilford Press.

Thompson, A. S., & Super, D. E. (Eds.) (1964). *The professional preparation of counseling psychologists.* New York: Teachers College, Columbia University.

Thoresen, C. (1969). The counselor as an applied behavioral scientist. *Personnel and Guidance Journal, 47,* 841–848.

Thoresen, C. (1978). Making better science, intensively. *Personnel and Guidance Journal, 56,* 270–282.

Walton, J. M. (1982). Research activity and scholarly productivity among counselor educators. *Counselor Education and Supervision, 21,* 305–311.

Chapter 17

PROFESSIONAL ETHICS AND THE MENTAL HEALTH COUNSELOR

SHARON E. ROBINSON KURPIUS AND DOUGLAS R. GROSS

For the novice mental health counselor (MHC) and even for his/her counterpart with years of experience, determining what is or is not ethical behavior is often a perplexing dilemma. While the numerous branches of the helping professions have provided practitioners with a plethora of guidelines and codes for ethical behavior, confusion still exists (Gross & Capuzzi, 1994). Representative codes include the *Codes of Ethics* and Standards of Practice (1988 with proposed 1995 adoption of revised edition*) published by the American Counselors Association (ACA); *AMHCA Code of Ethics* (1987) published by the American Mental Health Counselors Association (AMHCA) and supported by the National Academy for Certified Clinical Mental Health Counselors (NACCMHC); *Ethical Principles of Psychologists and Code of Conduct* (1992) published by the American Psychological Association (APA); *Code of Professional Ethics for Marriage and Family Therapists* (1991) published by the American Association for Marriage and Family Therapy (AAMFT); *Code of Ethics* (1989) published by the National Board for Certified Counselors (NBCC); and *Ethical Guidelines for Group Counselors* (1989) published by the Association for Specialists in Group Work (ASGW). Not only have these professional groups provided ethical guidelines for their members, but many state associations and credentialling boards are now adopting their own ethical standards.

Although intended to be helpful, these numerous codes, standards, and guidelines often result in more questions than answers. This is particularly true if one examines the documents for parameters of ethical conduct in light of the various roles/functions an MHC might perform. Most MHCs consider their primary role as providing direct therapy to individuals, to groups, or to families. Secondary role responsibilities might include consultation as an indirect service, research attempting to evaluate service or to answer clinical questions, and supervision of counselor trainees or subordinates. Regardless of whether MHCs view themselves primarily providing direct service through therapy or functioning in another role, they must be cognizant of ethical responsibilities to the client or client system and to their profession. Certain ethical issues such as counselor responsibility, counselor competence, confidentiality, and client welfare are relevant regardless which role the MHC might choose to enact.

The Mental Health Counselor as Therapist

A review of the various ethical codes/guidelines indicate that these have been primarily formulated in terms of a therapeutic relationship consisting of one counselor and one client. As comprehensive as these codes/guidelines may seem, questions remain and the situation becomes more complex when the MHC is faced with multiple client systems. This section attempts to draw attention to the ethical issues encountered by the mental health professional in interactions with either individual clients or multiple client systems. Questions are raised, and answers are sought by a review of two documents, the *AMHCA Code of Ethics* (1987) and the NBCC *Code of Ethics* (1989). Ethical issues for mental health counselors are discussed as they relate to responsibility, competence, confidentiality, and client welfare.

The Mental Health Counselor and Responsibility

At the core of all ethical behavior is the personal responsibility of MHCs to determine what ethical conduct means both philosophically and behaviorally and to incorporate these meanings into their professional practice. The standards provided by the various professional groups serve only as guides or benchmarks to enable MHCs continually to evaluate not only their ethical behaviors but also those of colleagues. While such standards serve as the foundation upon which the structure of ethical behavior rests, responsibility for maintaining this structure is in the hands of each MHC.

Questions basic to the concept of responsibility are present with every client seen by the MHC. Regardless of the presenting problem, the following questions need to be addressed:

1. To whom are MHCs responsible—the client, the referral agency, the social/family system of the client, society, the institution for which the MHC works, or all of the above?
2. Does the concept of responsibility change when the MHC moves from individual to multiple client systems?

At first glance, the answer to the question "To whom are MHCs responsible . . . ?" seems obvious. Of course, their major responsibility is to their client. The NBCC *Code of Ethics* (1989) specifically states that "the primary obligation of certified counselors is to respect the integrity and promote the welfare of a client, regardless of whether the client is assisted individually or in a group relationship." (Section B: Counseling Relationship, No. 1). However, a perusal of the documents reviewed in this chapter indicate that the concept of responsibility is broader than that related just to the client. According to the 1987 *AMHCA Code of Ethics*, the MHC has responsibility in several domains:

> As practitioners, mental health counselors know they bear a heavy social responsibility because their recommendations and professional actions may alter the lives of others. They, therefore, remain fully cognizant of their impact and alert to personal, social, organizational, financial or political situations or pressures which might lead to misuse of their influence (p. 2).
> As employees of an institution or agency, mental health counselors have the responsibility of remaining alert to institutional pressures which may distort reports of counseling findings or use them in ways counter to the promotion of human welfare (p. 1).
> When serving as members of governmental or other organizational bodies, mental health counselors remain accountable as individuals to the *Code of Ethics* of the American Mental Health Counselors Association (p. 1).

In the NBCC *Code of Ethics* (1989), the following reference is made regarding responsibility:

> Certified counselors have a responsibility to the clients they are serving and to the institutions within which the services are being performed. Certified counselors also strive to assist the respective agency, organization, or institution in providing the highest caliber of professional service (Section A: General, No. 1).

After careful consideration of these ethical guidelines, it would seem that the best answer to the question "To whom are MHCs responsible . . . ? would be "all of the above." Their responsibility goes beyond the client. This is further substantiated by a review of the *Ethical Principles of Psychologists and Code of Conduct* (1992) and the ACA's *Codes of Ethics and Standards of Practice* (1988/Proposed 1995 adoption).

Added dimensions of responsibility are found as one attempts to answer question two, "Does the concept of responsibility change when the MHC moves from individual to multiple client systems?" A review of the *AMCHA Code of Ethics* (1987) and the *NBCC Code of Ethics* (1989) yields little specificity regarding the differences between individual and multiple client systems with respect to responsibility. Although work with groups and families are discussed, one is left to interpret statements made regarding responsibility for the individual as having equal applicability when the MHC is faced with more than one client. A more definitive statement is found in the ACA *Codes of Ethics and Standards of Practice* (1988/Proposed 1995 adoption). In discussing responsibility, it states:

> When counselors agree to provide counseling services to two or more persons who have a relationship (such as husband and wife, or parents and children), counselors clarify at the outset which person or persons are clients and the nature of the relationships they will have with each involved person. If it becomes apparent that counselors may be called upon to perform potential conflicting roles, they clarify, adjust, or withdraw from roles appropriately (p. 21).

Even this degree of specificity seems to be only the tip of the iceberg. In discussing the ethical and legal considerations in marital and family therapy, Margolin (1982) stated, "Yet difficult ethical questions confronted in individual therapy became even more complicated when a number of family members are seen together in therapy" (p. 788). Multiple client systems bring into play a variety of issues which are touched upon only superficially in existing standards. It would be safe to say that the answer to question two regarding responsibility in multiple client systems is yes, but the ramifications to this answer still are not fully articulated nor understood.

What meaning does all of this have for MHCs? How do they decide the appropriate division of responsibility? What guidelines are available to aid them in making such ethical decisions? As mentioned previously, the adopted standards of ethical behavior provide the foundation, but it is up to each MHC to determine the structure within which he or she will ethically operate. The review of the various ethical standards provides benchmarks, not answers, which must be taken into consideration each time responsibility becomes an issue. The following factors need to be considered when defining parameters of counselor responsibility:

1. Age of the client.
2. Legal statutes established within your state.

3. Relevant constitutional and case law.
4. Policies and procedures of the employing agency.
5. Referral sources.
6. Client rights and privileges.
7. Ethical standards of the profession.
8. Individual versus multiple-client systems.

The Mental Health Counselor and Competence

The concept of competence is a second generic component of all professional statements regarding ethical behavior. Competence seems to be broken down into the following basic aspects related to MHCs: (1) accurate representation of professional qualifications; (2) professional growth through involvement in continuing education; (3) providing only those services for which qualified; (4) maintaining accurate knowledge and expertise in specialized areas; and (5) seeking assistance in solving personal issues which could impede effectiveness or lead to inadequate professional services or harm to a client.

A review of these aspects and the fact that they consistently appear in codes of ethics leads one to assume that this area of ethical behavior has been clearly defined and that evaluation of competence is a relatively simple task. In reality, however, this is not the case. Ethical review boards, certification boards, and licensing committees spend a significant percentage of time and financial resources attempting to determine degree of competence of practitioners. Efforts are devoted to reviewing professional qualifications, tabulating continuing education credits, processing complaints from consumers regarding issues of misrepresentation and misconduct, and determining qualifications to perform various services.

The knowledge aspect of competence is also addressed by these same boards and committees. The boards oversee the administration of certification and licensing examinations to document the applicant's degree of academic knowledge in the fields of mental health counseling and psychology.

If effort expended correlates with degree of importance, then the area of competence is very high in the priority listing of ethical issues. Few, if any, of the other areas of ethical behaviors are witness to the reviewing, processing, evaluating, examining, and screening that characterize this area. This may be viewed in several ways. Perhaps due to the specificity of the characteristics of competence, evaluation in this area is more easily accomplished than in the other areas. Perhaps quality efforts applied to determining competence will assure greater compliance with other aspects of the ethical standards. Perhaps competence is the core of professionalism and, therefore, the major variable in assuring ethical behavior. Perhaps it is the only area of ethical behavior which is open to quantifiable measurement. Or perhaps the policing and enforcement of ethical standards is such a complex task that this is the one area where professional and governmental bodies can have an impact.

It is interesting to note that of the five aspects defining the concept of competence only four are open to formal review and evaluation. The fifth, which deals with the personal aspects of the MHC, is seemingly left to the individual's discretion. If a MHC has personal issues which impede effectiveness, the ethical standards recommend that he or she seek assistance in solving these issues. Such a directive seems weak when compared with the strong valuative measures for the other aspects of competence.

For MHCs, the concept of competence must be viewed from both an internal and an external frame of reference. From an internal perspective, MHCs do all they can to gain the skills and knowledge basic to the profession. They continue to grow through reading and attending to new and developing trends, through attaining post graduate education, and through attending seminars and workshops aimed at sharpening and increasing both knowledge and skill bases. Each MHC takes full responsibility for adhering to the rules and regulations of the profession which address the concepts of proper representation of professional qualifications, for providing only those services for which he or she has training, and for seeking assistance with personal issues that are barriers to providing effective service.

From an external perspective, it is important for the MHC to realize that processes such as reviewing, evaluating, examining, and screening will continue to be handled by forces external to self. The best advice which can be given to the MHC in dealing with this situation is to exercise the responsibilities and controls from an internal perspective, to develop the highest level possible of competence, and to be alert to the established criteria utilized in external evaluations. If the MHC conscientiously attends to these aspects of competence, the end result should be highly positive.

The Mental Health Counselor and Confidentiality

A third generic component of ethical standards found in all statements regarding ethical behavior centers on confidentiality. The following statement, taken from the *AMHCA Code of Ethics* (1987), can be found in one form or another in most adopted standards of ethical behavior:

> Mental health counselors have a primary obligation to safeguard information about individuals obtained in the course of teaching, practice, or research. Personal information is communicated to others only with the person's written consent or in those circumstances where there is clear and imminent danger to the client, to others or to society. Disclosures of counseling information are restricted to what is necessary, relevant, and verifiable (Principle 5.).

Inherent in such statements is the concept of the mental health professional's responsibility to protect the right of clients to have information disclosed in therapy remain confidential. Clients should be informed that they have privileged communication only if their MHC is state certified or licensed (Robinson Kurpius, in press). While confidentiality is a professional concept, privileged communication is a legal concept which protects the client from having his or her disclosures revealed in a court of law. This privilege belongs to the client, not to the MHC, and covers both verbal disclosures and records of therapy sessions. Only a judge can force a MHC to break the privilege and this is usually only in circumstances where the best interests of society are deemed to outweigh the interests of an individual client.

The various ethical guidelines are fairly specific about the parameters of confidentiality regardless of the setting, the presenting problem, or whether the practitioner is dealing with an individual or a multiple client system. These directives, as presented in the *AMCHA Code of Ethics* (1987), are as follows:

a. All materials in the official record shall be shared with the client who shall have the right to decide what information may be shared with anyone beyond the immediate provider of service and to be informed of the implications of the materials to be shared (p. 5).

b. The anonymity of clients served in public and other agencies is preserved, if at all possible, by withholding names and personal identifying data. If external conditions require reporting such information, the client shall be so informed (p. 5).

c. Information received in confidence by one agency or person shall not be forwarded to another person or agency without the client's written permission (p. 5).

d. Service providers have a responsibility to insure the accuracy and to indicate the validity of data shared with their parties (p. 5).

e. Case reports presented in classes, professional meetings, or in publications shall be so disguised that no identification is possible unless the client or responsible authority has read the report and agreed in writing to its presentation or publication (p. 6).

f. Counseling reports and records are maintained under conditions of security and provisions are made for their destruction when they have outlived their usefulness. Mental health counselors insure that privacy and confidentiality are maintained by all persons in the employ or volunteers, and community aides (p. 6).

g. Mental health counselors who ask that an individual reveal personal information in the course of interviewing, testing or evaluation, or who will allow such information to be divulged, do so only after making certain that the person or authorized representative is fully aware of the purposes of the interview, testing or evaluation and of the ways in which the information will be used (p. 6).

h. Sessions with clients are taped or otherwise recorded only with their written permission or the written permission of a responsible guardian. Even with guardian written consent one should not record a session against the expressed wishes of a client (p. 6).

i. Where a child or adolescent is the primary client, the interests of the minor shall be paramount (p. 6).

j. In work with families, the rights of each family member should be safe guarded. The provider of service also has the responsibility to discuss the contents of the record with the parent and/or child, as appropriate, and to keep separate those parts which should remain the property of each family member (p. 6).

Undergirding each of these directives is the MHC's duty to ensure that a client's right to confidentiality is safeguarded. The mandate seems clear since to breach a client's confidentiality without just cause is legally viewed as an invasion of the client's constitutional right of privacy (Everstine et al., 1980). Just causes such as when the client is a clear and imminent danger to self or others (see Tarasoff v. Regents of the University of California, 1974, 1976; Gross & Robinson, 1987) and in certain situations involving abuse of minors or incapacitated adults require the breaking of confidentiality. Even in these situations, however, the client is informed of the action to be taken and every effort made to obtain the best professional advice and to act accordingly. If at all possible, a client should be informed of the parameters of confidentiality before commencing a therapeutic relationship so that there is fully informed consent regarding disclosures made in the process of therapy (Pope & Vasquez, 1991).

Several operational guidelines can be of assistance as the MHC faces the complex issues surrounding confidentiality. The following are offered for consideration:

1. Inform clients of the confidential nature of the relationship and your responsibilities as these relate to situations in which violations of confidentiality may need to occur.
2. Assure clients that they will always be informed of actions prior to implementation and that their consent will be sought.
3. Encourage clients to raise questions regarding confidential issues. This will aid in clarifying the MHC's position, strengthen the equality of the relationship, and generally lead to a more informed clientele.
4. Consistently review adopted standards and state laws relating to the issue of confidentiality.

Ethical issues surrounding confidentiality are some of the most problematic for mental health professionals (Pope & Vetter, 1992). Being fully informed of constitutional law, case law, and state statutes regarding privileged relationships can help the MHC make informed decisions regarding when and how to appropriately handle ethical dilemmas involving the potential breaching of client confidentiality.

The Mental Health Counselor and Client Welfare

The concept of client welfare is so highly interrelated with the other ethical aspects under discussion in this chapter that it is difficult to separate specific issues from discussion. For example, the concepts discussed under counselor responsibility and competence have as their basis the protection of the client's welfare. The directives presented under confidentiality are all directed at maintaining the rights and welfare of clients. An issue which has not been addressed but is of increasing concern to the mental health profession is dual relationships between counselors and their clients.

According to Robinson Kurpius (in press), dual relationships has become an area of frequent ethical complaints and litigation. Dual relationships occur when professionals assume two or more roles simultaneously or sequentially with a person seeking counseling (Herlihy & Corey, 1992). These relationships include a professional relationship and a secondary relationship such as a friendship, social or business relationships, an intimate relationship, or financial relationship. In each of these, the secondary relationship conflicts with the primary therapeutic relationship and can be hurtful to the client. It should always be remembered that there is a power differential between the MHC and the client, that there is a differential of expectations and responsibilities, and that the natural boundaries of the fiduciary relationship are voided when a secondary relationship occurs (Robinson Kurpius, in press).

This is particularly true when an intimate relationship develops between the MHC and client. When sexual involvement becomes part of the therapeutic relationship, "the expectation of trust, fundamental to the professional relationship, has been violated" (Thoreson, Shaughnessy, Heppner, & Cook, 1993, p. 429). While it is recognized that attraction occurs between a MHC and his or her client, the ethical problem arises when this attraction is not confronted as a therapeutic issue and instead is acted upon. MHCs should be aware that in many states, sexual contact between a mental health professional and a client is illegal.

Keith-Spiegel and Koocher (1985) noted that the profile of the therapist who becomes sexually involved with clients resembles that of an impaired helper. They usually have severe personal problems and are trying to get their needs for love and affection met through their relationships with their clients. Typically, these therapists are men in their forties and fifties who exploit young, attractive female clients. Perhaps the best guide for MHCs who find themselves becoming involved with clients is to ask themselves whether they must hide what they are thinking or doing with a client. If the answer is yes, they need to seek consultation and/or supervision immediately and to stop the behaviors which must be hidden (Weiner & Robinson Kurpius, 1995).

The various ethical codes are very specific regarding dual relationships. For example, Principle 6. Welfare of the Consumer, of the *AMHCA Code of Ethics* (1987) states that:

> Mental health counselors are continually cognizant both of their own needs and of their inherently powerful position "vis-a-vis" clients, in order to avoid exploiting the client's trust and dependency. Mental health counselors make every effort to avoid dual relationships with clients and/or relationships which might impair their professional judgement or increase the risk of client exploitation. Examples of such dual relationships include treating an employee or supervisor, treating a close friend or family relative and sexual relationships with clients.

Principle 3. Moral and Legal Standards, makes even a stronger statement that sexual relationships are explicitly prohibited. "Sexual conduct, not limited to sexual intercourse, between mental health counselors and clients is specifically in violation of this code of ethics."

The NBCC *Code of Ethics* (1989) also specifically addresses dual relationships in Section A: General, No. 9 and 10, respectively:

> Certified counselors are aware of the intimacy in the counseling relationship, maintain respect for the client, and avoid engaging in activities that seek to meet their personal needs at the expense of the client. Certified counselors do not condone or engage in sexual harassment which is defined as deliberate or repeated comments, gestures, or physical contact of a sexual nature.

In addition to dual relationships, there are many other areas of client welfare which must be of concern to MHCs. The *AMHCA Code of Ethics* (1987) lists 14 issues relevant to the Welfare of the Consumer.

As can be seen from the above, responsibility for protecting the welfare of clients rests squarely with the counselor. The MHC must be cognizant of the complex nature of the counseling relationship, guard against aspects which can jeopardize client welfare, and be willing to take any steps necessary to alleviate this situation. The following suggestions are offered:

1. Check to be sure that you are working in harmony with any other mental health professional also seeing your client.
2. Develop clear, written descriptions of what clients may expect with respect to therapeutic regime, testing and reports, record keeping, billing, scheduling, and emergencies.
3. Share your professional code of ethics with your clients and prior to beginning therapy discuss the parameters of a therapeutic relationship.
4. Know your own limitations and do not hesitate to utilize appropriate referral sources.
5. Be sure that the approaches and techniques utilized are appropriate for the client and that you have the necessary expertise for their utilization.
6. Consider all other possibilities before establishing a counseling relationship which could be considered a dual relationship.
7. Evaluate the client's ability to pay and when the payment of the usual fee would create a hardship. Either accept a reduced fee or assist the client in findings needed services at an affordable cost.

8. Objectively evaluate client progress and the therapeutic relationship to determine if it is consistently in the best interests of the client.

The most recent version of the *AMHCA Code of Ethics* (1987) added a section on client rights. Rights of clients include the right to be treated with consideration and respect, to expect quality service, to receive informed consent, to be given information about their case record, to be involved in treatment planning, to confidentiality, to discuss fees, and to refuse recommended services. These rights are essential for the full welfare of the client to be protected.

The Mental Health Counselor as Consultant

A second role enacted by many MHCs is that of consultant. Although consultation is gradually evolving as an alternative to direct service therapy, there has been relatively little written on the ethics of doing consultation as a MHC.

Gallessich (1982) was one of the first to write on the ethics of consultation, and her ideas were expanded by Robinson and Gross (1985). Since then, many more authors have addressed this complex area in attempt to shed light and understanding on this arena of professional functioning. This discussion will focus on the welfare of the consultee/client, relationship issues, and consultant competence.

Welfare of Consultee/Client

Discussing the ethical concerns regarding the best interests and welfare of consultees, Newman and Robinson (1991) identified four basic issues. These issues include identification of the "client", a client's right to informed consent, ethical issues in assessment, and mediating individual and system interests.

Who Is the Client? Unlike therapy, consulting consists of a triadic relationship among consultees, their clients or client systems, and the consultant. Since consultation often has an indirect impact on the client/client system (often referred to as the hidden clients), identification of "the client" becomes complex. This is particularly true when consulting with organizations which are comprised of diverse individuals and groups whose needs, interests, and views of organizational goals may be very diverse. In addition, there are tremendous power differentials, and therefore, personal investment in the outcomes of consultation varies. Gallessich (1982) stressed that the client must ultimately be the chief executive officer (CEO) who has the power to interpret the interests of the organization. Newman (1993) points out that consultation involves multiple parties and complex relationships which create ethical dilemmas, especially in trying to identify the client and to whom the consultant is ultimately responsible. Identifying "the client" in consultation is not an easy process and often presents ethical problems, particularly for the novice MHC doing consultation.

Informed Consent. Providing clients/consultees with informed consent becomes difficult when working within an organization. Traditionally, informed consent should be voluntary, fully informed, and given by a competent individual and have the provision that the individual can withdraw consent at any time. In consultation, individuals often are expected to take part in the intervention as part of their work responsibilities. To refuse is to put themselves at risk. The MHC functioning as a consultant must find a way to avoid employee coercion and co-optation while still getting the type of cooperation which is essential for the success of the consulting endeavor (Newman & Robinson, 1991). Kelman (1969, cited in Gallessich, 1982) proposed that consultants could reduce the likelihood of manipulation by openly discussing their own biases and values, emphasizing consultees' values over their own, and including freedom of choice as a central goal in consultation.

Assessment. Informed consent and confidentiality are also key to the problems involved in assessment in organizations. Again, coercion must be a major concern as well as who will have access to the assessment data, whether it will be confidential, and how will it be utilized. The consultant must balance the individual employee's needs with those of the organization while taking into consideration the goals of the consulting project. It is generally agreed upon that data gathered in consultation are confidential and only aggregate data are used for decision making. To avoid ethical problems in this area, consultants should clearly specify in their contract the type of data to be gathered, how it will be used, limits of confidentiality, how it will be reported, and who owns the raw data.

Client v. System Welfare. The fourth issue identified by Newman and Robinson (1991), the welfare of the individual versus the system, could be seen as paralleling that of individual client versus society welfare. However, often the choice in consultation is between greater productivity and higher profits for the system versus a better quality of work life for the employees. The skillful consultant may be able to mediate a compromise which will result in both being realized. More often, however, the consultant must meet the goals of the consultee who is responsible for the organization. What may serve the organization well may not be in the best interests of all employees. There are no easy solutions for this dilemma, other than trying to clarify this possibility before accepting the consulting contract. The NBCC *Code of Ethics* (1989) provides MHCs working as consultants with this guideline: "In the consulting relationship, the certified counselor and client must understand and agree upon the problem definition, subsequent goals, and predicted consequences of interventions selected" (Section E: Consulting, No. 2).

Relationships Within Consultation

Relationship issues in consulting also have the potential of becoming ethical dilemmas. Newman and Robinson (1991) and Newman (1993) discussed concerns about confidentiality, informed consent, power, and dual relationships.

Confidentiality and Informed Consent. Ethical guidelines consistently tell MHCs to protect the confidentiality of their clients and to provide them with informed consent for participation. However, these issues are not addressed when referring to consulting relationships. The NBCC *Code of Ethics* (1989) section on consulting fails to mention confidentiality and informed consent and only states that "Certified counselors in a consulting relationship must encourage and cultivate client adaptability and growth toward self-direction." (Section E. Consulting, No. 4). How to do this within the confines of confidentiality and informed consent is left to the consultant.

In considering how to provide consultees with confidentiality and informed consent, the MHC functioning as a consultant should be aware of these special circumstances:

 (a) in organizational contexts, maintenance of confidentiality depends not only on the consultant, but on the cooperative efforts of perhaps many organizational members as well;

 (b) levels of participation by members are often variable and so, too, must access to information be variable;

 (c) selective access to information in organizational consultation must be ensured even in light of long-term patterns of relationships that existed before consultation began;

(d) this selective confidentiality must be maintained in a system that is structured to facilitate open communication flow;

(e) because they are selective, parameters of confidentiality are not inherent in given relationships, but must be negotiated;

(f) those parameters must be publicly delineated to ensure that all parties know who has access to what information; and

(g) while consultants have an ethical responsibility to ensure confidentiality, in reality, they often have very limited control over the information and the participants in consultation (Newman & Robinson, 1991, p. 27).

While consultants cannot guarantee confidentiality nor informed consent, they should ensure that the limits of confidentiality are clearly and universally understood by all participants and that participants are afforded as much freedom of choice as possible.

Power. Further complicating the issue of confidentiality and informed consent is the abuse of power in organizations where power is typically distributed unevenly. For example, when the MHC is hired as an expert, the consultation can elicit dependence, resentment, or resistance from participants within the organization (Gallessich, 1982). Blatant misuse of consultant power includes fostering dependency to meet the consultant's needs for power or status or prolonging the relationship in order to enhance financial gains. Consultants need to realize that they by nature of their position have power to influence participants. When fostering the growth of the consultee or client system, the "certified counselor must . . . not become a decision maker for clients or create a future dependency on the consultant" (NBCC *Code of Ethics*, 1989, Section E: Consulting, No. 4).

Because of their structure, organizations have power differentials. Some members have self-determination and others do not. It is not the role of the consultant to change this, although careful consideration of power uses and abuses is an ethical responsibility. Merrell (1991) recommends that consultants educate executives in constructive ways to use their power to elicit cooperation from and involvement of employees and for strengthening their commitment to organizational goals.

Dual Relationships. Like any other helping relationship, dual relationships in consulting involve the professional working relationship and a secondary relationship with the consultee. Often a MHC will receive an invitation to provide consultation based on a previous relationship with someone within the organization. Whether this will hamper the consulting process will depend on the extent to which the person who made the referral is involved with the consultation and whether this person influences the objectivity and honesty of the consultant (Robinson, 1993).

Often when a consultant works closely with consultees over time, a working bond develops (Groder, 1991). Indeed, those writing in the field of corporate psychology encourage the development of this bond. Somerville (1991) stressed that if the consulting "relationship has an impact on the very soul of the chief executive, much of the potential for influence on the client company, as well as the CEO as an individual, cannot be achieved" (p. 22). He does note, however, that when the CEO discusses personal issues that are not work related, it is inappropriate and unethical for the consultant to do therapy and referral is needed (Somerville, personal communication, August 1993).

When the consultant has a close working bond or relationship with the consultees, the question to be answered is whether this new relationship impacts the professional judgment and actions of the consultant. If the answer is yes, then this relationship has become an ethical concern and could limit the consultant's ability to work within the organization. Levinson (1991) cautioned against friendships within the consulting relationship and stated that consultants must live with "his or her own loneliness" (p. 13). Maintaining professional distance, however, is especially difficult when working with CEOs since they are usually on a first name basis with the consultant and become familiar as they work closely together. As Goodstein (1991) noted, "the ordinary professional distance that one maintains in psychotherapeutic and other clinical relationships simply cannot be maintained" when working with a CEO (p. 20).

Our ethical codes do not provide guidance related to this other than to warn that the "Focus of the consulting relationship must be on the issues to be resolved and not on the person(s) presenting the problem" (NBCC *Code of Ethics*, 1989, Section E: Consulting, No. 1). Therefore, consultants must be constantly aware of the impact of their relationships potentially have on their ability to perform their duties effectively (Newman, 1993). Ultimately the consultant bears sole responsibility for establishing and maintaining appropriate boundaries which allow the consultation process to be effective.

Consultant Competencies

The NBCC *Code of Ethics* (1989) states that "certified counselors, acting as consultants, must have a high degree of self awareness of their own values, knowledge, skills, limitations, and needs in entering a helping relationship that involves human and/or organizational change" (Section E: Consulting, No. 1). It further notes that "Certified counselors must be reasonably certain that they, or the organization represented, have the necessary competencies and resources for giving the kind of help that is needed or that may develop later, and that appropriate referral resources are available to the consultant" (Section E: Consulting, No. 3). No other specifics regarding skills, knowledge or competencies are given.

Robinson and Gross (1985) did, however, identify three areas of counselor competence needed when functioning as a consultant. These areas include appropriate education and training, ability to identify client, and fulfilling client needs and purposes versus one's own. The last two issues have been discussed above, while training and education still needs to be addressed.

While many graduate programs in counseling do not offer coursework in consultation, most graduates eventually find themselves involved in consulting relationships. Being a good MHC is not justification enough for expanding one's services to include consultation. Nor is reading a book on the topic sufficient. If a MHC wants to do consultation and to be ethical in the process, he or she needs to be knowledgeable in the various theories of consultation, techniques and assessment procedures to meet consultation goals, and skills necessary for effective interventions. In addition, a practicum or internship in consultation would help transfer knowledge into practice. To offer to do consulting without special educational and training would be unethical.

Although there is some overlap between the skills needed for therapy and those used in consultation, several professional organizations including the ACA and the APA have appointed special task forces to develop formal standards for training consultation. In two 1993 special issues of the *Journal of Counseling and Development* (Kurpius & Fuqua, 1993a, 1993b) focusing on consultation, issues of education and training were also addressed. As Dougherty (1995) notes, however, training is currently haphazard. Hopefully, the ongoing efforts toward specifying standards for education and training will help to ensure that MHCs offering consultation services do so in an ethical and competent manner.

The Mental Health Counselor as Researcher

A third role enacted by some MHCs is that of researcher. While almost all codes of ethics address the topic of research, the *AMHCA Code of Ethics* (1987) is particularly applicable to MHCs who are researchers. Research is undertaken "to contribute to counseling and to human welfare . . . with respect for the people who participate and with concern for their dignity and welfare" (Principle 9. Pursuit of Research Activities). As Robinson and Gross (1986) pointed out, counselor researchers make judgments about the individual therapeutic value of their research while weighing the cost-benefit ratio of the value of the research to society. When deciding to proceed, issues of competence, responsibility, and confidentiality become relevant.

Researcher Competence

Prior to beginning any research project, the MHC must objectively determine his or her competence to conduct the given study. In doing this self-evaluation, questions such as the following need to be answered:

1. Do I have a theoretical foundation for this study?
2. Do I have the ability to judge the psychometric properties of the tests/instruments which will measure the variables of interest?
3. Am I competent to design and administer the treatments or interventions?
4. Am I aware of possible negative side effects to participants and am I prepared to handle them? and
5. Do I have the knowledge to analyze and interpret my data in a meaningful way?

If the answers to these questions are positive, the MHC should proceed with the study. If the answer to any is negative, he or she should seek competent help and advice before proceeding.

Researcher Responsibility

In addition to analyzing competence to conduct the proposed study and the motive behind doing the study, the MHC doing research must also be concerned about the welfare of the research participants. Issues such as invasion of privacy and informed consent become central. Any researcher's primary responsibility is to safeguard the participants. This begins with objectively evaluating the study's ethical acceptability, weighing scientific and humane values of the study, and perhaps having a Human Subjects Committee review the research proposal (*AMHCA Code of Ethics,* 1987, Principle 9a. Pursuit of Research Activities). A second step occurs during the recruitment of participants. In order for participants to give informed consent for involvement, they need to know "all features of the research that reasonably might be expected to influence willingness to participate" (Principle 9c) and to inform the participant of potential physical and mental discomfort, harm, and danger (Principle 9g). To meet these requirements, full disclosure is required. When this would contaminate findings, it is essential that the MHC doing research debrief participants as soon after the completion of the study as possible (Principles 9d and 9h). Since the primary responsibility of any researcher is to protect the welfare of participants while generating knowledge, the clients must be protected from harmful consequences when involved in any research study.

Confidentiality

As in any other encounter with clients, the verbal and written information given to a MHC doing research is governed by the ethic of confidentiality. Researchers would do well to remember that even answering questions on a measurement device can constitute an invasion of one's privacy; therefore, every effort should be made to protect the privacy and confidentiality of participants. As with client case notes, research data should be kept in a locked file cabinet and if possible in a locked office to ensure security.

When discussing or reporting results, all identifying information must be removed. It is simply not enough to remove names to protect client privacy. For example, often clinical research consists of a small sample whose personal characteristics make participants identifiable. In instances such as this, as well as in other research endeavors, it is the researcher's responsibility to determine whether the privacy of participants is being unduly invaded, if they are being protected from harm, and whether confidentiality and anonymity is secure.

The Mental Health Counselor as Supervisor

Acting as a clinical supervisor is the fourth function often performed by MHCs. Kurpius, Gibson, Lewis, and Corbet (1991) defined supervision as a "teaching procedure in which an experienced person aids a less experienced person in the acquisition of a body of knowledge and experience that will foster competence and skill in handling therapeutic situations" (p. 48). Supervision is a triadic relationship involving the client, the supervisee/counselor and the supervisor. The ultimate goal is to provide the best possible clinical service to the client as well as promotion of the professional development of the supervisee/counselor.

In light of the professional demand for supervision both before and after a counselor receives a masters degree, it is surprising that the *AMHCA Code of Ethics* (1987) and the NBCC *Code of Ethics* (1989) say almost nothing about appropriate supervisory behavior. The AMHCA code simply warns that MHCs acting as supervisors "accord recipients informed choice, confidentiality, and protection from physical and mental harm" (Principle 6.c) and that MHCs cannot serve as counselors to an individual if they already have a supervisory relationship (Principle 6.1). The NBCC code merely says that a counselor providing information to a supervisor should ensure that the information is general in order to protect client identity. The responsibility of the supervisor is not discussed at all.

Clearly there is a tremendous need for the counseling professional association to attend to the ethics and legalities of providing supervision. To meet this need, the Governing Council for the American Association for Counseling and Development (now the American Counselors Association) in 1989 adopted *Standards for Counseling Supervisors.* The rationale statement for these standards points out that "supervision of professional counseling is essential from the first moments of pre-service training to the continuing practice of experienced counselors in all employment settings" (p. 7).

The *Standards for Counseling Supervisors* (AACD, 1989) specifies 11 core areas of knowledge and competency. These include:

1. Professional counseling supervisors are effective counselors whose knowledge and competencies have been acquired through training, education, and supervised employment experience (p. 8);
2. Professional counseling supervisors demonstrate personal traits and characteristics that are consistent with the role (p. 8);

3. Professional counseling supervisors are knowledgeable regarding ethical, legal and regulatory aspects of the profession, and are skilled in applying this knowledge (p. 8);
4. Professional counseling supervisors demonstrate conceptual knowledge of the personal and professional nature of the supervisory relationship and are skilled in applying the knowledge (p. 8);
5. Professional counseling supervisors demonstrate conceptual knowledge of supervision methods and techniques, and are skilled in using this knowledge to promote counselor development (p. 9);
6. Professional counseling supervisors demonstrate conceptual knowledge of the counselor developmental process and are skilled in applying this knowledge (p. 9);
7. Professional counseling supervisors demonstrate knowledge and competency in case conceptualization and management (p. 9);
8. Professional counseling supervisors demonstrate knowledge and competency in client assessment and evaluation (p. 9);
9. Professional counseling supervisors demonstrate knowledge and competency in oral and written reporting and recording (pp. 9–10);
10. Professional counseling supervisors demonstrate knowledge and competency in the evaluation of counseling performance (p. 10); and
11. Professional counseling supervisors are knowledgeable regarding research [in] counseling and counselor supervision and consistently incorporate this knowledge into the supervision process (p. 10).

The *Standards* (AACD, 1989) also notes that "Counseling supervision is a distinct field of preparation and practice" (p. 11); therefore, special education and training of supervisors is necessary for effective performance. Most frequently this training occurs as advanced graduate education.

In 1993, the Association for Counselor Education and Supervision adopted *Ethical Guidelines for Counseling Supervisors.* Three board issues are addressed: Client welfare and rights; supervisory role; and programs administration. Unlike other ethical guidelines, this document spells out the duties of supervisors to ensure the client's welfare and to promote the growth of the counselor/supervisor.

Functioning as a supervisor is not an easy task. The supervisor bears a heavy responsibility for the welfare of the client and often has direct legal liability. The legal doctrine, respondeat superior, refers to this vicarious liability for the client's welfare (Cormier & Bernard, 1982). While safeguarding the trainee's interest, the supervisor must ensure that the client is receiving the same standard of care as that which would be provided by a licensed professional (Harrar, VandeCreek, & Knapp, 1990). This standard of care includes aspects such as informed consent, confidentiality, and protection from harm. It would be well for MHCs contemplating doing supervision that "supervisors ultimately bear the legal responsibility for the welfare of those clients who are counseled by their trainees" (Corey, Corey, & Callanan, 1988, p. 156).

Supervisors need to be familiar with all cases of their supervisees, to be involved actively in supervision, to assess progress being made by the client, and to give the supervisee feedback on progress being made in counseling. In order to fulfill these responsibilities, there must be full disclosure to the supervisor. The supervisor, as well as the counselor/supervisee, is ethically obligated to maintain the client's confidentiality.

In addition to responsibilities to clients, supervisors have an ethical obligation not to become involved in dual relationships with their supervisees. The same standards for relationships which occur between the client and counselor are appropriate for relationships between supervisor and supervisee. A supervisor's ability to function objectively as a teacher, evaluator, and therapist is severely impaired by intimate, sexual relationships with supervisees. As a result, the client becomes secondary to this relationship. Yet this is one of the most violated ethical guidelines in our profession (Pope, Schover, & Levenson, 1980).

It is highly evident that a MHC functioning in a supervisory capacity needs to be aware of the legal and ethical parameters surrounding supervision. Supervision is a professional activity which can be highly rewarding, but being a triadic relationship, it is fraught with ethical pitfalls.

Summary

Regardless of what hat is being worn—therapist, consultant, researcher, or supervisor—MHCs need to govern their behavior so that it falls within the established legal and ethical guidelines of our profession. As mentioned previously, numerous codes of ethics are available as standards by which to judge one's own and others' behaviors. As a professional group, MHCs have a compelling responsibility to abide by their code of ethics. It is also their responsibility to monitor the behavior of their peers. As stated in the *AMHCA Code of Ethics* (1987), "As practitioners, mental health counselors know that they bear a heavy social responsibility because their recommendations and professional actions may alter the lives of others." (Principle 1.e). This responsibility demands respect and obedience of the ethical standards which bind us as professionals.

Endnote

*The American Counselors Association is currently preparing the final version of its *Codes of Ethics and Standards of Practice* and indicates a 1995 adoption.

REFERENCES

American Association for Counseling and Development (1989). Standards for Counseling Supervisors, *ACES Spectrum Newsletter, 49,* 7–10.

American Association for Marriage and Family Therapists (1991). *Code of professional ethics for marriage and family therapists* (rev. ed.). Washington, DC: Author.

American Counselors Association (1988/1995). *Codes of ethics and standards of practice* (rev. ed.). Alexandria, VA: Author.

American Mental Health Counselors Association (1987). *AMHCA Code of ethics.* Alexandria, VA: Author.

American Psychological Association (1992). *Ethical principles of psychologists and code of conduct* (rev. ed.). Washington, DC: Author.

Association for Counselor Education and Supervision (1993). Ethical guidelines for counseling supervisors, *ACES Spectrum, 53,* 2–5.

Association for Specialists in Group Work (1989). *Ethical guidelines for group counselors.* Alexandria, VA: Author.

Corey, G., Corey, M.S., & Callanan, P. (1988). *Issues and ethics in the helping professions* (3rd Ed.). Monterey, CA: Brooks/Cole.

Cormier, L.S., & Bernard, J.M. (1982). Ethical and legal responsibilities of clinical supervisors. *Personnel and Guidance Journal, 60,* 480–491.

Dougherty, A.M. (1995). *Consultation: Practice and perspectives in school and community settings* (2nd ed.). Monterey, CA: Brooks/Cole.

Everstine, L., Everstine, D.S., Hayman, G.M., True, R.H., Frey, D.H., Johnson, H.G., & Seiden, R.H. (1980). Privacy and confidentiality in psychotherapy. *American Psychologist, 35,* 828–840.

Gallessich, J. (1982). *The profession and practice of consultation.* San Francisco, CA: Jossey-Bass.

Goodstein, L.D. (1991). Loneliness at the top: Opportunities for consultation. *Consulting Psychology Bulletin, 43,* 19–21.

Groder, M.G. (1991). A grand viler: Every chief executive needs one. *Consulting Psychology Bulletin, 43,* 4.

Gross, D.R., & Capuzzi, D. (1994). *Counseling and Psychotherapy: Theories and Applications.* Columbus, OH. Macmillan.

Gross, D.R., & Robinson, S.E. (1987). Ethics and violence: Hear no evil, see no evil, speak no evil. *Journal of Counseling and Development, 65,* 334–344.

Harrar, W.R., VandeCreek, L., & Knapp, S. (1990). Ethical and legal aspects of clinical supervision. *Professional Psychology: Research and Practice, 21,* 37–41.

Herlihy, B., & Corey, G. (1992). *Dual relationships in counseling.* Alexandria, VA: American Association for Counseling and Development.

Keith-Spiegel, P., & Koocher, G.P. (1985). *Ethics in psychology: Professional standards and cases.* New York: McGraw-Hill.

Kurpius, D.J., & Fuqua, D.L. (1993a). Consultation I. *Journal of Counseling and Development, 71.*

Kurpius, D.J., & Fuqua, D.L. (1993b). Consultation II. *Journal of Counseling and Development, 72.*

Kurpius, D.J., Gibson, R.G., Lewis, J., & Corbet, M. (1991). Ethical issues in supervising counseling practitioners. *Counselor Education and Supervision, 31,* 48–57.

Levinson, H. (1991). Counseling with top management. *Consulting Psychology Bulletin, 43,* 10–15.

Margolin, G. (1982). Ethical and legal considerations in marital and family therapy. *American Psychologist, 37,* 788–801.

Merrell, D.W. (1991). Back to basics: Things you have always known about consulting but tend to forget in the heat of battle. *Consulting Psychology Bulletin, 43,* 64–68.

National Board for Certified Counselors (1989). *Code of Ethics.* Alexandria, VA: American Association for Counseling and Development.

Newman, J.L. (1993). Ethical issues in consultation. *Journal of Counseling and Development, 72,* 148–156.

Newman, J.L., & Robinson, S.E. (1991). In the best interests of the consultee: Ethical issues in consultation. *Consulting Psychology Bulletin, 43,* 23–29.

Pope, K.S., Schover, L.R., & Levenson, H. (1980). Sexual behavior between clinical supervisors and trainees: Implications for professional standards. *Professional Psychology, 10,* 157–162.

Pope, K.S., & Vasquez, M.J.T. (1991). *Ethics in psychotherapy and counseling: A practical guide for psychologists.* San Francisco, CA: Jossey-Bass.

Pope, K.S., & Vetter, V.A. (1992). Ethical dilemmas encountered by members of the American Psychological Association: A national survey. *American Psychologist, 47,* 397–411.

Robinson, S.E. (1993). *Dual relationships in consultation.* Paper presented at the American Psychological Association Annual Meeting, Toronto, Canada, August.

Robinson Kurpius, S.E. (in press). Current ethical issues in the practice of psychology. *Directions in Clinical Psychology.*

Robinson, S.E., & Gross, D.R. (1986). Counseling research: Ethics and issues. *Journal of Counseling and Development, 64,* 331–333.

Robinson, S.E., & Gross, D.R. (1985). Ethics of consultation: The Canterville Ghost. *The Counseling Psychologist, 13,* 444–465.

Somerville, K.E. (1991). Corporate psychology and the soul of the CEO. *Consulting Psychology Bulletin, 43,* 22–24.

Tarasoff v. Regents of the University of California. 118 Cal., Rptr. 129.529 P.2d. 533 (Cal. 1974).

Tarasoff v. Regents of the University of California. 113 Cal., Rptr. 14.551 P.2d. 334 (Cal. 1976).

Thoreson, R.W., Shaughnessy, P., Heppner, P.P., & Cook, S.W. (1993). Sexual contact during and after the professional relationship: Attitudes and practices of male counselors. *Journal of Counseling and Development, 71,* 429–434.

Weiner, N., & Robinson Kurpius, S.E. (1995). *Shattered innocence: A practical guide for counseling women survivors of childhood sexual abuse.* Washington, DC: Taylor & Francis.

HIGHLIGHT SECTION

BEHAVIORAL MEDICINE/HEALTH COUNSELING

MOLLY VASS

The interest in health issues in our society has increased dramatically over the last ten years. One of the major factors for this is the mounting research that links lifestyle factors such as stress, diet, exercise, smoking, and alcohol consumption to degenerative diseases. Nearly half of the American people suffer from some form of degenerative disease with over 50 percent of these attributed to heart disease (Kalita, 1977). There are also great numbers of people who seek medical care for unspecified symptoms such as low energy, headaches, insomnia, and appetite problems. Some doctors estimate that 50 percent or more of the people they see as outpatients have no discernible illness. Many times these problems are labeled psychosomatic illnesses and these people are referred to mental health professionals for assistance. Because of the epidemic proportion of problems related to lifestyle factors and the escalating health care costs, a new interdisciplinary field called Behavioral Medicine has emerged. Behavioral Medicine ties the disciplines of medicine, sociology, psychology, anthropology, biochemistry, biology, and nutrition together to more effectively deal with health issues (Matarazzo & Carmody, 1983).

This new field of study has had a great impact on the mental health profession. A new counseling speciality has emerged from Behavioral Medicine called Health Counseling. It is based on the philosophy that the mind and body are integrally related and need to be treated as such.

In reviewing the literature pertaining to Health Counseling, the following five areas stand out as having the greatest impact on the mental health profession:

1. Nutrition and Health
2. Stress Management and Pain Control
3. Exercise and Health

378

4. Environment and Health
5. Addictive Habits

Nutrition and Health

There is a growing body of literature that addresses the effect of nutrition on human functioning (Lesser, 1980; Pearson & Shaw, 1982; Pritikin & McGrady, 1979). This literature can be broken down into two major categories that are important to the mental health professional. First, there has been a great deal of attention given to the effect of nutrition on behavior. A new medical speciality called Orthomolecular Psychiatry has developed to study the unique nutrient needs of individuals. When the molecular balance is upset there can be serious physiological and psychological responses, such as depression, schizophrenia, and psychosis (Pauling, 1968; Hoffer & Walker, 1978; Pfeiffer, 1975). This has led to considerable study of vitamin and mineral deficiencies as a cause for behavioral abnormalities.

Another area that comes under this category is the connection between allergies and behavior. Rapp (1981) has demonstrated in double-blind studies that certain foods will cause allergic reactions that range from mild fatigue to severe hyperactivity and learning disabilities. In the book, *Brain Allergies* (Philpott & Kalita, 1975), Dr. William Philpott also suggests a direct relationship between allergies and depression, schizophrenia and psychosis in adults. From his own psychiatric practice, Philpott gives the following statistics on the number of patients that have major symptoms upon exposure to commonly consumed foods and chemicals. Out of 250 emotionally disturbed patients:

> Ninety-two percent (92%) of those classified as schizophrenic developed symptoms of maladaptive reactions to foods and chemicals, sixty-four percent (64%) manifested symptom formation on exposure to pasteurized whole cows' milk. Approximately seventy-five percent (75%) of the schizophrenics manifest symptom formation to tobacco. Approximately thirty percent (30%) developed symptoms on exposure to petrochemical hydrocarbons. Some of the reactions in this group were so severe as to precipitate suicidal attempts. (Philpott, 1975, p. 16)

It is information like this that has caused mental health professionals to become more knowledgeable in the area of nutrition in order to not misdiagnose symptoms as behavioral problems when in actuality they are ecologic or organic in nature.

Another area of nutrition and behavior that has been linked to mental health problems is the effect of blood sugar abnormalities on psychological functioning. The term most widely used is hypoglycemia or low blood sugar. This abnormality has been proposed as the possible cause for mood swings, manic-depressive disorders, and other types of behavioral problems. Clients with blood sugar abnormalities will frequently experience inconsistent fluctuations in levels of energy and temperament. Alcoholism has also been linked to blood sugar problems. Counselors are now being trained to identify signs and symptoms of possible nutritional problems so these clients can be referred to the appropriate professional(s).

The second major category of Nutrition and Health is the effect of diet on degenerative diseases such as heart disease, cancer, and diabetes. This has led to efforts to educate children and adults to make healthier choices in terms of diet. The new U.S. dietary guidelines indicate the necessity for the reduction of fat, sugar, alcohol, caffeine, and food additives to improve the health of society. It is not uncommon for children as young as twelve years old to have the beginning symptoms of heart disease or diabetes related to high fat, high sugar diets (Brentlinger, 1980). Mental health professionals are becoming part of the educating process to help people change dietary habits and develop healthier lifestyles.

Stress Management and Pain Control

Stress and pain control were the first areas to be developed in Behavioral Medicine. This came about partly as the result of the pioneering work by Hans Selye on stress (Selye, 1974). In his landmark book, *Stress Without Distress,* he provides an explanation of the systemic response to stress in our lives. As an outgrowth of his work, there has been a burgeoning of stress management techniques and programs. They range from progressive relaxation methods to the utilization of biofeedback, meditation, hypnosis, and visual imagery. Within the counseling process all of these can be utilized to work towards the goal of monitoring and controlling physiological responses in order to reduce stress and pain. There is also a growing body of literature supporting the idea that people can mobilize their inner resources to assist themselves in recovering from severe diseases. An example of this is the work of Stephanie and Carl Simonton with cancer patients. They have found that some cancer patients can mobilize their inner resources to help combat the growth of cancer and heal themselves (Simonton, Mathews-Simonton, & Creighton, 1978).

The biofeedback movement has had an impact on the field of mental health by involving counseling professionals in medical problems such as migraine headaches, backaches, back pain, sexual dysfunctioning, and many other chronic disabilities. Biofeedback has been used successfully by therapists to assist people in reducing chronic pain and stress induced illnesses (Danskin & Crow, 1981).

Exercise and Health

There is a growing interest in exercise and fitness in our society. This has resulted in extensive research on the role exercise plays in prevention of degenerative diseases such as cardiovascular disease, diabetes, and cancer. The importance of exercise has also taken on a new dimension because of research done on the positive effects of exercise in the treatment of depression and low self concept (Rimm, Hannaford & Atkins, 1981). With the growing number of people viewing exercise as an important aspect of their life, counselors have been compelled to become more aware of the literature addressing the role of exercise in mental health and assisting clients in working towards their own goals of integrating exercise into a balanced lifestyle.

Environment and Health

Concerns with environmental problems, such as toxic chemical pollution and noise pollution, have caused health care professionals to look more closely at their impact on human functioning. Alexander Schauss (1980) in his book, *Diet, Crime and Delinquency,* cites evidence that high levels of lead in children and adults can cause behavioral disorders and learning disabilities. There are a number of studies on children which have shown that levels of lead impair normal functions and produce symptoms such as hyperkinesis, aggressive behaviors, and poor learning ability (Needleman, 1972; Marlowe et al., 1982).

Another facet of the environment that is under study is the effect of noise on people. As our environment continues to become more highly industrialized, one of the consequences is an increase in the level of noise to which we are exposed in our daily lives. Cohen, Evans, Krantz and Stokols (1980) studied the effect of aircraft noise on children living and going to school in close proximity to an airport. The study was concerned with the impact of noise on children's attention, feelings of personal control, and physiological processes. Their findings indicated that noise factors had the greatest impact on elevated blood pressures and that the children from the highest noise areas were more likely to fail on cognitive tasks and to give up before the time to complete the task had elapsed. These types of findings have important implications for mental health professionals.

Addictive Habits

Addictive habits such as smoking, drinking, and over-eating are of major concern to many people. Approximately 12 million Americans have problems with alcohol, 50 million Americans smoke cigarettes regularly, and three fourths of our population are at least ten pounds overweight (Edlin & Golanty, 1982).

The amount of money, time, and energy spent in an attempt to control these habits is astounding. For example, last year alone, ten billion dollars was spent on attempts to lose weight. Yet, only two percent of the people who lost weight will keep it off for five years. Because addictive habits often involve both chemical and psychological dependency, counselors become an important part of the treatment process to break the habit. Professionals use a variety of approaches to assist people in their efforts to stop destructive habits. Some of these include educational approaches, support groups, and various theoretical methods such as social-learning theory (modeling) and behavioral management programs. When the habits get to a point of severity that they are impairing the person's daily living, the counselor will often encourage their client to consider a residential treatment program. These programs offer controlled environments where clients do not have the opportunity to continue the habit and are taught new ways to deal with the addiction. There are residential treatment programs for drug and alcohol problems, eating disorders, and other addictive habits throughout the country. Also springing up are health spas and fitness centers that provide programs to assist people in changing nonhealthy habits into healthy ones before they get to the point of impairing a person's life.

Health counseling is an exciting new dimension to the mental health profession. The trend seems to indicate that this will be one of the most expanding areas of study and practice for some time to come.

REFERENCES

Brentlinger, W. (1980). An Oklahoma study reveals our kids' killer diets. *Let's Live*, 34–37.

Cohen, S., Evans, G., Krantz, D., & Stokols, D. (1980). Physiological, motivational and cognitive effects of aircraft noise on children. *American Psychologist, 34*(3), 231–243.

Danskin, D., & Crow, M. (1981). *Biofeedback: An introduction and guide.* Palo Alto, CA: Mayfield Publishing.

Edlin, G., & Golanty, E. (1982). *Health and wellness.* Boston: Science Books International.

Hoffer, A., & Walker, M. (1978). *Orthomolecular nutrition.* New Canaan, CT: Keats Publishing.

Kalita, D. (1977). Orthomolecular medicine: We command nature by obeying her. In R. J. Williams & D. F. Kalita (Eds.), *A physicians handbook on orthomolecular medicine* (1–3). New York: Pergamon Press.

Lesser, M. (1980). *Nutrition and vitamin therapy.* New York: Grove Press.

Marlowe, M., Folio, R., Hall, D., & Errera, J. (1982). Increased lead burdens and trace mineral status in mentally retarded children. *The Journal of Special Education, 16*(1), 87–99.

Matarazzo, J., & Carmody, T. (1983). Health psychology. In M. Hersen, A. Kazdin, & A. Bellack (Eds.), *The clinical psychology handbook* (657–682). New York: Pergamon Press.

Needleman, H., Orhan, C., & Shapiro, I. (1972). Lead levels in deciduous teeth of urban and suburban American children. *Nature, 235,* 111–112.

Pauling, L. (1968). Orthomolecular psychiatry. *Science, 160,* 265–271.

Pearson, D., & Shaw, S. (1982). *Life extension.* New York: Warner Books.

Pfeiffer, C. (1975). *Mental and elemental nutrients.* New Canaan, CT: Keats Publishing.

Philpott, W., & Kalita, D. (1975). *Brain allergies.* New Canaan, CT: Keats Publishing.

Pritikin, N., & McGrady, P. (1979). *The Pritikin program for diet and exercise.* New York: Grosset and Dunlap.

Rapp, D. (1981). *Allergies and the hyperactive child.* New York: Simon and Schuster.

Rimm, D., Hannaford, C., & Atkins, K. (1981). Treatment of depression through physical exercise. *The Behavioral Counselor, 2*(1), 23–29.

Schauss, A. (1980). *Diet, crime and delinquency.* Berkeley, CA: Parker House.

Selye, H. (1974). *Stress without distress.* New York: New American Library.

Simonton, O., Matthews-Simonton, S., & Creighton, J. (1978). *Getting well again.* Los Angeles, CA: Tarcher.

Additional Resources

Vass, M. (1983). The holistic health movement: Its impact on the counseling profession, *Wyoming Personnel and Guidance Journal, 30*(2), 11–16.

Vass, M. (1983). Nutrition, environment and behavior: The missing link in counseling approaches. *The International Journal of Biosocial Research, 4*(1), 19–24.

Chapter 18

CURRICULUM INNOVATION IN THE EDUCATION AND TRAINING OF MENTAL HEALTH COUNSELORS

GARY SEILER

Curriculum development molds the future of mental health counseling. How a profession trains its constituents and defines itself have a direct bearing on how they fare in the job market. As the job market undergoes shifts and changes, so do the role relationships of the various disciplines represented in counseling and therapy to each other (e.g., psychiatry, psychology, social work, mental health counseling, etc.). Counselor education programs are a powerful contributor to the balance of functions of various mental health professionals.

The fundamental knowledge and skills of mental health counselors (MHCs) are first acquired during their academic training. Since most mental health counselors are trained in counselor education graduate programs, the curricula of these programs provide the orientation for knowledge and skills that counselors develop during and after graduate education. Curriculum shapes the professional image that these helpers will project.

This chapter will discuss the role of the interrelationships between training curriculum, professional identity, and career opportunities. In addition, the chapter will evaluate how the status of training curricula can help counselors maintain an edge in the current job market for mental health professionals. The concept of "curriculum" includes supervised field experience. Field experience is a critical component of the graduate education of MHCs and provides new counselors with their transition from academia to the job market. A major professional obligation of counselor education programs is to facilitate that transition.

Changing Professional Identity

Mental health counseling is a relatively new profession, and as discussed in Chapter 3, is suffering growing pains associated with establishment of identity. From their beginnings in the 1970s, organizations have struggled with an appropriate definition for this professional group. In 1979, Seiler and Messina offered the following definition:

> Professional mental health counseling is an interdisciplinary, multifaceted, holistic process of the (1) promotion of healthy lifestyles, (2) identification of individual stressors and personal levels of functioning, and (3) preservation or restoration of mental health (p. 6).

This generic definition is consistent with the traditional view of prevention, diagnosis, and treatment of mental health problems. However, more recently, federal and state governments have deemphasized the preventive and developmental issues related to mental health, as evidenced by funding patterns and lack of support for agency and/or program initiatives in this area. Governmental bodies have focused funding, and continue to focus, on treatment and therapy. Hence, more and more MHCs find themselves involved in direct therapeutic mental health services to clients, rather than preventive or developmental activities.

The chief professional organization of MHCs, the American Mental Health Counselors Association (AMHCA), is committed to the philosophic principles of mental health enhancement and problem prevention, as evidenced by its support of holistic and wellness points of view. Although most MHCs deal with severe or chronic psychological problems to some extent, an ideological commitment continues the support of preventive and developmental counseling.

Ideally, there should be congruence between how a profession defines itself, career patterns, and the curricula by which its professionals are trained. The educational institution that turns out these professionals should be committed to providing competently trained individuals as well as to developing programs that meet the needs of society. Also, educational programs must meet their obligations to their students, making certain that they are being trained to meet the real-life conditions awaiting them in the employment market. Both academic advisors and field supervisors need to join hands in guiding students in mental health counseling to capitalize on both societal needs and existing job conditions.

History of Counselor Education Programs

The U.S. Office of Health, Education, and Welfare provided leadership in the development of counselor education as a specialty in graduate education. As a result, counselor education programs began to emerge in this country in the 1950s, responding to society's need for school guidance counselors. Their role was to help schools deal with problems arising from the burgeoning school population resulting from the postwar baby boom. However, as these children passed through the school system, the demand for school counselors waned due to dwindling school enrollments. As a result, in the 1970s counselor education programs began to train MHCs in order to survive.

Interestingly, during this same period, programs for other mental health professionals, such as social workers and marriage and family therapists, began to gain in popularity. They responded to the federal government's growing emphasis on human and social service programs. It happened that during this time the American Psychological Association (APA) began to focus on doctoral level training of psychologists, with a deemphasis of master's level training, thus leaving many master's level psychologists feeling displaced, without a professional "home." In fact, many of the early original members of AMHCA were M.A. psychologists.

As all aspects of the human services system began to mushroom, it became apparent that the system required large numbers of mental health professionals who offered greater cost-effective services than the high-salaried and limited number of psychologists and psychiatrists. The first group to attempt to fill this void were social workers followed by other mental health professionals, such as marriage and family therapists and psychiatric nurses.

By the early 1970s, the human services field was experiencing an almost exponential growth pattern due to heavy federal funding. This phenomenon was creating an array of mental health personnel who could no longer be neatly categorized. To offer structure as well as needed training, counselor education programs began producing master's level counselors for community agency settings. Since human services employers evidenced no reluctance to hire master's level graduates, society's needs and counselor education programs' responses were mutually beneficial.

As state colleges and universities began to include community counseling in counselor education programs, there evolved an informal standard training period of one academic year, or approximately 30 semester hours. The other mental health professions such as social work opted for two-year training models.

It was not until the early 1970s that Dr. Robert Stripling, under the auspices of the Association of Counselor Education and Supervision (ACES), developed a set of standards for the preparation of counselors. Under these standards, preparation programs would be two years in length, with significantly more hours of supervised field experience than were standard in existing programs. These original standards were modified and adopted by the American Association for Counseling and Development's (AACD) Counsel for Accreditation of Counseling and Related Educational Programs (CACREP). The Council was created as an independent body to implement training standards. As of May 1983, 22 programs had received full or provisional approval in one or more program areas. CACREP accreditation, as a voluntary evaluation process, provides for the review of counselor education programs by extramural groups of professionals, who examine compliance to professional training standards. The evaluation process includes qualifications of faculty, faculty-student ratios, and training facilities. Accreditation also deals with the scope of counseling courses and supervised field experience.

An example of the drastic changes taking place in counselor education occurred in 1976. At that time, the faculty of the University of Florida's Counselor Education Department decided not only to implement the standards recommended by the ACES, but also to offer an expanded 72-semester-hour, counselor education curriculum. This new program fulfilled all of the requirements of the ACES standards and added its own supplementary field experience requirements. The typical curriculum was subdivided into 42 hours of core curriculum courses (basic courses such as Counseling Theory and Practice), 9 hours minimum of specialization (which would prepare the student with a minimal level of expertise in a focus area), and additional 12 hours of electives, bringing the total to 72 hours, or two full calendar years of preparation.

Problems of Curriculum Compliance

Many graduate programs for counselor education remain at one academic year of study with approximately 30 semester hours. These degree programs, for better or for worse, are still the most common training format, although the 1973 ACES standards advocated a two-year program of roughly 60 semester hours. The current standards of CACREP require a two-year, 48 semester hour minimum. One of the difficulties with standards for counselor education training programs is that the program **chooses** to be reviewed for program accreditation. Another is that compliance to standards is voluntary. Perhaps the only vehicle in the future for mandatory compliance would be standards used by the regional accreditation associations for schools and colleges or the National Council for Accreditation of Teacher Education, since most counselor education departments are located in schools or colleges of education.

Historically, until ACES and CACREP developed standards for counselor education programs, the programs themselves were the sole purveyors of standards. There was no forum for the programs to ally with one another and create a framework for standards. Even now, CACREP has no authority to enforce standards, and adherence is by voluntary compliance. Unfortunately, most programs still do not abide by the profession's standards of training.

Students seeking exemplary programs should consider such factors as CACREP accreditation, the eminence and national visibility of faculty to assist in networking for employment, and the required number of hours of training and supervised field experience. The minimum semester hours of academic work recommended in the Training Standards of the American Mental Health Counselors Association is 60 hours. Their guidelines recommend a minimum of 1000 hours of supervised field experience. When looking at counselor education programs, prospective graduate students should be alert for evidence that a program expresses a desire to upgrade its program to meet current or future training standards.

Curriculum Courses

In 1973, ACES developed standards for training that were later modified to the current CACREP standards. These standards divide proposed curricula into three distinct components: (1) core courses, (2) environmental emphasis courses, and (3) specialized studies.

Generic core courses provide a foundation for all aspects of counselor training, whether the area be school counseling, community agency work, or private mental health counseling. They include: Human Growth and Development, Social and Cultural Foundations. The Helping

Relationship, Groups, Lifestyle and Career Development, Appraisal of the Individual, Research and Evaluation, and Professional Orientation.

Environmental emphasis courses are intended to train the counselor education student for the general setting in which he/she will work after graduation. For most MHCs, this is the community setting. These courses, either by title or description, refer to the relationship between the community and mental health services. Examples include such courses as Mental Health Counseling in Community Settings, Community-Based Mental Health Services, or Community Psychology.

The specialized studies area is intended to provide a focus that will enable the student to explore in depth one particular aspect of mental health counseling. Examples of specialized studies include gerontology, substance abuse, and minority counseling.

Supervised Field Experience: Practicum and Internship

Supervised field work is the bridge between theory and practice. Field experience gives trainees the opportunity to apply and develop the skills they learned in graduate training. Few counselor education programs provide the minimum 1000 hours of supervised field experience recommended by AMHCA in the early 1980s.

The concept of supervision includes a commitment to monitoring the performance of a trainee, giving ongoing feedback, and offering regular consultation to enhance counseling skill development. The 1973 ACES standards and now CACREP's standards indicate that supervision should include three distinct professional components: (1) the host or on-site supervisor, (2) the individual supervisor from the counselor education program, and (3) the group supervisor from the counselor education program.

The host supervisor functions in the field placement setting. He/she is responsible for overseeing the trainee's performance on-site. The individual supervisor is usually a counselor educator associated with the on-campus training faculty. This person holds an hourly meeting on a weekly basis with the trainee. During this time, audio- or videotape samples of counseling sessions are reviewed and critiqued. The individual supervisor may also visit the student's field site to observe his/her skills directly.

The group supervisor meets weekly with a small group of trainees (usually from six to ten) who are clustered together by virtue of their environmental emphasis area, or even specialized studies. Although some time in this small group may be devoted to reviewing taped material from counseling sessions, the majority of time is spent in discussing cases and consulting each other on problem areas.

Employment Patterns

The evolution of mental health counseling as a discipline has occurred largely in response to changes in the employment market. Counselor education programs have attempted to accommodate to expanding employment opportunities by diversifying their specialized study areas.

The multifaceted and interdisciplinary definition of mental health counseling gives latitude to the areas of specialized study that can be made available to MHCs in training. The counselor education faculty need not have background experience or training in all specialized areas, since interrelationships with other university programs may be desirable. Thus, students can take courses in other university departments or study in community settings when the counselor education program lacks some courses not responsive to particular needs. For example, a student interested in business and industrial mental health could take courses in business administration. Community resources might include crisis centers and spouse abuse facilities.

Students themselves often display a sensitivity to the changing job market. For example, enrollment in teacher training dropped precipitously in the early 1970s, at the same time that the job market for teachers declined significantly. And now that the economy has strengthened and the business climate has become more encouraging, students are applying to master's of business administration (MBA) programs.

The faculty of counselor education programs certainly have an ethical obligation to prepare students for the current and future job market. To train students for shrinking job opportunities seems indefensible. Counselor educators need to stay abreast of new fields of work, for areas where growth is likely, and for career paths that seem to be limited in opportunity or declining. For example, one of the fastest-growing human services job markets seems to be gerontological counseling. Another rapidly expanding area for MHCs is business and industrial mental health. This is also referred to as organizational development, or training and development. Health counseling, offered in medical and health-related settings has emerged as another important mental health discipline. It seems likely that the present "high tech" era will bring to light new mental health needs, as people in the marketplace become more separated from each other in their work. In this post-industrial high tech era, computers are assuming functions that were formerly performed on an interpersonal level. The "high touch" skills of the MHC will help the workforce deal with problems of alienation and rapid change, emphasizing human relationships as an enduring value.

Curriculum Innovation 1985–1995: A Decade of Progress

In the 1980s, counselor education programs began seriously courting the discipline of marriage and family as their newest curricular interest. At that time, most programs accredited by the American Association of Marriage and Family Therapists (AAMFT) were housed outside of colleges and schools of education. Counselor education programs seemed to have the ability to move swiftly into new specialty disciplines, perhaps as a measure to keep programs or departments expanding.

AMHCA was ready to maintain its innovative posture by being the first of the counseling organizations to officially recognize marriage and family counseling as a specialty area for MHCs. In 1988, AMHCA approved training standards in the marriage and family area and published a monograph by Seiler, Isenhour, and Driscoll (1988) entitled "Training Standards for Mental Health Counselors with a Specialty Practice in Marriage/Couple and Family Counseling. This publication set forth the essential knowledge and skills necessary for MHCs to specialize in this area of counseling.

Another influential development of the late 1980s was the evolution of general training standards for the entire profession of mental health counseling. Training standards crystalize a specific body of knowledge by which a profession distinguishes itself. This body of knowledge then establishes the foundation for curriculum development and suggests a course of study for the training of MHCs.

In the mid 1980s, Seiler (1986) conceived and drafted what would be labeled by some as the "Cadillac" of training standards within the counseling profession. Later these standards were adopted by AMHCA as the "official" training standards for MHC's. They were edited and reported by Seiler, Brooks and Beck (1987) in the *Journal of Mental Health Counseling* as "Training Standards of the American Mental Health Counselors Association: History, Rationale, and Implications" and reprinted for wider distribution throughout the other helping professions as an AMHCA monograph (1988).

The evolution of AMHCA's training standards set the scene for the 1990s. Moving toward ever increasing professional and governmental approval, the field of mental health counseling emerged as a "recognized" mental health care provider.

Curriculum Innovations for the Future

The constantly changing health care scene in the 1990s provided both challenge and opportunity for the mental health counseling profession. The various cost containment measures such as the health maintenance organization, the preferred provider, managed care, and various proposals of government-sponsored universal health care all began to influence the mental health delivery system.

Two significant events occurred in the mid 1990s which could set the pace for future curriculum development and training of MHCs: The development of the Orlando Project and the establishment of the National Commission for Mental Health Counselor Training (NCMHCT) has the potential of revitalizing and reshaping the education and training of MHCs. Both of these projects were sponsored by AMHCA, which provided "seed" money for their development.

The purpose of the Orlando Project was to identify the competencies, including those for internship and residencies, needed for MHC's to compete in the job markets of the future. The NCMHCT has been identified as the "guardian" of the Orlando Model and to promote further quality clinical training. Some of the projects of the Commission include consultation, publications, and continuing education through competency-based workshops and institutes.

Conclusion

Despite the fact that professional training standards for counselor education programs have been in place for over a decade, training curricula for MHCs nationally continue to lack consistency and scope. Part of the difficulty has arisen from the need for continuing redefinition of the profession as it has evolved in the 1970s and 80s. Rapid changes in the profession have made it difficult to solidify commitment to its identity through training curricula. The identity issue must be clarified at all levels of mental health counseling, but particularly as it is translated at the level of graduate training programs.

Counselor education programs should be encouraged to become accredited, to bring more stability to the training of MHCs. Training program accreditation as the rule, instead of the exception, would bring with it across-the-board upgrading of the profession.

Suggestions that would enhance consistent, high standards for counselor education programs and high-quality students seeking applications include the following:

1. Students investigating graduate programs in counselor education should select only schools that have met CACREP training and accreditation standards.
2. Counselor education programs that have met CACREP and/or AMHCA training standards should be acclaimed as models of excellence for other graduate programs and the profession itself.
3. Students who have graduated from accredited schools should enter this fact on their resumes and curriculum vitaes.
4. Approved programs should advertise their accreditation.
5. Doctoral graduates preparing to be counselor educators should be encouraged to take positions at CACREP-approved programs.

Quality training standards are one major step toward successful competition in the human services job market. The mental health counseling profession must continue to define itself, support improvements in training programs, and make certain that its constituency remains sensitive and responsive to the ever-changing employment market.

REFERENCES

Hollis, J. W., & Wantz, R. A. (1984). *Counselor preparation 1983–85: Programs, personnel, trends.* Muncie, IN: Accelerated Development, Inc.

Program standards. (1985) Council for the Accreditation of Counseling and Related Educational Programs (Rev. ed.). Alexandria, VA: AACD Press.

Seiler, G. (1986) MHC Training Standards: Final Draft. Gainesville, FL.

Seiler, G. D., Brooks, D. K., & Beck, E. S. (1987). Training standards of the American Mental Health Counselors Association: History, rationale, and implications. *Journal of Mental Health Counseling, 9* (4), 199–209.

Seiler, G. D., Brooks, D. K., & Beck, E. S. (1988). *Training standards for mental health counselors,* Alexandria, VA: American Mental Health Counselors Association.

Seiler, G. D., Isenhour, G. E., & Driscoll, R. M. (1988). *Training standards for mental health counselors with a specialty practice in marriage/couples and family counseling.* Alexandria, VA: American Mental Health Counselors Association, 1988.

Seiler, G. D., & Messina, J. J. (1979). Toward professional identity: The dimensions of mental health counseling in perspective. *American Mental Health Counselor Association Journal, 1* (3), 3–8.

Stripling, R. O. (1983). Building on the past: A challenge for the future. In G. R. Waltz & Benjamin, L. (Eds.), *Shaping counselor education programs for the next five years: An experimental prototype for the counselor of tomorrow* (pp. 205–209). Ann Arbor, MI: ERIC Counseling and Personnel Services Clearinghouse.

HIGHLIGHT SECTION

THE MENTAL HEALTH COUNSELOR'S ROLE IN PREVENTION

ARTIS J. PALMO

The concept of prevention as a major component of mental health care services began in the very early 1970s as an outgrowth of the community psychology movement (Goodyear, 1976). Today, as in the early beginnings, the concepts of prevention psychology (Landsman, 1994) are based in the medical model, focused upon the prevention of dysfunction or illness rather than upon the development or "Promotion of positive mental health . . . " (p. 1086). Mental health counselors have had a significant impact upon the development of programs that assist the general population in building upon personal strengths and abilities, rather than focusing upon "illness" and cures (Goodyear, 1976; Hershenson & Strein, 1991). MHCs have played major roles in the establishment of prevention programs in schools, agencies, communities, colleges, and industrial settings.

Although there are various interpretations of prevention programs, the following description and definition should provide the reader with a basic conception of prevention. Goodyear's (1976) original article utilizing the tripartite model of Caplan and Cowen continues to be the best description of the concepts of prevention. There are three levels of intervention involved in prevention. First, **primary prevention** " . . . consists of working to prevent dysfunction . . . " (p. 513) through special programs and activities aimed at the population in general. **Secondary prevention** involves direct services (crisis counseling, marriage counseling, brief therapy) to clients who may be suffering from " . . . mild disorders and/or crises" (p. 514). Finally, **tertiary prevention** is oriented toward rehabilitating the client who has suffered severe and chronic problems. Tertiary services are generally viewed as beyond the commonly-held notion of prevention.

In mental health today, prevention means to intervene early in the sequence of stages of the development of a problem (Drum, 1984), although many professionals (Landsman, 1994), including mental health counselors, believe that this definition continues to be a "front" for the medical model. Cowen (1984), one of the professionals responsible for much of the writing on prevention, stated that primary preventions are targeted primarily for "well people" (p. 485) before maladjustment occurs with the intent of supporting an "adjustment-enhancing rationale" (p. 485). For mental health counselors today, the focus is upon an emphasis on the healthy, or as Landsman (1994) has stated, it is important for professionals to examine " . . . what makes life worth living for the healthy earth dweller . . . " (p. 1087), moving away from the focus on the unhealthy.

When examining primary prevention interventions, Cowen (1984) cites a five-step process. Altering Cowen's wording to match a more up-to-date interpretation of prevention, the five steps include: (1) Identifying the normal developmental milestones faced by all individuals in the targeted population to be served; (2) Translating the normal developmental milestones into basic concepts to guide the program; (3) Developing practical, behavioral, and manageable programs grounded in the basic concepts; (4) Operating the programs to reach the largest number of individuals and groups possible; and (5) Assessing the effectiveness of the prevention program.

Any prevention program involves several important elements taken from the writings of Cowen (1982): (1) The program must not only inform the community of the potential problems that exist, but also provide information about the normal developmental hurdles to be faced in day-to-day living; (2) The program has to be directed toward the largest population possible, while at the same time providing a personal message that is attractive for individuals; and (3) The program, through a sound research effort, should be proven to work and be adaptable to the community in which it is implemented.

Prevention Programs

Throughout the literature (Hatfield & Hatfield, 1992; Heller, 1993; Myers, 1992; Shaw, 1986; Westbrook, Kandell, Kirkland, Phillips, Regan, Medvene, & Oslin, 1993; Wittmer & Sweeney, 1992) are examples of prevention programs directed at many and varied groups, but none more prominent than programs aimed at the issues surrounding adolescent development. Prevention programs have aimed to resolve such issues as youth crime, violence, drug use, family disintegration, AIDS, and a plethora of topics. However, no programming has taken more energy than those programs directed at halting the significant increase in adolescent suicide. Suicide prevention programs have been developed at all three levels—primary, secondary, and tertiary.

One of the active state groups is an organization in Wisconsin named, the Marinette and Menominee County Youth Suicide Prevention (Harper, 1994), or for short, **MMCYSP.** This group, organized to help provide a direct focus on the issues faced by adolescents, was formed by a collection of mental health professionals, including an active core of MHCs. **MMCYS** has developed materials and programs aimed to prevent the growth of adolescent suicide. The programs include newsletters, speakers, support groups, conferences, and books that are made available to all groups having contact with adolescents.

One of the successful programs that has been developed by **MMCYS** is the **Life-Saver Week,** a program developed specifically for the schools. MHCs and school counselors make presentations and lead groups for children, parents, and school personnel on the issues facing today's children. Along with the activities, **MMCYS** has developed a packet of materials (Life-Saver Project Packets) for use by school personnel in organizing **Life-Saver Week.** Over the past several years, the activities and materials have been successful in making the population of students and parents more aware of the developmental issues and problems faced by adolescents.

In Pennsylvania, MHCs have made major contributions in the development of the Student Assistance Programs (**SAP**) throughout the schools and within the individual communities. **SAPs** have been developed to provide services to school students who have demonstrated behaviors that can be identified as at-risk (Pennsylvania Department of Education, 1987). At-risk students are defined as those " . . . who run(s) the risk of not acquiring the knowledge, skills, and attitudes needed to become successful adults . . . " (p. 1). In defining at-risk students so broadly, the development of prevention programs can be more broad-based, serving more students.

In the **SAPs,** the MHC has served in several capacities. First, within the school, the MHC has functioned in secondary prevention roles by offering groups for identified at-risk students or serving as consultants for parents trying to handle an at-risk child. Also, from within the school, MHCs have developed and operated primary prevention activities aimed at all students and parents with school in-service programs and community presentations. Second, some MHCs have functioned from the community to either assist in identifying at-risk students or providing directing counseling services to families and students. Many MHCs serve in the role as crisis counselors when the school is faced with students who have reached severe levels of dysfunction.

It is important to remember, within the prevention psychology movement, MHCs have taken a very active role in defining prevention in a positive fashion by viewing many problems within the context of normal growth and development. Normal development is wrought with the potential for dysfunction or at-risk behavior; however, for the MHC, viewing the individual as normal and not dysfunctional is very important. The goal for the MHC is to assist each person to examine themselves within the context of normal development. Therefore, the at-risk teenager may be an adolescent who is overwhelmed by normal pressures associated with growing older, rather than dysfunctional or "ill." For an MHC, prevention is based in normality, not dysfunctionality.

Future Directions

In a recent article (Coie, Watt, West, Hawkins, Asarnow, Markman, Ramey, Shure, & Long, 1993), some directions for the field of prevention psychology were presented as guidelines for the future. While the focus of the authors' presentation was directions for future research, the following are some thoughts taken from Coie et al. for MHCs to consider as they attempt to meet the demands of prevention in the future. Prevention psychology is a major building block in the foundation of mental health counseling, and MHCs need to carefully consider the direction prevention programs are to take in the future.

Future directions (Coie, 1993) for MHCs to consider with regards to prevention include: (1) Prevention models must consider the **normal developmental processes** and factors facing each individual as they occur from birth to death, and not focus on the dysfunctional dynamics; (2) Prevention models must consider the complex nature of the interactions of the individual with the various environments encountered each day and not be tempted to answer very complex problems with simple prevention programs; (3) Although prevention models are focused upon special groups or populations, all individuals are different, responding to developmental stressors in very individualistic fashions; (4) Satisfactory early childhood experiences provide the basis for sound adulthood experiences and general good health, meaning prevention programs aimed at the young can have lasting effects for a lifetime; and (5) Prevention programming should be at the center of the MHCs commitment to the field of mental health.

REFERENCES

Coie, J. D., Watt, N. F., West, S. G., Hawkings, J. D., Asarnow, J. R., Markman, H. J., Ramey, S. L., Shure, M. B., & Long, B. (1993). The science of prevention: A conceptual framework and some directions for a national research program. *American Psychologist, 48,* 1013–1022.

Cowen, E. L. (1984). A general structural model for primary prevention program development in mental health. *The Personnel and Guidance Journal, 62,* 485–490.

Cowen, E. L. (1982). Primary prevention research: Barriers, needs, and opportunities. *Journal of Prevention, 2,* 131–137.

Drum, D. J. (1984). Implementing theme-focused prevention: Challenge for the 1980s. *The Personnel and Guidance Journal, 62,* 509–514.

Goodyear, R. K. (1976). Counselors as community psychologists. *The Personnel and Guidance Journal, 62,* 509–514.

Harper, J. M. (1994). 1995 Life-Saver week: March 5–11. *Suicide Prevention Link, 1*(3), 3.

Hatfield, T., & Hatfield, S. R. (1992). As if your life depended on it: Promoting cognitive development to promote wellness. *Journal of Counseling and Development, 71,* 164–167.

Heller, K. (1993). Prevention activities for older adults: Social structures and personal competencies that maintain useful social roles. *Journal of Counseling and Development, 72,* 124–130.

Hershenson, D. B., & Strein, W. (1991). Toward a mentally healthy curriculum for mental health counselor education. *Journal of Mental Health Counseling, 13,* 247–252.

Landsman, M. S. (1994). Needed: Metaphors for the prevention model of mental health. *American Psychologist, 49,* 1086–1087.

Myers, J. E. (1992). Wellness, prevention, development: The cornerstone of the profession. *Journal of Counseling and Development, 71,* 136–139.

Pennsylvania Department of Education. (1987). *Achieving success with more students: Addressing the problem of students at risk, K–12.* Harrisburg, PA: Author.

Shaw, M. C. (1986). The prevention of learning and interpersonal problems. *Journal of Counseling and Development, 64,* 624–627.

Westbrook, F. D., Kandell, J. J., Kirkland, S. E., Phillips, P. E., Regan, A. M.,

Medvene, A., & Oslin, Y. D. (1993). University campus consultation: Opportunities and limitations. *Journal of Counseling and Development, 72,* 684–688.

Wittmer, J. M., & Sweeney, T. J. (1992). A holistic model for wellness and prevention over the life span. *Journal of Counseling and Development, 71,* 140–148.

Chapter 19

THE FUTURE OF
MENTAL HEALTH COUNSELING

WILLIAM J. WEIKEL

Counseling, 1996. No, it's not a course title or graduate catalogue course number. It's the reality of being a practitioner of an exciting profession as it reaches maturity. Twenty-five years ago, when I entered this field, one was hard pressed to find individuals working as "counselors" other than in school settings. In my first job, I was a "therapeutic activity worker" and later a "group leader," while friends with the same degree in other settings were called "psychological assistants," "therapist," and psych technicians.

Psychiatrists, nurses, psychologists, social workers, and paraprofessionals all did "counseling," but a counselor was frequently thought of as someone who worked at summer camp and blew a whistle! Counseling in general, and mental health counseling in particular, came into its own in the later 1970s and early 1980s. Today, pick up a telephone directory in any American city or town and you are apt to find several listings for mental health counselors or professional counselors.

In the past twenty years, MHCs have founded a major professional organization of about 12,000 members, instituted a code of ethics, passed licensure or registry laws in 41 states, and established a national certification process administered through the National Board for Certified Counselors. This does not mean, however, that the profession is "home free." Competition for the provision of mental health care services is still intense and MHCs are by no means universally recognized as mental health care providers. Some see MHCs as losing ground in the fight for recognition and the provision of therapeutic services and relegated to the role of psychoeducational and career counselors.

Credentialing

The 1980s were the decade of counselor licensure and certification. In 1976, Virginia became the first state to license counselors. By late 1995, counselors have been credentialed (licensed, registered) in 41 states and the District of Columbia. A major problem has been the lack of uniformity of the credentialing acts. For example, some states have a counselor registry, others only protect the title (e.g., Licensed Professional Counselor or LPC) and others have a full "scope of practice" law, defining who counselors are and what they can do. States that regulate the title and practice of counselors (Morrissey, 1995) are: Alabama, Arkansas, California, the District of Columbia, Florida, Georgia, Louisiana, Maine, Michigan, Mississippi, Missouri, Nebraska, New Jersey, New Mexico, North Carolina, North Dakota, Ohio, Tennessee, Texas, Utah, Virginia, West Virginia, and Wyoming. In 1993, Georgia, Nebraska, North Carolina, Texas, and Wyoming upgraded title protection laws into stronger scope of practice and title laws (Morrissey, 1995). This has been the goal for counselors in all states.

The acceptance of voluntary certification has also been strong. The Commission on Rehabilitation Counselor Certification (CRCC) led the way in the 1970s with the initiation of certification procedures for the Certified Rehabilitation Counselor (CRC). In 1979, the American Mental Health Counselors Association (AMHCA) created the national Academy of Certified Clinical Mental Health Counselors (NACCMHC) which established rigorous procedures for the Certified Clinical Mental Health Counselor (CCMHC) credential. The National Board for Certified Counselors (NBCC) was established in 1982, by the American Personnel and Guidance Association (APGA), now known as the American Counseling Association (ACA). They began testing and certification in January of 1983 and as of this writing, are the parent certification group for mental health counselors, career counselors, and marriage and family counselors.

These certifications are voluntary and are not substitutes for a state license. In many, but not all instances, they demonstrate that a counselor has chosen to go beyond minimal standards established for practice of the profession. As predicted in 1986 (Weikel, 1986), licensure and certification have flourished. An NBCC letterhead in front of me, for example, lists: John Doe, Ph.D., NCC, CCMHC, NCC, CRC, LMHC. Translation: John Doe, Doctor of Philosophy (degree), National Certified

Counselor, Certified Clinical Mental Health Counselor, National Certified Career Counselor, and Certified Rehabilitation Counselor (voluntary certifications) and finally Licensed Mental Health Counselor (state license). Eventually, economic constraints will take over, and many counselors will self limit to a state license and perhaps one or two of the most relevant certifications.

In 1986, I wrote that the better known certifications would likely survive, since counselors had invested thousands of hours and millions of dollars to attain and maintain them, but that " . . . the smaller, more specialized certifications will most likely become specialties under the NBCC . . . " This is exactly what has happened. As state licensure becomes universal, especially with strong scope of practice laws, voluntary certification will diminish in popularity. The possible salvation for speciality certification is that as more and more practitioners vie for a limited pool of clients, this will be one way of demonstrating enhanced skills in a particular area. Another possibility is that future legislation may specify a state license plus a speciality certification to be reimbursed under a particular program.

New Delivery Systems

Mental health counseling has been increasingly moving to the private sector. Numerous surveys throughout the 1980s showed that MHCs were becoming established in group and individual practices offering services directly to the public. Many opt for a part-time practice, often with shared office space and support services while maintaining the security of a full-time public, governmental, or university position. Others are in full-time, private practice, often with full staffs that include psychologists and even psychiatrists in their employ. Many practices are interdisciplinary with partners representing several of the helping professions. Such practices offer comprehensive diagnostic, treatment, and follow-up services, frequently covered by a client's health insurance and provide a viable alternative to the client preferring private care versus the services of their local mental health center.

The escalation of health care service costs above the consumer price index of inflation led to the development of Health Maintenance Organizations (HMOs) and Preferred Provider Organizations (PPOs). By the mid-1980s, MHCs were seeking contracts or employment with these groups, and have met, at best, limited success. HMOs are geared towards the prevention of physical and mental illness and should be a perfect match with the psychoeducational preventative model espoused by many counselors. PPOs offer a discount to insurance carriers for contracting exclusive services and can account for substantial reductions in premiums, although most carriers are reluctant to reimburse for mental health services without the presence of a clearly diagnosed "mental illness." Employee Assistance Programs (EAPs) have a strong preventive philosophy and are well entrenched throughout the United States. Many employ in-house counselors while others refer to community-based practitioners.

Many insurers express reluctance to include MHCs or LPCs in existing policy benefits, citing increased costs. Actual data from a Texas Department of Insurance study (Throckmorton, 1995a) reveal that Texas LPCs account for only .08 percent or eight cents for every $100 paid in medical benefits. The study also demonstrated that although insurers were allowed to charge an additional premium for the inclusion of mandating LPCs, due to the negligible claims effects, 95 percent of the respondents did not charge this premium. Throckmorton (1995a) cites other research suggesting that mandates for providers of benefits widely available result in increased competition among professional groups. Other studies suggest that mandates do not cause an increase in utilization of mental health services, but a shift in the market share of the various vendors.

In another article by Throckmorton (1995b), it was reported that 80 percent of the managed care companies in the 1994 Business Insurance survey either employ or contract with licensed/professional mental health counselors. This was a significant increase from 1992 when only 44 percent of the respondents listed MHCs as network providers. Throckmorton adds, "A tally of companies including counselors revealed the widespread recognition and suggests that mental health counselor eligibility is becoming an industry standard." Unfortunately, the same survey noted that among the largest managed care companies, MHC participation ranged from 2 percent to 9.1 percent of total mental health network providers. With the consolidation now taking place in the managed care industry, MHCs and their professional associations need to establish strong relationships with these large providers to insure wholesale inclusion of MHCs.

MHCs can be found working in a large variety of counseling settings including: hospitals; clinics; private practices; schools; colleges and universities; community agencies; community mental health centers;

business and industry; and state, federal, and local governments. Traditionally, the largest percentage of AMHCA members are employed in private practices, followed by colleges and universities, community mental health centers, and community agencies. Many employers have found that they can hire competent master's-level MHCs at a rate much cheaper than clinical social workers or psychologists. A continuing problem, however, centers around eligibility for reimbursement. Until MHCs are universally reimbursed by third-party payors, the other core professionals will have an employment edge. MHCs in the private sector also tend to charge less than psychologists and psychiatrists, but the difference in fees does not appear to be as pronounced as it was in the 1980s.

Political Climate

In the 1986 writing of this chapter, I said, " . . . for the immediate future, accountability, justification, and cost containment will be important to any program's chances of survival." This is still the case. The Republican controlled Congress is not likely to expand any social program or to include MHCs in existing programs until they are convinced it would be a prudent fiscal move. As we get closer to the 1996 presidential election, there is a chance that things may "loosen up" and that MHCs and counselors in general may make some progress towards reaching their legislative goals.

We do know that millions of Americans continue with psychiatric problems and are not being treated. A National Institute of Mental Health survey quoted in *U.S. News and World Report* (1984) found that "nearly 1 in 5 Americans suffered from a psychiatric problem" and "fewer than 1 of every 5 persons with psychiatric problems received any treatment during the six-month survey period." This twelve-year-old survey of 9000 respondents estimated that 13 million persons were affected by anxiety disorders; 10 million were dependent or abused drugs and alcohol; 9.5 million suffered severe depression and manic depression; 1.5 million were crippled by schizophrenia and 1.4 million had antisocial personalities leading to behavior that caused serious conflicts with others. This survey predated the crack cocaine epidemic that has helped to inflate our national prison and jail population to over a million incarcerated persons . . . with a disproportionate number of young, black males. Our social problems persist and seem to beg for a national intervention, yet all attempts at a national or universal mental health insurance plan have failed. Sooner or later we must realize that we need to invest in preventive and treatment programs for our citizens or the country will crumble. MHCs need to continue to be at the forefront of the battle for universal mental health services and to insure that Americans have the freedom to choose among service providers.

Treatment Approaches

Imagine for a moment that you were sick or injured and needed the services of a physician, and that he/she began treatment using the tools and procedures of the World War I era. Absurd? Maybe, yet it is still possible to find analysts using the classic approaches developed in the early twentieth century. New approaches to counseling and psychotherapy have been both few and far between. The nondirective approaches of Carl R. Rogers were first presented in 1942 (*Counseling and Psychotherapy*) and 1951 (*Client Centered Therapy*). Bandura presented *Principles of Behavior Modification* in 1951; Perls, *Gestalt Therapy* also in 1951, and Ellis, *Reason and Emotion in Psychotherapy* in 1962.

Certainly none of these approaches has been static, yet there has not been much in the way of new developments in the counseling field per se. Multimodal and brief treatment approaches simply build on traditional theories. Where are the original thinkers and the researchers needed to develop the methods and ideas that may improve upon our current rates of success? There are those who believe that most of the advances in the understanding and control of human behavior will come from psychobiological and pharmacological researchers, yet we must all strive, through research and "theory building," to provide the profession with the best possible tools.

Perhaps the paucity of research directly relating to the efficacy of mental health counseling can be blamed on the National Institute of Mental Health (NIMH) or its satellites. Or perhaps counselors themselves have been too eager to jump on any bandwagon of psychological "mumbo jumbo" and "psychobabble" without examining the effectiveness and demanding empirical research on new therapeutic approaches. Lindenberg (1984) wrote that counselors were " . . . long on ideas and short on proofs of outcome. If in fact the techniques that we invoke with our clients produce behavioral change, there must be a way to measure outcomes quantitatively or qualitatively, either through traditional research paradigms or innovative quasi-experimental designs" (p. 11).

In the past ten years, AMHCA has encouraged and funded research and their *Journal of Mental Health Counseling* has become the premier outlet for the dissemination of findings relevant to the field. However, pressure must be exerted on NIMH and private foundations to sponsor and fund comprehensive studies nationwide.

Crystal Ball: The Mental Health Counselor in the 21st Century

Oh, for a crystal ball or a friendly Oracle at Delphi to forecast the future of the field. My pessimistic colleagues see counselors losing the battles for recognition and, in doing so, losing all rights to third-party reimbursements and eventually their jobs. The optimistic ones see full recognition of the profession and universal acceptance of MHCs as the fifth core mental health care providers. Realists, such as I, see continued struggles and slow, hard-won victories in a piecemeal fashion. In the last fifteen to twenty years, mental health counseling has become a recognized speciality within the counseling field and has grown in acceptance outside of the field. MHCs are better educated and prepared to address job demands than they were a generation ago and, in most states, have at least some legislative recognition of their profession. Yet they still must compete with the older more established professions for job openings or clients and their reimbursability for services continues in many instances to be an important issue.

Hollis and Wantz (1993) have noted the increase in specialization among counselors, most recently in the number of new masters programs in marriage and family therapy/counseling. They also note the growing trends towards program accreditation in response to factors such as the need for "professional acceptance by other mental health providers, educators, third-party payment providers and the public . . . " (p. 27).

Generally speaking, the accreditation bodies " . . . have an important influence upon what and how much curriculum content areas are taught, where and for how long clinical experiences occur, and what degree is accepted as an entry level for professional practice . . . " (Hollis and Wantz, 1993, p. 28). It seems that counseling as a profession is in a much stronger position and more firmly entrenched than it was twenty years ago. According to Hollis and Wantz (1993), there are 205 Master's Degree programs in Community Counseling, 102 in Marriage and Family Counseling/Therapy, 85 in Mental Health Counseling, 84 in Rehabilitation Counseling, 343 in School Counseling and 128 in "other counseling specialties." At the doctoral level, there are 65 programs in Counseling Psychology, 61 in Counselor Education and 33 in "other counseling specialties." A handful of other schools offer the Specialist in Education degree or post master's/doctoral training.

What might the MHC of the 21st century look like? How about a true professional who has obtained a bachelor's degree in counseling (rare now) or a closely related field, followed by a 60-hour master's degree or even a doctorate in mental health or "community" counseling. A person who is licensed by their state and possesses at least one national or speciality certification. An active member of a strong state and national association that spearheads lobbing efforts and promotes research and processes information for the profession. A person who is well versed in the latest effective intervention strategies, and well-grounded in classical theories. A person who has a strong foundation in counseling, consultation, legal and ethical issues, assessment, diagnosis, prevention and human development throughout the lifespan. A person who is caring and sensitive to the needs of all humans and is free of all prejudice or bias. A person who can serve as a member of an interdisciplinary health care team, comfortable with his/her defined "turf," and cooperative in areas of mutual concern and competence. A community-based professional who provides contract services to business and industry, education institutions, churches, the military, and other social groups. A person who sees private clients and routinely receives third-party reimbursements from a variety of governmental and private insurance programs.

This author's advice to the aspiring student would be to shop around for the best academic program you can find. Look at the current line-up of professors who will be teaching your classes. Look at certifications of the faculty and program accreditation. See where recent graduates have been employed and at what salaries. Join your professional association (most offer excellent student rates) and become an active member at both the state and national level. Read your journals and newsletters, and prepare yourself for "lifelong learning." Apply for certification and licensure as soon as you qualify and behave in an ethical and professional manner at all times. You represent the future of this young and growing profession and it is you who will shape that future.

REFERENCES

Hollis, J. W., & Wantz, R. A. (1993). *Counselor preparation 1993–95.* Muncie, IN: Accelerated Development.

Lindenberg, S. P. (1984). Mental health counseling: Approaching the 21st century. *Counseling and Human Development, 16*(7), 1–12.

Mental disorders: 1 in 5 is a victim. (1984, October 15). *U.S. News and World Report,* p. 18.

Morrissey, M. (1995, March). Persistence and patience named as keys to achieving licensure. *Counseling Today,* pp. 16–19.

Throckmorton, W. (1995a, March/April). Texas study on costs of insurance mandates. *The Advocate,* p. 5.

Throckmorton, W. (1995b, March/April). 80% of managed care companies include MHCs. *The Advocate,* p. 5.

Weikel, W. J. (1986). Future trends in mental health counseling. In A. J. Palmo & W. J. Weikel (Eds.), *Foundations of mental health counseling* (pp. 353–367). Springfield, IL: Charles C Thomas.

NAME INDEX

411

SUBJECT INDEX

Charles C Thomas
PUBLISHER • LTD.

Leader In Behavioral Sciences Publications

▶ denotes new publication

▶ Landy, Robert J.—**HOW WE SEE GOD AND WHY IT MAT-TERS: A Multicultural View Through Children's Drawings and Stories.** '01, 230 pp. (8 x 1/2 x 11), 55 il. (40 in color).

▶ Racino, Julie Ann—**PERSONNEL PREPARATION IN DIS-ABILITY AND COMMUNITY LIFE: Toward Universal Approaches to Support.** '00, 350 pp. (7 x 10), 3 il., 36 tables, $69.95, cloth, $51.95, paper.

▶ Mercier, Peter J. & Judith D. Mercier—**BATTLE CRIES ON THE HOME FRONT: Violence in the Military Family.** '00, 238 pp. (7 x 10), 8 il., 66 tables, $43.95, cloth, $29.95, paper.

▶ Sumerall, Scott W., Shane J. Lopez and Mary E. Oehlert—**COM-PETENCY-BASED EDUCATION AND TRAINING IN PSYCHOLOGY: A Primer.** '00, 130 pp. (6 1/2 x 9 1/2), 1 il., 12 tables, $19.95, paper.

▶ Moser, Rosemarie Scolaro & Corinne E. Frantz—**SHOCKING VIOLENCE: Youth Perpetrators and Victims—A Multidisciplinary Perspective.** '00, 230 pp. (7 x 10), 1 il., 2 tables, $50.95, hard, $33.95, paper.

▶ Bellini, James L. & Phillip D. Rumrill, Jr.—**RESEARCH IN REHABILITATION COUNSELING: A Guide to Design, Methodology, and Utilization.** '99, 252 pp. (7 x 10), 5 tables, $47.95, cloth, $34.95, paper.

▶ Boy, Angelo V. & Gerald J. Pine—**A PERSON-CENTERED FOUNDATION FOR COUNSELING AND PSYCHOTHER-APY. (2nd Ed.)** '99, 274 pp. (7 x 10), 1 il., 1 table, $57.95, cloth, $41.95, paper.

▶ Lantz, Jim—**MEANING-CENTERED MARITAL AND FAMI-LY THERAPY: Learning to Bear the Beams of Love.** '99, 166 pp. (7 x 10), 12 il., $38.95, cloth, $24.95, paper.

▶ Berger, LeslieBeth—**INCEST, WORK AND WOMEN: Understanding the Consequences of Incest on Women's Careers, Work and Dreams.** '98, 234 pp. (7 x 10), 3 tables, $51.95, cloth, $37.95, paper.

▶ Malouff, John & Nicola Schutte—**GAMES TO ENHANCE SOCIAL AND EMOTIONAL SKILLS: Sixty-Six Games that Teach Children, Adolescents, and Adults Skills Crucial to Success in Life.** '98, 218 pp. (8 1/2 x 11), 3 il., $35.95 spiral (paper).

▶ Weikel, William J. & Artis J. Palmo—**FOUNDATIONS OF MEN-TAL HEALTH COUNSELING. (2nd Ed.)** '96, 446 pp. (7 x 10), 7 il., 1 table, $93.95, cloth, $71.95, paper.

▶ Paton, Douglas & John Violanti—**TRAUMATIC STRESS IN CRITICAL OCCUPATIONS: Recognition, Consequences and Treatment.** '96, 260 pp. (7 x 10), 1 il., 13 tables, $65.95, cloth, $43.95, paper.

▶ Ponterotto, Joseph G. & J. Manuel Casas—**HANDBOOK OF RACIAL/ETHNIC MINORITY COUNSELING RE-SEARCH.** '91, 208 pp. (7 x 10), 18 tables, $43.95, cloth, $31.95, paper.

▶ Aiken, Lewis R.—**PERSONALITY: Theories, Assessment, Research, and Applications.** '00, 476 pp. (7 x 10), 24 il., 23 tables, $89.95, cloth, $64.95, paper.

▶ Thomas, R. Murray—**MULTICULTURAL COUNSELING AND HUMAN DEVELOPMENT THEORIES: 25 Theoretical Perspectives.** '00, 252 pp. (6 1/4 x 9 1/4), $39.95, hard, $26.95, paper.

▶ Thorson, James A.—**PERSPECTIVES ON SPIRITUAL WELL-BEING AND AGING.** '00, 230 pp. (7 x 10), $45.95, cloth, $31.95, paper.

▶ Knauer, Sandra—**NO ORDINARY LIFE: Parenting the Sexually Abused Child and Adolescent.** '00, 188 pp. (7 x 10), $41.95, hard, $25.95, paper.

▶ St. John, Iris—**CREATIVE SPIRITUALITY FOR WOMEN: Developing a Positive Sense of Self Through Spiritual Growth Exercises.** '00, 180 pp. (8 1/2 x 11) , 1 table, $26.95, spi-ral paper.

Gandy, Gerald L., E. Davis Martin, Jr. & Richard E. Hardy—**COUNSELING IN THE REHABILITATION PROCESS: Community Services for Mental and Physical Disabilities. (2nd Ed.)** '99, 358 pp. (7 x 10), 9 il., $60.95, cloth, $46.95, paper.

Dixon, Charlotte G. & William G. Emener—**PROFESSIONAL COUNSELING: Transitioning into the Next Millennium.** '99, 194 pp. (7 x 10), 2 il., 1 table, $38.95, cloth, $25.95, paper.

Dennison, Susan T. & Connie M. Knight—**ACTIVITIES FOR CHILDREN IN THERAPY: A Guide for Planning and Facilitating Therapy with Troubled Children. (2nd Ed.)** '99, 302 pp. (8 1/2 x 11), 201 il., 12 tables, $47.95, spiral (paper).

Bryan, Willie V.—**MULTICULTURAL ASPECTS OF DIS-ABILITIES: A Guide to Understanding and Assisting Minorities in the Rehabilitation Process.** '99, 300 pp. (7 x 10), 19 tables, $60.95, hard, $47.95, paper.

Parker, Woodrow M.—**CONSCIOUSNESS-RAISING: A Primer for Multicultural Counseling. (2nd Ed.)** '98, 328 pp. (7 x 10), 2 il., 3 tables, $65.95, cloth, $49.95, paper.

Everstine, Louis—**THE ANATOMY OF SUICIDE: Silence of the Heart.** '98, 170 pp. (7 x 10), 6 il., $44.95, cloth, $29.95, paper.

Dennison, Susan T.—**ACTIVITIES FOR ADOLESCENTS IN THERAPY: A Handbook of Facilitating Guidelines and Planning Ideas for Group Therapy With Troubled Adolescents. (2nd Ed.)** '98, 264 pp. (7 x 10), 16 tables, $41.95, spiral (paper).

Chubon, Robert A.—**SOCIAL AND PSYCHOLOGICAL FOUNDATIONS OF REHABILITATION.** '94, 274 pp. (7 x 10), $57.95, cloth, $39.95, paper.

Geldard, David—**BASIC PERSONAL COUNSELING: A Training Manual for Counselors.** '89, 214 pp. (7 x 10), 28 il., $42.95, paper

Books sent on approval • Shipping charges: $5.95 U.S. / $6.95 Canada • Prices subject to change without notice

Contact us to order books or a free catalog with over 800 titles

Call 1-800-258-8980 or 1-217-789-8980 or Fax 1-217-789-9130
2600 South First Street • Springfield • Illinois • 62704
Complete catalog available at www.ccthomas.com • books@ccthomas.com